THE EMT-INTERMEDIATE EXAM REVIEW

The EMT-Intermediate Exam Review

•

Bob Elling, MPA, REMT-P

Kirsten M. Elling, BS, REMT-P

THOMSON

DELMAR LEARNING

Australia Canada Mexico Singapore Spain United Kingdom United States

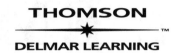

The EMT-Intermediate Exam Review
by Bob Elling and Kirsten Elling

Vice President,
Health Care Business Unit:
William Brottmiller

Editorial Director:
Matthew Kane

Acquisitions Editor:
Maureen Rosener

Senior Product Manager:
Darcy M. Scelsi

Marketing Director:
Jennifer McAvey

Marketing Coordinator:
Chris Manion

Technology Director:
Laurie Davis

Technology Project Manager:
Carolyn Fox

Production Director:
Carolyn Miller

Production Manager:
Barbara A. Bullock

Content Project Manager:
Kenneth McGrath

Library of Congress Cataloging-in-Publication Data

Elling, Bob.
  The EMT-intermediate exam review / Bob Elling, Kirsten M. Elling.
    p. cm.
  Includes bibliographical references and index.
  ISBN 1-4180-0610-6 (alk. paper)
  1. Emergency medical technicians--Examinations, questions, etc. 2. Emergency medicine--Examinations, questions, etc. I. Elling, Kirsten M. II. Title.
  RC86.9.E42 2007
  616.02'5076--dc22
                              2006014319

NOTICE TO THE READER

Dedications

Dedicated to my daughters, Laura and Caitlin, and my lovely wife, Kirsten. May you each maintain humility as your accomplishments reach the clouds!

—BOB ELLING

This book is dedicated to my husband, Bob, who is always there to encourage me in my educational and writing efforts.

—KIRT ELLING

Contents

PREFACE   viii

ACKNOWLEDGMENTS   ix

ABOUT THE AUTHORS   x

SECTION I   PREPARATORY   1

CHAPTER 1 • FOUNDATIONS OF EMT-INTERMEDIATE   3

CHAPTER 2 • OVERVIEW OF HUMAN SYSTEMS   12

CHAPTER 3 • EMERGENCY PHARMACOLOGY   20

CHAPTER 4 • VENOUS ACCESS AND MEDICATION ADMINISTRATION   24

CHAPTER 5 • AIRWAY MANAGEMENT AND VENTILATION   28

CHAPTER 6 • HISTORY TAKING   36

SECTION II   PATIENT ASSESSMENT   39

CHAPTER 7 • TECHNIQUES OF PHYSICAL EXAMINATION   41

CHAPTER 8 • PATIENT ASSESSMENT   48

CHAPTER 9 • CLINICAL DECISION MAKING   55

SECTION III   TRAUMA   59

CHAPTER 10 • COMMUNICATIONS   61

CHAPTER 11 • DOCUMENTATION   65

CHAPTER 12 • TRAUMA SYSTEMS AND MECHANISM OF INJURY   69

CHAPTER 13 • HEMORRHAGE AND SHOCK   72

CHAPTER 14 • BURNS   77

CHAPTER 15 • THORACIC TRAUMA   84

SECTION IV   MEDICAL/BEHAVIORAL EMERGENCIES AND OBSTETRICS/GYNECOLOGY   89

CHAPTER 16 • RESPIRATORY EMERGENCIES   91

CHAPTER 17 • CARDIOVASCULAR EMERGENCIES   95

CHAPTER 18 • DIABETIC EMERGENCIES   101

CHAPTER 19 • ALLERGIC REACTIONS   105

CHAPTER 20 • POISONING/OVERDOSE EMERGENCIES   109

CHAPTER 21 • NEUROLOGICAL EMERGENCIES   112

CHAPTER 22 • NONTRAUMATIC ABDOMINAL EMERGENCIES   115

CHAPTER 23 • ENVIRONMENTAL EMERGENCIES   118

CHAPTER 24 • BEHAVIORAL EMERGENCIES   123

CHAPTER 25 • GYNECOLOGICAL EMERGENCIES   126

CHAPTER 26 • OBSTETRICAL EMERGENCIES   129

SECTION V   INFANTS, CHILDREN, AND GERIATRICS   133

CHAPTER 27 • NEONATAL RESUSCITATION   135

CHAPTER 28 • PEDIATRICS   140

CHAPTER 29 • GERIATRICS   151

CHAPTER 30 • ASSESSMENT-BASED MANAGEMENT   155

APPENDIX A • ANSWERS WITH RATIONALES   160

APPENDIX B • TIPS FOR PREPARING FOR A PRACTICAL
SKILLS EXAMINATION   213

Preface

Today, instructors may choose from many books, magazines, videos, workbooks, and Web sites for use in preparing their students for EMS work in the streets. We sincerely hope you will agree that this book, *The EMT-I Examination Review*, is a valuable tool to help students review and prepare for state and national examinations.

Previously, together with our colleague Mikel Rothenberg, MD, we completed a book titled *Why-Driven EMS Enrichment* and its companion text, *The Paramedic Review*. *The EMT-B Examination Review* followed as the second in a series of review books designed to follow the organizational chapter format of the DOT curriculum. Now you have found *The EMT-Intermediate Exam Review*. The *Enrichment* book was designed for all levels of EMS providers, whereas the information and tests in each review book in the series are specifically tailored for each level of EMS provider.

The EMT-Intermediate Exam Review consists of multiple-choice questions covering all topics and objectives (both cognitive and affective) in the current EMT-I DOT National Standard Curriculum. The chapter order follows that of the standard curriculum, for ease of reference and use. *The EMT-Intermediate Exam Review* is the perfect resource for preparing for the National Registry written exam. The CD that accompanies the text has enough material to make up two full-length simulated practice examinations that mimic typical state and national exam formats.

Included in this book are appendices with the National Registry EMT-Intermediate level skills examination, as well as advice on how to prepare for each important skill. Blank answer forms are included at the end of each chapter.

Early in this project, we decided to use only multiple-choice questions, in the standard format of three distracters and one correct answer to each question. Because this book can be used to prepare for both state and national EMT-I examinations, it makes the most sense to use the format and style of questions used in these exams.

At the end of this book, in Appendix A, you will find an answer key listing the letter of the correct answer, accompanied by a corresponding rationale for the answer. If you would like a more detailed explanation of the material in this book, as well as enrichment for advanced objectives, we suggest that you purchase the companion text, *Why-Driven EMS Enrichment* (ISBN 0-7668-2507-8).

For each question, there is only one correct answer. Always read through all four choices and then select the best answer; you can use a process of elimination if you have difficulty, to narrow your choices. There are more than 1110 questions in this book and another 360 on the CD. That's more questions than any other EMT-I review text currently on the market. We suggest that you tackle a chapter at a time; after taking each exam, check the answer key and mark the material on which you need more review.

We sincerely hope that you will enjoy *The EMT-Intermediate Exam Review* and benefit from the test-taking review as you expand your knowledge base. After all, the real test occurs in the field, where our patients rely on us to be prepared.

See you in the streets!

—*Kirt and Bob*

Acknowledgments

Special Thanks

Our deepest thanks to our close friend and colleague Mikel A. Rothenberg, MD, for all his hard work, insight, and guidance during the development of the companion text, *Why-Driven EMS Enrichment.*

Thank you to all of the editorial and production personnel who have contributed to this project, especially Maureen Rosener, Elizabeth Howe, and Darcy Scelsi.

Thank you to our reviewers for their invaluable feedback:

Milton Ray Dillard, MEd, EMT-LP
Program Chair
Associate Professor
Texas State Technical College
Abilene, Texas

M. Jane Pollock, EMT-P, CEN, Level II, EMD
Adjunct Clinical Instructor
Education and Training Specialist
Brody School of Medicine, East Carolina University
Department of Emergency Medicine, Division of EMS
Greenville, North Carolina

J. Penny Shutts
AEMT, NREMT-B, CIC
Educator
Sandy Creek, New York

Mike Kennamer, EMT-P, MPA,
Director of Adult Education and Skills
Northeast Alabama Community College
Rainesville, Alabama

About the Authors

Bob Elling, MPA, REMT-P, has been involved in EMS since 1975. He is a full-time clinical instructor for Albany Medical Center, working in the Hudson Valley Community College Paramedic Program. He is also an active paramedic with the Town of Colonie (New York), Pepsi Arena, national faculty for the AHA, and regional faculty for the New York State Bureau of EMS. Bob is also a Professor of Management for the Andrew Jackson University. He has served as a paramedic and lieutenant for NYC EMS, a paramedic program director, Associate Director of the NYS EMS program, and the education coordinator for *PULSE: Emergency Medical Update.*

He is an author/coauthor of: *Emergency Care Workbook, EMT-Achieve, Essentials of Emergency Care, First Responder Achieve, First Responder: Exam Preparation and Review, MedReview for the EMT-B, Paramedic Care: Principles & Practice Workbook* (vol. 5), *Paramedic: Anatomy and Physiology, Paramedic: Pathophysiology, Pocket Reference for the EMT-B and First Responder, Principles of Assessment in EMS, The Paramedic Review,* and *Why-Driven EMS Enrichment.*

He was also a co-author of the National First Responder, Paramedic, and EMT-Intermediate curricula, as well as a co-author of the *Guidelines 2005* and *Winter Currents 2005.*

Kirsten (Kirt) M. Elling, BS, REMT-P, is a career paramedic who works for the Town of Colonie in upstate New York. She began EMS work in 1988 as an EMT/firefighter and has been a National Registered paramedic since 1991. She has been an EMS educator since 1990, teaching basic and advanced EMS programs at the Institute of Prehospital Emergency Medicine in Troy, New York. Kirt serves as Regional Faculty for the NYS DOH, Bureau of EMS and the American Heart Association. She has written numerous scripts for the EMS training video series *PULSE: Emergency Medical Update,* is a co-author of *Why-Driven EMS Enrichment, The Paramedic Review, Principles of Assessment, Paramedic: Anatomy & Physiology,* and *Paramedic: Pathophysiology,* contributing author of the IPEM *Paramedic Lab Manual,* and an adjunct writer for the 1998 revision of the National Highway Traffic Safety Administration, EMT-Paramedic and EMT-Intermediate: National Standard Curricula.

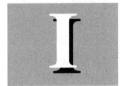
Preparatory

CHAPTER

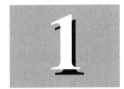

Foundations of EMT-Intermediate

1. An organized approach to providing emergency care to the sick and injured is defined as a/an:
   a. assessment plan of action.
   b. role of the local government.
   c. system of hospital categorization.
   d. Emergency Medical Service System.

2. The attributes of an emergency medical technician-intermediate (EMT-I) should include each of the following, except:
   a. genuine interest and pride in one's service.
   b. concern for patient welfare and safety.
   c. the ability to work well as a member of the health care team.
   d. a sense of complacency and the ability to not show one's feelings.

3. The process by which a governmental agency grants permission to an EMT-I to practice within the state, after ensuring that the individual is competent, is called:
   a. certification.
   b. verification.
   c. authorization.
   d. continuing education.

4. To help assure the public and medical community that quality patient care is being delivered, many states require some form of:
   a. written protocol examination(s).
   b. continuing education for the EMT-I.
   c. call documentation review by the public.
   d. emergency medical service (EMS) system response time interval studies.

5. It is important that the EMT-I be familiar with:
   a. the reciprocity requirements for each state.
   b. the treatment protocols for each region of the state.
   c. all the rules and regulations for both in-hospital and out-of-hospital care.
   d. the education, certification, and licensure requirements in his or her state.

6. An EMT-I is well groomed and wears a uniform appropriate for the job. This is an example of professional behavior referred to as:
   a. self-confidence.
   b. patient advocacy.
   c. diplomacy and respect.
   d. appearance and personal hygiene.

7. Which of the following activities constitutes appropriate professional behavior for an EMT-I?
   a. being courteous to other responders on the scene
   b. answering any question about patient-related activities
   c. smoking in the cab of the ambulance during a transport
   d. wearing a uniform when going out to a pub after a shift

8. When an EMT-I is off duty, it is important that he avoid:
   a. wearing his uniform in drinking establishments.
   b. speaking out for health-related causes as an advocate.
   c. participating in continuing medical education programs.
   d. reading medical journals or trade magazines.

9. The primary responsibility of the EMT-I who is responding to a call is to:
   a. ensure her own safety and that of her coworkers.
   b. take over control of the scene and management of resources.
   c. interact with first responders who are already on the scene.
   d. drive the emergency vehicle to the scene in a timely and lawful manner.

10. Why is quality EMS research important to the future of EMS?

   a. It helps to bring more personnel into the EMS agency through grant funding.

   b. The companies sponsoring the research provide lots of equipment to your service.

   c. It will help physicians make decisions about the efficiency and effectiveness of the care we provide to patients.

   d. In the future, all decisions will be based on research models.

11. Why is it important for the EMT-I to have a good working relationship with the EMS physician who provides medical direction?

   a. State law requires it.

   b. The EMT-I cannot practice without a physician's approval.

   c. Mutual respect and understanding of each other's capabilities will lead to better patient care.

   d. If you tell the medical direction physician what he or she wants to hear, you will get more orders.

12. Having a committee of physicians and providers review protocols on a regular basis is an example of the:

   a. benefit of offline medical direction.

   b. benefit of online medical direction.

   c. quality improvement requirements of OSHA.

   d. need for continuing education.

13. The EMT-I is on the scene, for an adult male patient complaining of chest pain, when the patient's family physician arrives at the residence. How should the EMT-I handle any differences between the treatment protocols and the feelings of the patient's physician?

   a. Remove the patient from the scene as soon as possible.

   b. Tell the physician that the EMT-I must follow the service's standing orders.

   c. Most systems suggest that the family physician be put in touch with online medical direction to discuss the case.

   d. Ignore the patient's physician, because he or she is probably not aware of the region's EMT-I treatment protocols.

14. Call review, analysis of response time intervals, and focused studies of specific types of patient complaints are all examples of activities of a/an:

   a. continuing education certification.

   b. disciplinary hearing on competency.

   c. original training program for the provider.

   d. continuous quality improvement program.

15. When the EMT-I is confronted with a patient who has a fever of unknown origin, it is important to employ:

   a. body substance isolation (BSI) practices.

   b. wound precaution procedures.

   c. complete isolation procedures.

   d. all of the above.

16. If the EMT-I suspects that a patient may have a disease that can be transmitted by the airborne route, what personal precautions should be taken?

   a. Place an oxygen mask with oxygen flowing on the patient.

   b. Place a HEPA or N-95 mask on the patient.

   c. Place disposable gloves and an eye shield on the patient.

   d. Place oxygen masks on yourself and assisting crew members.

17. When treating a patient, the EMT-I failed to immediately place a sharp from a venipuncture directly into the appropriate container. A crew member managed to cut himself with the sharp later in the call. Is this considered an exposure?

   a. No, because the needle was originally sterile.

   b. Yes, and it should be reported to the emergency department (ED) right away.

   c. Yes, but washing the cut with soap and water is adequate.

   d. No, an exposure would require the injection of a large quantity of blood.

18. A journal article discusses the number of patients who died from a preventable injury. Such deaths are often referred to as the:

   a. morbidity.

   b. mortality.

   c. socioeconomic impact.

   d. incidence or occurrence.

19. Spinal injuries caused by entering a shallow pool head first are considered:

   a. lethal injuries.

   b. preventable illnesses.

   c. preventable injuries.

   d. trauma that is not avoidable.

20. An EMT-I is reading a journal article discussing the financial costs of a preventable injury and illness. These costs are usually referred to as the:

   a. future impact.

   b. human impact.

   c. environmental impact.

   d. socioeconomic impact.

21. Your EMS medical director develops a program whereby the service helps citizens learn how to use child car seats properly in their vehicles. This is an example of an EMT-I being involved in:
    a. a public health crisis.
    b. patient care advocacy.
    c. an injury prevention activity.
    d. an expanded scope of practice.

22. Which of the following is an example of a strategy for the implementation of an EMS-related illness and injury prevention program in the community?
    a. assigning crews to do citizen cardiopulmonary resuscitation (CPR) training courses
    b. planning quicker response routes in the community
    c. conducting continuing education lectures on a regular basis
    d. reviewing call documentation for specific types of complaints

23. What is the value of identifying health hazards and potential crime areas within your district?
    a. There is no value in this type of planning.
    b. It helps in planning for call volume and crew safety.
    c. Extra resources should be expended within those areas.
    d. The providers should avoid those areas as much as possible.

24. Which of the following is an example of a local municipal or community resource that the EMT-I should be aware of for assisting with physical and socioeconomic crises?
    a. Child protective services can be helpful in cases of accidental injury.
    b. Many communities have programs to help feed the homebound elderly.
    c. Some communities have mobile crisis teams that can provide permanent housing to homeless individuals.
    d. All community hospitals have programs to help assist the elderly with taking medications.

25. In a negligence case, the plaintiff must prove four elements to be successful. Which of the following is not one of those elements?
    a. The patient sustained an injury.
    b. The EMT-I had a duty to act.
    c. An act or omission was the direct cause of the patient's injury.
    d. The number of times the patient was transported for similar complaints.

26. Putting on a "slow-code," whereby the EMT-I provides only part of the normal resuscitation procedures until the patient is removed from the residence, is considered:
    a. an unethical act.
    b. appropriate for the situation.
    c. an illegal action.
    d. a violation of the standard operating procedure.

27. Because the EMT-I may be involved in the interhospital transfer of patients, it is important to understand the provisions of the:
    a. FOIL law.
    b. OSHA law.
    c. COBRA law.
    d. mental health law.

28. The utterance of false statements by the EMT-I that have the potential to damage another's reputation is against the law and is referred to as:
    a. assault.
    b. slander.
    c. battery.
    d. prejudice.

29. When a patient has an altered level of consciousness and is unable to make life-or-death decisions, the EMT-I relies on a specific form of consent referred to as:
    a. implied consent.
    b. informed consent.
    c. express consent.
    d. emancipated consent.

30. In most states, the EMT-I is required to report which of the following situations when found or suspected on a call?
    a. child abuse or neglect
    b. an injury in a private residence
    c. a call involving any toxic substance
    d. an adult patient who refuses medical attention

31. If an EMT-I fails to obtain the appropriate consent from a conscious adult patient to transport that patient to the hospital, the EMT-I could be charged with the crime of:
    a. breach of duty.
    b. assault and battery.
    c. false imprisonment.
    d. breach of confidentiality.

32. The description of what assessment and management the EMT-I may legally perform is referred to as the:
    a. standard of care.
    b. regional protocol.
    c. scope of practice.
    d. offline medical direction.

33. The process of delegating practice to the EMT-I by a physician is usually referred to as:

    a. licensure.

    b. medical direction.

    c. a standing order.

    d. the standard of care.

34. A law pertaining to a private or public wrong or injury that occurs due to a breach of a legal duty or obligation is called a:

    a. tort.

    b. regulation.

    c. stipulation.

    d. criminal event.

35. When treating a patient with a suspected spinal injury, it is essential to document movement and sensation in all four extremities before and after immobilization. If the EMT-I fails to document this on the prehospital care report (PCR), it could help the plaintiff's case in proving:

    a. that there was a breach of duty.

    b. that the EMT-I had a duty to the patient.

    c. that an injury was actually present.

    d. a relationship between the injury and who may have caused the injury.

36. The medical director has certain responsibilities regarding the EMT-I's practice. With respect to the medical care provided at the scene of an emergency, why should the EMT-I pay close attention to the care being provided by the first responders and EMT-Basics (EMT-Bs)?

    a. The EMT-I will need to do all the documentation for the calls.

    b. The EMT-I has no responsibility for the care provided by others.

    c. The EMT-I may be held liable for the medical supervision of other providers.

    d. It is not necessary for the EMT-I to worry about care given by other providers.

37. Some states have Good Samaritan statutes and governmental immunity protection for EMT-Is. In general, though, it is best not to rely on these laws for legal protection and to always:

    a. be respectful to patients and their families.

    b. do the right care within your scope of practice.

    c. document all your assessment and management clearly on the PCR.

    d. each of the choices listed here is good advice.

38. For many years, EMS providers have been taught to keep medical information about patients confidential. Aside from the ethical issues, what law now makes it illegal to share confidential information about patients?

    a. the NFPA rules

    b. the HIPAA law

    c. the general tort clause

    d. the OSHA privacy rule

39. What steps should be taken if a patient refuses care?

    a. Clearly explain the best-case scenario of not going, and have the patient sign the refusal form.

    b. Do not involve family members in helping to convince the patient to go to the hospital.

    c. Avoid calling medical direction once a patient has decided to refuse treatment and transport.

    d. Make sure you have a credible witness to the documented refusal, as well as to what you said to the patient.

40. An EMT-I turns over a patient to the EMT-Bs when the patient should have had advanced life support (ALS) care. This could be considered:

    a. patient abuse.

    b. misdiagnosis.

    c. abandonment.

    d. a breach of confidentiality.

41. In which of the following circumstances would it be appropriate for the EMT-I to consider the use of force to restrain a patient?

    a. when the police are present to witness the EMT-I's actions

    b. as long as the family is not present when the patient is restrained

    c. whenever the patient gets argumentative

    d. in a state where it is legal for a physician to order removal for a mental health evaluation and the EMT-I has the appropriate paperwork to do so

42. When you arrive at the home of a very sick patient who is being treated for a terminal illness, the family tells you she has an advance directive. What is important for the EMT-I to ask the family?

    a. whether the patient will want an IV

    b. whether the patient care surrogate will be riding in the ambulance

    c. whether all family members agree on the specific care plans

    d. whether the patient has signed a prehospital do not attempt resuscitation (DNAR) form

43. You are on the scene with a young male in critical condition, who was thrown from his motorcycle onto his head. The patient has been in cardiac arrest for the past 10 minutes and you are ready to transport. If the patient has injuries that are not survivable, what else is a consideration?

    a. A young trauma victim may be a potential organ donor.
    b. The ED may need the patient to practice a new surgical technique.
    c. Patients in asystole often survive after aggressive fluid resuscitation.
    d. The police may want the body removed from the crime scene by EMS.

44. EMT-Is are occasionally called to testify in court cases as to what they did and what the patient said at the time of a tragic accident. Why is it important to complete an accurate and legible PCR after each call?

    a. The PCR will keep you from having to go to court.
    b. The patient may ask for you to make him a copy after the call.
    c. Your PCR may be the best way to refresh your memory about the incident.
    d. The hospital will not have to document what you have already written down.

45. For the PCR to be an effective legal document, the EMT-I should make sure that it is:

    a. legible.
    b. biased.
    c. subjective.
    d. mostly complete.

46. Which of the following is a premise that should underlie the EMT-I's ethical decisions in out-of-hospital care?

    a. Avoid ethical decisions as much as possible.
    b. Remember that there are no ethical decisions, just protocols to follow.
    c. Treat all patients the way you would want your own family to be treated.
    d. Make sure you would feel comfortable about having your treatment decisions scrutinized.

47. When the EMT-I follows the provisions in the state EMS Code, the EMT-I is making a/an:

    a. judgment call.
    b. legal decision.
    c. ethical decision.
    d. clinical decision.

48. The form of advance directive most frequently used in out-of-hospital resuscitation decisions is called a:

    a. living will.
    b. standard will.
    c. DNR or DNAR.
    d. health care proxy.

49. In most states, for an EMT-I to follow the provisions of an advance directive, the patient will need to have a:

    a. prehospital DNR or DNAR form.
    b. videotape specifying his or her wishes.
    c. living will on file with your service.
    d. bracelet stating the name of the surrogate.

50. Which of the following is not an example of how an EMT-I can serve as a role model for others by displaying professionalism in EMS?

    a. Avoid using seat belts while off duty.
    b. Wear a helmet whenever biking or skiing.
    c. Write letters to the editor promoting CPR training.
    d. Help teach your neighbors what to do in an emergency.

51. The best EMT-Is serve as advocates for patients with:

    a. special needs.
    b. alternative lifestyles.
    c. diverse cultural backgrounds.
    d. all of the above.

52. Continuing medical education courses are important for the EMT-I because:

    a. continuing education is a requirement in all states.
    b. there is no other way to recertify.
    c. all medical directors feel the need to require it.
    d. skills will decay and you need to keep up to date.

53. How can the EMT-I help to advance the future of EMS and potentially expand treatment options?

    a. Save as much data as possible on each call.
    b. Take online training programs to upgrade your skills.
    c. Advocate for and support research efforts in your agency.
    d. Encourage your medical director to purchase new equipment.

54. Which of the following is not an example of personal attitudes and demeanor that may distract from the EMT-I's professionalism?

    a. referring to patients with derogatory terms or pet names
    b. taking a personal interest in and talking with elderly patients
    c. speaking to each patient like a child who does not understand
    d. standing over the patient with arms crossed while questioning

55. Emphasizing the need for injury prevention directly with a patient while treating her, in a nonthreatening manner, is referred to as a/an:

    a. teachable moment.
    b. prevention strategy.
    c. element of management.
    d. documentation component.

56. After delivering a patient to the ED, you are changing the linen on the stretcher. You notice a $10 bill that must have fallen out of the patient's pocket onto the stretcher. Finding the patient to return the money is an example of the professional behaviors of the EMT-I called:
    a. integrity and honesty.
    b. respect and empathy.
    c. self-motivation and diplomacy.
    d. patient advocacy and teamwork.

57. Which of the following is not an important benefit to the EMT-I in working toward the goal of total personal wellness?
    a. feeling better about yourself
    b. performing better under stress
    c. having more time to sleep or watch television
    d. living longer because of appropriate weight

58. How can the EMT-I serve as a role model for other EMS providers in regard to a total wellness lifestyle?
    a. Bet your partner that she can't quit smoking.
    b. Exercise regularly and watch what you eat.
    c. Constantly remind coworkers if they are overweight.
    d. Distribute information on obesity to all employees.

59. Before the EMT-I can serve as a role model for wellness, he or she must remember that:
    a. most coworkers are simply not interested.
    b. most coworkers do not have time for wellness.
    c. wellness begins with an assessment of one's own lifestyle.
    d. most coworkers cannot afford to eat health foods at work.

60. Mentioning to patients that they should be going for a walk every day or limiting their intake of fried foods is an example of:
    a. overstepping your bounds.
    b. invading patients' privacy.
    c. practicing medicine without a license.
    d. teaching wellness concepts in your role as an EMT-I.

61. When asked, most dying patients agree that they would like to be treated by health care providers:
    a. with dignity.
    b. with respect.
    c. as individuals.
    d. all of the above.

62. In respect to cultural diversity, the EMT-I should:
    a. treat everyone exactly the same.
    b. learn just enough about each group to get by.
    c. understand her prejudices and leave them at the door.
    d. avoid getting too close to people she does not understand.

63. The EMT-I can improve his or her personal, physical well-being by:
    a. participating in regular exercise.
    b. maintaining proper body weight.
    c. paying attention to proper nutrition.
    d. all of the above.

64. When dealing with a patient who is dying, and the patient's family members, the EMT-I should always try to:
    a. respect their emotional needs.
    b. help control their decision making.
    c. tell them everything will be all right.
    d. eliminate the need for them to make decisions.

65. At all collision scenes, the EMT-I should be a good role model and:
    a. take control of the extrication.
    b. practice the use of personal safety precautions.
    c. tell the rescue personnel how to do their jobs.
    d. have all members of the public removed from the scene.

66. The EMT-I can help other EMS providers on a call scene to develop good habits by:
    a. showing off how smart he is.
    b. advocating and serving as a role model by practicing BSI.
    c. assuring the patient's family that the patient will be all right.
    d. using correct medical terminology, especially when talking to patients.

67. To be most effective in defending the tenets of prevention for patients and the communities she serves, the EMT-I should:
    a. tell everyone she treats.
    b. make prevention a personal value.
    c. give talks to community groups when asked.
    d. make sure she has the newest equipment available.

68. Prevention programs are most successful when an employer values the employees':
    a. experience in the field.
    b. personal commitment.
    c. broad knowledge base.
    d. respect of coworkers.

69. An experienced EMT-I:
    a. is able to take over all incident scenes.
    b. never gets frazzled or stressed on the job.
    c. can tell patients news they do not want to hear.
    d. shows respect for the rights and feelings of patients.

70. When confronted by the news media after a car crash involving a celebrity, the EMT-I should always remember that:
    a. the story will get told sooner or later.
    b. the public has a right to know the details.
    c. the news media do lots of favors for your agency.
    d. protecting the patient's confidentiality is very important.

71. Upon arrival at a scene involving a patient who is terminally ill, you find the first responders doing CPR. The family arrives and presents a valid prehospital DNAR. What should you do next?
    a. Tell the family that once CPR has been started, you cannot stop the care.
    b. Immediately take the patient to the hospital while doing CPR.
    c. Tell the responders they were wrong to begin CPR.
    d. Contact medical direction to see if it is appropriate to stop the care.

72. If friends, neighbors, or patients ask about the role of advance directives, the EMT-I should consider advising that:
    a. advance directives are rarely used.
    b. they are needed only if the patient is dying.
    c. they are used only if the family is wealthy.
    d. all adults should seriously consider making advance directives for medical care.

73. Advance directives or living wills are best when prepared by the patient, the patient's physician, and the patient's surrogate, because:
    a. it is most cost-effective this way.
    b. all parties will have witnessed the document.
    c. the courts will not recognize a directive if the patient was not directly involved in making it.
    d. they can reinforce the patient's autonomy in the decision-making process.

74. If the physician orders therapy over the radio but the EMT-I feels that the therapy is totally inappropriate, the EMT-I should:
    a. find another hospital.
    b. tell the physician he refuses to follow the order.
    c. go ahead and follow the order even though he knows it is wrong.
    d. discuss his concerns so they are clearly understood by both parties.

75. A physician gives you an order to administer 10 times the standard dose of a medication to a patient. What should you do when talking to the physician on the radio?
    a. Refer to your EMT-I textbook.
    b. Know and mention all the doses listed in the *Physician's Desk Reference.*
    c. Know your protocols and remind the physician of the standard dose.
    d. It makes no sense to try to argue with a physician about a medical order.

Chapter 1 Answer Form

	A	B	C	D			A	B	C	D
1.	❏	❏	❏	❏		26.	❏	❏	❏	❏
2.	❏	❏	❏	❏		27.	❏	❏	❏	❏
3.	❏	❏	❏	❏		28.	❏	❏	❏	❏
4.	❏	❏	❏	❏		29.	❏	❏	❏	❏
5.	❏	❏	❏	❏		30.	❏	❏	❏	❏
6.	❏	❏	❏	❏		31.	❏	❏	❏	❏
7.	❏	❏	❏	❏		32.	❏	❏	❏	❏
8.	❏	❏	❏	❏		33.	❏	❏	❏	❏
9.	❏	❏	❏	❏		34.	❏	❏	❏	❏
10.	❏	❏	❏	❏		35.	❏	❏	❏	❏
11.	❏	❏	❏	❏		36.	❏	❏	❏	❏
12.	❏	❏	❏	❏		37.	❏	❏	❏	❏
13.	❏	❏	❏	❏		38.	❏	❏	❏	❏
14.	❏	❏	❏	❏		39.	❏	❏	❏	❏
15.	❏	❏	❏	❏		40.	❏	❏	❏	❏
16.	❏	❏	❏	❏		41.	❏	❏	❏	❏
17.	❏	❏	❏	❏		42.	❏	❏	❏	❏
18.	❏	❏	❏	❏		43.	❏	❏	❏	❏
19.	❏	❏	❏	❏		44.	❏	❏	❏	❏
20.	❏	❏	❏	❏		45.	❏	❏	❏	❏
21.	❏	❏	❏	❏		46.	❏	❏	❏	❏
22.	❏	❏	❏	❏		47.	❏	❏	❏	❏
23.	❏	❏	❏	❏		48.	❏	❏	❏	❏
24.	❏	❏	❏	❏		49.	❏	❏	❏	❏
25.	❏	❏	❏	❏		50.	❏	❏	❏	❏

	A	B	C	D			A	B	C	D
51.	❏	❏	❏	❏		64.	❏	❏	❏	❏
52.	❏	❏	❏	❏		65.	❏	❏	❏	❏
53.	❏	❏	❏	❏		66.	❏	❏	❏	❏
54.	❏	❏	❏	❏		67.	❏	❏	❏	❏
55.	❏	❏	❏	❏		68.	❏	❏	❏	❏
56.	❏	❏	❏	❏		69.	❏	❏	❏	❏
57.	❏	❏	❏	❏		70.	❏	❏	❏	❏
58.	❏	❏	❏	❏		71.	❏	❏	❏	❏
59.	❏	❏	❏	❏		72.	❏	❏	❏	❏
60.	❏	❏	❏	❏		73.	❏	❏	❏	❏
61.	❏	❏	❏	❏		74.	❏	❏	❏	❏
62.	❏	❏	❏	❏		75.	❏	❏	❏	❏
63.	❏	❏	❏	❏						

CHAPTER 2

Overview of Human Systems

1. The study of the normal structures of the human body is called:
   a. anatomy.
   b. pathology.
   c. physiology.
   d. pathophysiology.

2. Of the following statements, which best describes the levels of organization of the body in order of simplest to more complex?
   a. tissues, cells, organelles
   b. cells, organs, organ systems
   c. organelles, cells, tissues, organs
   d. tissues, organelles, organ systems

3. What is homeostasis?
   a. all the cellular processes of a cell that are unstable
   b. the study of anatomy associated with a particular body region
   c. the study of the body's functions in an abnormally functioning cell
   d. the body's ability to maintain a stable internal physiologic environment

4. The anatomical term for the upper part of the body (as opposed to the lower part) is:
   a. superior.
   b. anterior.
   c. distal plane.
   d. dorsal surface.

5. An EMT-I is describing the location of an injury on the inside surface of the right thigh. It is helpful to call this location:
   a. anterior knee.
   b. posterior femoral area.
   c. midshaft, lateral femur.
   d. midshaft, medial femur.

6. The EMT-I uses the term _____ to describe an injury that is closer to the elbow joint than to the shoulder joint.
   a. distal
   b. inferior
   c. superior
   d. proximal

7. The major body cavity that contains the kidneys is called the:
   a. thorax.
   b. abdomen.
   c. retroperitoneal space.
   d. subdiaphragmatic region.

8. The anatomical plane that cuts an imaginary line through the body from the head down, splitting it into two equal parts, is called the:
   a. frontal plane.
   b. medial plane.
   c. sagittal plane.
   d. transverse plane.

9. The cecum and appendix are found in the _____ abdominal quadrant.
   a. left upper
   b. left lower
   c. right lower
   d. right upper

10. The movement of a solvent through a semi-permeable membrane from an area of low solute concentration to an area of high concentration is called:
    a. osmosis.
    b. oncotic force.
    c. phagocytosis.
    d. facilitated diffusion.

11. The destructive chemical processes that take place in the body to break down larger molecules into smaller molecules is called:
    a. anabolism.
    b. catabolism.
    c. metabolism.
    d. homeostasis.

12. Food that enters the body is broken down into primary sugars, amino acids, and fatty acids. These substances ultimately are metabolized in the _____ to produce large amounts of _____.
    a. liver; ATP
    b. kidneys; RNA
    c. mitochondria; ATP
    d. small intestine; DNA

13. A type of tissue that covers all the external surfaces of the human body is called:
    a. skeletal tissue.
    b. nervous tissue.
    c. adipose tissue.
    d. epithelial tissue.

14. The human skin is divided into three layers. The outermost layer is called the:
    a. dermis.
    b. epidermis.
    c. sebaceous gland.
    d. subcutaneous tissue.

15. The human skeleton provides the essential function(s) of:
    a. temperature regulation.
    b. support and movement.
    c. protection against disease.
    d. fluid and electrolyte balance.

16. Bones are classified according to their:
    a. weight.
    b. shape.
    c. density.
    d. amount of marrow.

17. An example of a saddle joint is the joint in the:
    a. hip.
    b. knee.
    c. thumb.
    d. vertebrae.

18. A smooth muscle may also be described as:
    a. a voluntary muscle.
    b. an involuntary muscle.
    c. an accessory muscle.
    d. a resistant-type muscle.

19. The three types of muscle are smooth,:
    a. cardiac, and skeletal.
    b. skeletal, and voluntary.
    c. cardiac, and involuntary.
    d. involuntary, and voluntary.

20. The unique ability of cardiac cells to generate impulses is called:
    a. conduction.
    b. automaticity.
    c. pacemaking.
    d. electromagnetism.

21. The function of the nervous system is to:
    a. control body functions.
    b. communicate with the environment.
    c. act as a shock absorber for the body.
    d. allow electricity to be transmitted throughout the body.

22. The nervous system is divided into the:
    a. brain and spinal cord.
    b. central and peripheral divisions.
    c. autonomic and sympathetic systems.
    d. spinal and parasympathetic systems.

23. The space between the neurons is called the:
    a. synaptic cleft.
    b. synaptic vesicles.
    c. nodes of Ranvier.
    d. postsynaptic terminal.

24. Projections from a nerve cell that make connections with adjacent nerve cells are called:
    a. axons.
    b. afferent tracts.
    c. action potentials.
    d. accessory nerves.

25. Spinal and cranial nerves are _____ types of nerves.
    a. central
    b. specific
    c. automatic
    d. underutilized

26. The clear fluid that is produced in the ventricles of the brain and circulated around the coverings of the brain and spinal cord is called _____ fluid.
    a. cervical
    b. synovial
    c. lymphatic
    d. cerebral spinal

27. The state or process of returning to the resting state that occurs after a cell has allowed electrical activity to occur, or flow through, is referred to as:
    a. renewal.
    b. polarization.
    c. repolarization.
    d. depolarization.

28. The central nervous system includes the spinal cord and the:
   a. brain.
   b. cerebrum.
   c. spinal column.
   d. peripheral nerves.

29. The layer of membrane that covers the outside of the brain and spinal cord is called the:
   a. pia mater.
   b. dura mater.
   c. cranial mater.
   d. arachnoid mater.

30. The autonomic nervous system is further broken down into the:
   a. brain and spinal cord.
   b. white and gray matter.
   c. postganglionic and motor nerves.
   d. sympathetic and parasympathetic.

31. Glands located throughout the body secrete _____, which regulate body functions by traveling through the bloodstream to their target organs.
   a. sugars
   b. hormones
   c. acetylcholines
   d. prostaglandins

32. The pancreas secretes a hormone called _____, which helps the body process _____.
   a. gall; gallstones
   b. insulin; glucose
   c. adrenaline; energy
   d. antidiuretic hormone; urine

33. To help the body deal with a potential crisis, such as blood loss, the brain tells the adrenal glands to secrete a chemical. This chemical is called _____ and designed to _____.
   a. epinephrine; speed up the heart
   b. norepinephrine; speed up the heart
   c. epinephrine; dilate the blood vessels
   d. norepinephrine; slow down the heart

34. A straw-colored fluid that accounts for more than half of the total blood volume is called:
   a. plasma.
   b. antibodies.
   c. hemoglobin.
   d. red blood cells.

35. The primary function of white blood cells is to:
   a. fight infection.
   b. assist in blood clotting.
   c. carry oxygen to the cells.
   d. remove byproducts of cellular metabolism.

36. A patient who has a clotting problem is often deficient in which type of blood cells?
   a. platelets
   b. neutrophils
   c. erythrocytes
   d. red blood cells

37. What is hemostasis, and why is it important to the human body?
   a. Cessation of bleeding; without it the person could bleed to death.
   b. Elimination of infection; without it the person could die from sepsis.
   c. Flow of the blood to each of the cells; without it, electrolyte imbalance could result.
   d. None of the above.

38. Anatomically, the heart is located in the _____ of the chest under the _____.
   a. left, ribs
   b. right, ribs
   c. center, ribs
   d. center, sternum

39. The thick, fibrous membrane that surrounds the heart is called the:
   a. pleura.
   b. epidurum.
   c. pericardium.
   d. endocardium.

40. When blood flows through the heart, it enters the right _____ and exits the _____ before flowing to the rest of the body.
   a. ventricle; left atrium
   b. atrium; left ventricle
   c. ventricle; right atrium
   d. atrium; right ventricle

41. Freshly oxygenated blood returns to the left side of the heart through a vein. After the blood is collected in a chamber, it then is ejected through a valve into the final chamber of the heart before being pumped out to other parts of the body. What is the name of this valve?
   a. mitral valve
   b. tricuspid valve
   c. pulmonic valve
   d. semilunar valve

42. Blood ejected through the _____ valve enters the pulmonary circulation and travels to the lungs to pick up oxygen; the blood then return to the heart's _____ chamber.
   a. mitral; left ventricle
   b. aortic; right ventricle
   c. pulmonic; left atrium
   d. tricuspid; right atrium

43. The "dub" or S-2 sound of a patient's heart sounds is actually the:
    a. closing of the aortic and pulmonic valves at the end of systole.
    b. closing of the mitral and tricuspid valves at the start of systole.
    c. opening of the mitral and tricuspid valves at the beginning of systole.
    d. opening of the pulmonic and aortic valves at the beginning of systole.

44. A soft, low-pitched heart sound that occurs about one-third of the way through diastole is the _____ heart sound; it sounds like _____.
    a. S-1; "lub"
    b. S-2; "dub"
    c. S-3; "da"
    d. S-4; "bla"

45. An abnormal, whooshing sound heard over the heart that indicates turbulent blood flow within the heart is called a:
    a. bruit.
    b. thrill.
    c. trickle.
    d. murmur.

46. The mechanical pumping of the heart occurs only in response to an electrical stimulus. The heart's primary pacemaker is called the _____ and is located in the _____.
    a. bundle of His; right atrium
    b. Purkinje fibers; left ventricle
    c. sinoatrial node; right atrium
    d. atrioventricular node; center of the heart

47. The ability of cells to respond to electrical impulses is referred to as the property of:
    a. excitability.
    b. contractility.
    c. conductivity.
    d. automaticity.

48. The pressure in the aorta against which the left ventricle must pump blood is called:
    a. systole.
    b. diastole.
    c. the preload.
    d. the afterload.

49. The amount of blood pumped through the circulatory system in one minute is referred to as the:
    a. preload.
    b. stroke volume.
    c. cardiac output.
    d. ejection fraction.

50. The nervous system is responsible for regulating the heart's:
    a. pressure and volume.
    b. preload and stroke volume.
    c. ejection fraction and output.
    d. rate and force of contraction.

51. A drug with a "beta" effect, such as epinephrine, will have what effect on the heart?
    a. slow it down
    b. reduce the preload
    c. make it pump stronger
    d. decrease the need for oxygen

52. The middle layer of a blood vessel wall is composed of elastic tissue and smooth muscle cells that allow the vessel to expand and contract. This layer is called the:
    a. endothelium.
    b. tunica intima.
    c. tunica media.
    d. tunica adventitia.

53. Which type of blood vessels has a series of valves?
    a. veins
    b. arteries
    c. capillaries
    d. lymphatic vessels

54. The walls of the capillaries are thin and semi-permeable so that it is possible for:
    a. oxygen to diffuse from the capillaries to the cells.
    b. nutrients to pass from the capillaries to the cells.
    c. carbon dioxide to diffuse from the cells into the capillaries.
    d. all of the above.

55. Blood circulation between the heart and the lungs is referred to as the _____ circulation.
    a. aortic
    b. systolic
    c. pulmonic
    d. systemic

56. In its pathway through the body, the circulation returns to the heart through a/an _____, which is called the _____.
    a. artery; aorta
    b. vein; vena cava
    c. capillary; iliac vessel
    d. artery; pulmonary artery

57. What factor contributes to the patient's blood pressure?
    a. blood volume
    b. heart rate and force
    c. peripheral vascular resistance
    d. all of the above

58. If the blood volume drops and the body is unable to compensate, the blood pressure will likely:
   a. drop.
   b. increase rapidly.
   c. increase slowly.
   d. remain the same.

59. The blood pressure is regulated by the:
   a. skeletal system.
   b. systole of the heart.
   c. brain and nervous system.
   d. smooth muscles in the vessels.

60. What is lymph fluid formed from?
   a. drainoff of the CSF
   b. excess intestinal fluid
   c. interstitial or extracellular fluid
   d. kidney byproducts

61. Part of the immune response consists of the release of chemicals that promote the influx of cells and other chemicals to fight the foreign challenge. This process is referred to as a/an:
   a. diffusion response.
   b. immunity response.
   c. inflammatory response.
   d. compensation response.

62. When the body is able to recognize, respond to, and remember a particular substance, this is called _____ immunity.
   a. specific
   b. cell-altered
   c. phagocytosis
   d. basophil-mediated

63. The primary function of the respiratory system is to:
   a. help purify the blood.
   b. eliminate waste products from the organs.
   c. circulate oxygenated blood to the heart cells.
   d. exchange gases at the alveolocapillary membrane.

64. When a patient inhales normally, the EMT-I should realize that the _____ muscle contracts, creating a _____ pressure that results in air being pulled into the thorax.
   a. rib; positive
   b. chest wall; negative
   c. diaphragm; negative
   d. intercostal; positive

65. The process of moving air into and out of the lungs is called:
   a. inhalation.
   b. ventilation.
   c. respiration.
   d. cellular respiration.

66. Diffusion in the respiratory system occurs at the:
   a. blood-brain barrier.
   b. blood-vessel level.
   c. bronchial-tree level.
   d. alveolocapillary junction.

67. What is the essential purpose of the circulatory system, in relation to the respiratory system?
   a. Carbon dioxide regulates the speed at which the heart pumps.
   b. The waste products of the circulatory system are excreted by the respiratory system.
   c. Without a functioning circulatory system, the lungs would be oxygenated but the cells of the body would not be.
   d. All of the above.

68. Respiration is regulated by the functioning of chemoreceptors that communicate directly with the brain. In this normal relationship, if the _____ level is high, the respiratory rate _____.
   a. oxygen; increases
   b. oxygen; decreases
   c. carbon dioxide; increases
   d. carbon dioxide; decreases

69. Which of the following is not considered an organ or component of the gastrointestinal tract?
   a. nose
   b. colon
   c. mouth
   d. duodenum

70. Where in the digestive system does food get masticated?
   a. mouth
   b. stomach
   c. large intestine
   d. small intestine

71. What is the function of the gallbladder in the digestive system?
   a. It stores bile, which helps to break down fatty foods.
   b. It is a holding place for the byproducts of the kidneys.
   c. It stores the sugar that is broken down in the pancreas.
   d. It stores acids that break down protein in the stomach.

72. Where do the nutrients in food get absorbed into the body?
   a. in the stomach
   b. in the large intestine
   c. in the small intestine
   d. at the cellular level in the liver

73. The human body is mostly made up of water and other fluids. The fluid found within individual cells is called the _____ and constitutes approximately _____ percent of the total body weight.
    a. interstitial fluid; 10.5
    b. intravascular fluid; 4.5
    c. intracellular fluid; 40 to 45
    d. extracellular fluid; 15 to 20

74. The fluid balance within the body is maintained by the actions of a combination of water shifts and:
    a. thyroid hormone.
    b. diuretic hormone.
    c. work of the kidneys.
    d. all of the above.

75. The process by which water moves between body compartments is called:
    a. osmosis.
    b. active transport.
    c. passive transport.
    d. facilitated diffusion.

76. The functional unit of the kidney is called the _____. When this unit no longer functions properly, the patient may need _____.
    a. neuron; dialysis
    b. nephron; dialysis
    c. neuron; fluid infusion
    d. glomerulus; fluid infusion

77. Control of the kidneys involves two key chemicals, ADH and aldosterone. When the tubules in the kidney increase reabsorption of sodium from the filtrate and decrease reabsorption of potassium, water and sodium move from filtrate into the blood, and excess potassium is excreted. This action is caused by:
    a. increased ADH levels.
    b. decreased ADH levels.
    c. increased aldosterone levels.
    d. decreased aldosterone levels.

78. How does respiration affect the body's acid/base balance?
    a. Increasing the breathing rate helps to increase the pH.
    b. Decreasing the breathing rate helps to increase the pH.
    c. Increasing the breathing rate stimulates the brain to generate water.
    d. Decreasing the breathing rate stimulates the kidneys to work overtime.

79. One of the fastest-acting defenses against acid/base changes, providing almost immediate protection against changes in hydrogen ion concentration of the extracellular fluid, is the:
    a. renal system.
    b. buffer system.
    c. lymphatic system.
    d. respiratory system.

80. Acidosis is a condition in which the body's pH decreases, thereby affecting cellular metabolism. This condition can result from an exacerbation of which medical condition?
    a. COPD
    b. asthma
    c. drug overdose
    d. any of the above

Chapter 2 Answer Form

	A	B	C	D		A	B	C	D
1.	❏	❏	❏	❏	26.	❏	❏	❏	❏
2.	❏	❏	❏	❏	27.	❏	❏	❏	❏
3.	❏	❏	❏	❏	28.	❏	❏	❏	❏
4.	❏	❏	❏	❏	29.	❏	❏	❏	❏
5.	❏	❏	❏	❏	30.	❏	❏	❏	❏
6.	❏	❏	❏	❏	31.	❏	❏	❏	❏
7.	❏	❏	❏	❏	32.	❏	❏	❏	❏
8.	❏	❏	❏	❏	33.	❏	❏	❏	❏
9.	❏	❏	❏	❏	34.	❏	❏	❏	❏
10.	❏	❏	❏	❏	35.	❏	❏	❏	❏
11.	❏	❏	❏	❏	36.	❏	❏	❏	❏
12.	❏	❏	❏	❏	37.	❏	❏	❏	❏
13.	❏	❏	❏	❏	38.	❏	❏	❏	❏
14.	❏	❏	❏	❏	39.	❏	❏	❏	❏
15.	❏	❏	❏	❏	40.	❏	❏	❏	❏
16.	❏	❏	❏	❏	41.	❏	❏	❏	❏
17.	❏	❏	❏	❏	42.	❏	❏	❏	❏
18.	❏	❏	❏	❏	43.	❏	❏	❏	❏
19.	❏	❏	❏	❏	44.	❏	❏	❏	❏
20.	❏	❏	❏	❏	45.	❏	❏	❏	❏
21.	❏	❏	❏	❏	46.	❏	❏	❏	❏
22.	❏	❏	❏	❏	47.	❏	❏	❏	❏
23.	❏	❏	❏	❏	48.	❏	❏	❏	❏
24.	❏	❏	❏	❏	49.	❏	❏	❏	❏
25.	❏	❏	❏	❏	50.	❏	❏	❏	❏

	A	B	C	D			A	B	C	D
51.	❑	❑	❑	❑		66.	❑	❑	❑	❑
52.	❑	❑	❑	❑		67.	❑	❑	❑	❑
53.	❑	❑	❑	❑		68.	❑	❑	❑	❑
54.	❑	❑	❑	❑		69.	❑	❑	❑	❑
55.	❑	❑	❑	❑		70.	❑	❑	❑	❑
56.	❑	❑	❑	❑		71.	❑	❑	❑	❑
57.	❑	❑	❑	❑		72.	❑	❑	❑	❑
58.	❑	❑	❑	❑		73.	❑	❑	❑	❑
59.	❑	❑	❑	❑		74.	❑	❑	❑	❑
60.	❑	❑	❑	❑		75.	❑	❑	❑	❑
61.	❑	❑	❑	❑		76.	❑	❑	❑	❑
62.	❑	❑	❑	❑		77.	❑	❑	❑	❑
63.	❑	❑	❑	❑		78.	❑	❑	❑	❑
64.	❑	❑	❑	❑		79.	❑	❑	❑	❑
65.	❑	❑	❑	❑		80.	❑	❑	❑	❑

CHAPTER 3

Emergency Pharmacology

1. Pharmacokinetics is the study of the _____ in and excretion of a drug from the human body.
   a. absorption
   b. distribution
   c. metabolism
   d. all of the above

2. The rate of absorption is usually a function of the route of drug administration. Which route in the following list is the slowest?
   a. enteral
   b. pulmonary
   c. intravenous
   d. subcutaneous

3. The movement of a drug from the bloodstream into the tissues and fluids of the body is called:
   a. excretion.
   b. absorption.
   c. distribution.
   d. metabolism.

4. Drug standardization has been achieved through regulation and legislation by the federal government. Of the following laws concerning drugs, which was the first to establish federal control over the importation, manufacture, and sale of opium and coca plants and their compounds and derivatives?
   a. Narcotic Control Act
   b. Pure Food and Drug Act
   c. Controlled Substances Act
   d. Harrison Narcotic Act of 1914

5. The five schedules of drugs are a part of the federal law passed in 1970 and called the:
   a. Narcotic Control Act.
   b. Pure Food and Drug Act.
   c. Controlled Substances Act.
   d. Drug Enforcement Administration Act.

6. Drugs often have many names. The first name given to a drug is the _____ name. The drug is then given a _____ name. Both these names are outside the manufacturer's control and are considered nonproprietary.
   a. generic; trade
   b. trade; generic
   c. trade; chemical
   d. chemical; generic

7. Drug products are created by chemical synthesis in the laboratory. They can also be developed from sources such as:
   a. plants.
   b. animals.
   c. minerals.
   d. all of the above.

8. Most of the drugs that the EMT-I will use are given by injection, in liquid form. These drugs are referred to as
   a. enteral.
   b. intravascular.
   c. parenteral.
   d. rapid-administration.

9. If the EMT-I wants to know more about a drug before having to administer it in an emergency, she could use _____ as a source of information.
   a. a Broselow length-based tape
   b. the *Physician's Desk Reference*
   c. a pocket guide for drugs in the field
   d. the *North Atlantic Emergency Response Guidebook*

10. When giving a drug to an elderly patient, it is important to remember that:
    a. older people have faster metabolic processes.
    b. older people require double the dose of a middle-aged adult.
    c. age-related liver dysfunction will extend the breakdown time of the drug.
    d. age-related kidney dysfunction will shorten the excretion time of the drug.

11. Before administering a drug to a young, pregnant patient, the EMT-I should:

    a. remember that pregnant patients will need twice the regular dose.

    b. confirm that the fetus does not have an allergy to the medicine.

    c. verify with medical direction that it is safe to administer the drug to a pregnant patient.

    d. remember that pregnant patients have a much faster metabolism rate.

12. Because many medication doses are weight related, pediatric patients usually receive:

    a. twice the adult dose.

    b. about a tenth of the adult dose.

    c. very few medications by the IV route.

    d. a smaller dose than an adult's, based on their weight.

13. Before administering any drug, the EMT-I must know the drug's effect. Specifically, *drug effect* refers to which of the following?

    a. the cellular change effected by the drug

    b. the degree of physiologic change caused by the drug

    c. the movement of drugs through the body, including absorption, distribution, metabolism, and excretion

    d. none of the above

14. Before administering any drug, the EMT-I should review the specifics for that drug, including verifying if she has the right:

    a. time and date.

    b. dose and route.

    c. drug for a specific disease process.

    d. method of disposal for the empty container.

15. The EMT-I administers a drug that causes an effect that was not intended, such as a headache or dizziness. This effect is referred to as:

    a. a side effect.

    b. drug toxicity.

    c. a therapeutic effect.

    d. an anaphylactic reaction.

16. A drug combined with water and oil is called a/an:

    a. elixir.

    b. spirit.

    c. extract.

    d. emulsion.

17. Which of the following forms of medications is not considered a solid?

    a. lozenge

    b. capsule

    c. tincture

    d. ointment

18. During a patient assessment, the EMT-I notices that the patient has a nitro patch on his chest. This patch administers medication by the _____ route.

    a. sublingual

    b. transdermal

    c. intramuscular

    d. subcutaneous

19. The EMT-I has just given an injection into the fatty layer of tissue below the skin, by positioning the needle and syringe at a 45-degree angle to the skin. This medication is being delivered by the _____ route.

    a. intradermal

    b. intravenous

    c. intramuscular

    d. subcutaneous

20. The effects of a drug that is a parasympathetic blocker will include:

    a. increased heart rate.

    b. decreased heart rate.

    c. salivation and tearing.

    d. decreased effort of breathing.

21. When alpha-adrenergic receptors are stimulated by a drug that you administered to the patient, you should expect the patient to experience:

    a. vasodilation.

    b. vasoconstriction.

    c. bronchodilatation.

    d. a headache and tingling sensation.

22. When a beta-1 adrenergic stimulating medication is given to the patient, the EMT-I should expect to see:

    a. decreased inotropic effect.

    b. increased chronotropic effect.

    c. decreased dromotropic effect.

    d. increased parasympathetic effect.

23. When two or more drugs are taken simultaneously, and one drug prolongs or multiplies the effect of the other drug, this is referred to as:

    a. antagonism.

    b. synergism.

    c. potentiation.

    d. a cumulative effect.

24. An abnormal or unexpected reaction to a drug peculiar to a specific patient is called a/an:

    a. allergy.

    b. contraindication.

    c. hypersensitivity.

    d. idiosyncratic reaction.

25. Typically, many regions allow the EMT-I to administer which of the following medications when the patient presents with the appropriate clinical picture and the local medical direction approves?
    a. insulin
    b. Isuprel
    c. steroids
    d. albuterol sulfate

26. Security of controlled substances is important and highly regulated. Why is it so important for the EMT-I to strictly follow the mandated procedures?
    a. The supply of that substance to your agency could be decreased.
    b. Too many others have abused the privilege of handing controlled substances.
    c. The patient may ask questions about the use of narcotics.
    d. Failure to follow procedures could cause the loss of your medical director's license.

27. Medications should be stored:
    a. in a hot, dry location.
    b. in a sharps container.
    c. within the temperature ranges specified by the manufacturers.
    d. in the refrigerator so that they will last longer than the dates on the containers.

28. Before administering a medication, it is important to ensure that it is not:
    a. clear.
    b. outdated.
    c. absorbed too quickly.
    d. already prescribed for the patient's spouse.

29. The medication Dextrose 50% is usually supplied in a:
    a. plastic cup.
    b. large capsule.
    c. large barrel with syringe.
    d. can similar to those of diet supplements.

30. After administering any medication, it is important for the EMT-I to:
    a. prepare the next dose.
    b. tell the patient to sit still.
    c. administer high-concentration oxygen.
    d. do an ongoing assessment of the patient.

Chapter 3 Answer Form

	A	B	C	D		A	B	C	D
1.	❏	❏	❏	❏	16.	❏	❏	❏	❏
2.	❏	❏	❏	❏	17.	❏	❏	❏	❏
3.	❏	❏	❏	❏	18.	❏	❏	❏	❏
4.	❏	❏	❏	❏	19.	❏	❏	❏	❏
5.	❏	❏	❏	❏	20.	❏	❏	❏	❏
6.	❏	❏	❏	❏	21.	❏	❏	❏	❏
7.	❏	❏	❏	❏	22.	❏	❏	❏	❏
8.	❏	❏	❏	❏	23.	❏	❏	❏	❏
9.	❏	❏	❏	❏	24.	❏	❏	❏	❏
10.	❏	❏	❏	❏	25.	❏	❏	❏	❏
11.	❏	❏	❏	❏	26.	❏	❏	❏	❏
12.	❏	❏	❏	❏	27.	❏	❏	❏	❏
13.	❏	❏	❏	❏	28.	❏	❏	❏	❏
14.	❏	❏	❏	❏	29.	❏	❏	❏	❏
15.	❏	❏	❏	❏	30.	❏	❏	❏	❏

CHAPTER 4

Venous Access and Medication Administration

1. What anatomy is it important for the EMT-I to know when preparing to administer a medication?
   a. the location of the capillaries
   b. the length of a typical adult long bone
   c. the time it takes the large intestine to absorb food
   d. the layers of the skin for administration of medications by injection

2. What physiology is it important for the EMT-I to know when deciding on the route of administration for a drug?
   a. how many layers of skin must be punctured
   b. the rate at which the kidneys will metabolize the drug
   c. the speed with which the digestive system will absorb the drug
   d. how fast the bloodstream will be accessed by each route of administration

3. In mathematics, the number on the bottom of a fraction is called the:
   a. equal.
   b. multiplier.
   c. numerator.
   d. denominator.

4. Medications are often administered based on a patient's weight in kilograms, and the EMT-I will often have to convert the weight. When converting from kilograms to pounds, the number of pounds will appear to be:
   a. the same.
   b. half the size.
   c. double the size.
   d. slightly more (approximately 10% more) than double the size.

5. The drip chambers of three IV administration sets are designated by drip size (gtt): 10 gtt/ml, 15 gtt/ml, and 20 gtt/ml. Which of these sets delivers the largest size drop from the chamber?
   a. the 10 gtt/ml set
   b. the 15 gtt/ml set
   c. the 20 gtt/ml set
   d. they are all the same size when set at KVO

6. The basic unit of volume is a liter. How many milliliters are in one liter?
   a. 0.1
   b. 10
   c. 100
   d. 1,000

7. Medication doses may be administered in micrograms. One microgram is _____ of a gram.
   a. one-tenth
   b. one-hundredth
   c. one-thousandth
   d. one-millionth

8. On a very warm day in Phoenix, the temperature reached _____. In the northeast, it rarely gets that hot, but the Arizonans said that was typical for a May day!
   a. 100° Kelvin
   b. 100° Celsius
   c. 100° centigrade
   d. 100° Fahrenheit

9. The EMT-I may need to use a formula for simple drug calculation in the field. Which of the following is incorrect and should not be used?

   a. To convert pounds to kilograms, divide the number of lbs by 2.2.

   b. To convert Celsius to Fahrenheit, multiply by 9/5 and add 32.

   c. To convert Fahrenheit to Celsius, subtract 48 and multiply by 4/5.

   d. The formula for a drug dose is: dose ordered $\times$ unit measure/amount on hand.

10. Your patient weighs 110 lbs. She needs 5 mg per kg of an antidysrhythmic. How much should she receive?

   a. 50 mg

   b. 250 mg

   c. 500 mg

   d. 550 mg

11. Your patient is a 55-lb child. The medical control physician just ordered 10 mg per kg of a medication given by an IV bolus. How much should you inject?

   a. 50 mg

   b. 100 mg

   c. 250 mg

   d. 500 mg

12. You have just set up a macro drip administration set (15 gtt/ml) and are ordered to give the patient 100 ml over the next 30 minutes. How many drops per minute will you need to set the IV drip rate at to accomplish this?

   a. 25 gtt/min

   b. 50 gtt/min

   c. 100 gtt/min

   d. 150 gtt/min

13. Orders for medication administration can be received by the EMT-I from:

   a. a physician over the radio.

   b. a standing order in the local protocols.

   c. a medical control physician who is on the scene.

   d. any of the above.

14. Once a drug has been administered to the patient, it is the EMT-I's responsibility to document which of the following?

   a. the drug that was given

   b. the number of pills left in the bottle

   c. the time the drug was prepared for administration

   d. exactly who was present when the drug was administered

15. The "rights" of drug administration include each of the following, except the right:

   a. patient.

   b. route and dose.

   c. drug administered.

   d. size of syringe used.

16. Virtually no medical procedure is done in a 100 percent aseptic or sterile manner. Why is it important for the EMT-I to use the most sterile technique possible when administering an IV medication?

   a. It is on the exam that way.

   b. The protocols usually specify it.

   c. If this is not done, the patient may develop a serious infection.

   d. There is no need to use aseptic technique when starting an IV.

17. The EMT-I uses a iodine swab to clean the area where an IV will be started because iodine is a/an _____ agent.

   a. sterilizing

   b. cleansing

   c. antiseptic

   d. disinfecting

18. The minimal amount of personal protective equipment (PPE) the EMT-I should wear when starting an IV on a patient is:

   a. goggles.

   b. a gown.

   c. disposable gloves.

   d. a HEPA or N-95 mask.

19. When preparing to do a peripheral venous cannulation, which of the following items is not typically used?

   a. a 50-cc syringe

   b. adhesive tape

   c. Tegaderm™ or Veniguard®

   d. appropriate blood tubes

20. When setting up an IV administration set, it is important for the EMT-I to:

   a. flush all the air out of the line.

   b. flush all the fluid out of the line.

   c. completely fill the drip chamber.

   d. remove the cap at the end of the tubing.

21. An EMT-I is planning to administer fluid by the intraosseous (IO) route. Which of the following sites is a suitable location for injection of the IO needle?

   a. upper tibia

   b. lower femur

   c. midshaft femur

   d. upper humerus

22. In which of the following patients would it be appropriate for the EMT-I to consider the administration of fluid by the IO route?

   a. a 22-year-old asthmatic

   b. a 46-year-old male with chest pain

   c. a 3-year-old with circulatory collapse

   d. a patient with a crush injury to the lower extremities

23. Which medication is usually administered by the inhalation route?

    a. nitroglycerin
    b. albuterol
    c. dextrose
    d. morphine

24. To administer a medication by the inhalation route, the EMT-I should have _____ available.

    a. saline solution
    b. oxygen
    c. heat packs
    d. a humidifier

25. Oral medications can be given by which of the following doses?

    a. drop
    b. spray
    c. teaspoon
    d. all of the above

26. In small children, it may sometimes be appropriate to administer certain medications, such as diazepam, by the _____ route.

    a. nasal
    b. rectal
    c. gastric
    d. buccal

27. Which of the following medications is administered by the enteral route during emergency care?

    a. nitroglycerin
    b. aspirin
    c. albuterol
    d. morphine

28. Which of the following medications is administered by the parenteral route?

    a. Tylenol
    b. syrup of ipecac
    c. activated charcoal
    d. epinephrine 1:1000

29. Administration of a medication by injection is also described as:

    a. enteral.
    b. gastric.
    c. inhalation.
    d. percutaneous.

30. When preparing to start an IV on a patient, it is important that the EMT-I plan ahead and have a/an _____ at the patient's side.

    a. emesis basin
    b. sharps container
    c. pile of gauze bandages
    d. syringe with sterile saline

31. Proper disposal of a needle that has been used to administer a medication by the IM route includes:

    a. saving it for reuse.
    b. giving it to the nurse at the hospital.
    c. throwing it in the ambulance garbage can.
    d. placing it in a sharps container right away.

32. In what manner may understanding the pathophysiological principles of medication administration be helpful to the EMT-I?

    a. It helps the EMT-I remember the various names of each medication.
    b. It helps the EMT-I understand the methods of calculating the dose of a medication.
    c. It helps the EMT-I understand why certain routes of administration are better than others when the body is stressed.
    d. It helps the EMT-I understand why certain types of needles should be used for specific locations in the body.

33. When documenting the dose of a medication that you administered, be sure to note the:

    a. expiration date of the medication.
    b. exact dose of the medication.
    c. generic name of the medication.
    d. amount of medication left in the vial.

34. While starting an IV, you drop the IV catheter on the ground. You should:

    a. wipe it off with an alcohol prep.
    b. discard it and open another one.
    c. clean it off with alcohol and Betadine®.
    d. recleanse the IV site before sticking the patient.

35. When a medication is to be administered by the IM route in an adult, the most likely administration site is the:

    a. thigh.
    b. foot.
    c. deltoid.
    d. buttocks.

Chapter 4 Answer Form

	A	B	C	D		A	B	C	D
1.	❑	❑	❑	❑	19.	❑	❑	❑	❑
2.	❑	❑	❑	❑	20.	❑	❑	❑	❑
3.	❑	❑	❑	❑	21.	❑	❑	❑	❑
4.	❑	❑	❑	❑	22.	❑	❑	❑	❑
5.	❑	❑	❑	❑	23.	❑	❑	❑	❑
6.	❑	❑	❑	❑	24.	❑	❑	❑	❑
7.	❑	❑	❑	❑	25.	❑	❑	❑	❑
8.	❑	❑	❑	❑	26.	❑	❑	❑	❑
9.	❑	❑	❑	❑	27.	❑	❑	❑	❑
10.	❑	❑	❑	❑	28.	❑	❑	❑	❑
11.	❑	❑	❑	❑	29.	❑	❑	❑	❑
12.	❑	❑	❑	❑	30.	❑	❑	❑	❑
13.	❑	❑	❑	❑	31.	❑	❑	❑	❑
14.	❑	❑	❑	❑	32.	❑	❑	❑	❑
15.	❑	❑	❑	❑	33.	❑	❑	❑	❑
16.	❑	❑	❑	❑	34.	❑	❑	❑	❑
17.	❑	❑	❑	❑	35.	❑	❑	❑	❑
18.	❑	❑	❑	❑					

CHAPTER 5

Airway Management and Ventilation

1. A common problem associated with airway management in the patient requiring ventilation assistance is:
   a. improper seal of a bag mask.
   b. use of oral airways on patients who have a gag reflex.
   c. improper securing of an endotracheal tube.
   d. use of a nasal airway on patients with altered mental status.

2. The anatomical structure of the airway in which the vocal cords are located is the:
   a. carina.
   b. larynx.
   c. pharynx.
   d. bronchus.

3. The anatomical structure where the oxygen/carbon dioxide exchange with the bloodstream occurs is the:
   a. alveoli.
   b. larynx.
   c. bronchus.
   d. turbinates.

4. What is the function of the hairs in the nose?
   a. They act as a filter to catch impurities.
   b. They cool the air before it enters the lungs.
   c. They can cause constriction of the airway.
   d. They serve no function in the respiratory system.

5. Which of the following anatomical structures is a part of the upper airway?
   a. nares
   b. alveoli
   c. trachea
   d. carina

6. A patient has a reactive airway disease that causes constriction, inflammation, and audible wheezing. This pathology is mostly focused on the:
   a. trachea.
   b. bronchioles.
   c. mainstem bronchi.
   d. oropharynx and nasopharynx.

7. Each of the following statements is an example of the differences between adult and pediatric airway anatomy, except:
   a. the youngest pediatric patients are obligate nose breathers.
   b. the pediatric tongue is proportionately larger than the adult's.
   c. the smallest diameter in the pediatric airway is the cricoid ring.
   d. the pediatric trachea is more posterior than the adult trachea.

8. The normal tidal volume for an adult is:
   a. approximately 6–7 cc per kg.
   b. increased in an asthmatic patient.
   c. less than that of a pediatric patient.
   d. restricted when the patient has fully developed chest muscles.

9. When ventilating an infant with a bagmask, it is best to watch the chest for:
   a. improved color.
   b. visible chest rise.
   c. slight movement.
   d. constriction of the pupils.

10. When a patient does not exercise them by taking adequate-size breaths, the alveoli may collapse. This condition is referred to as:
    a. infection.
    b. atelectasis.
    c. pneumonia.
    d. consolidation.

11. The amount of oxygen that the EMT-I administers to a patient is often referred to as the:
    a. FiO_2.
    b. PCO_2.
    c. hematocrit.
    d. tidal volume.

12. When oxygen is inhaled into the body, how does it reach to the heart?

    a. by the coronary circulation
    b. through the systemic circulation
    c. through the pulmonary circulation
    d. through the alveolar membrane and venous system

13. Which of the following is unlikely to be associated with a decreased oxygen concentration in the blood?

    a. a lengthy submersion
    b. a pulmonary embolism
    c. elevated blood pressure
    d. carbon monoxide poisoning

14. The amount of carbon dioxide in the blood may be increased when the patient is:

    a. scuba diving.
    b. hypoventilating.
    c. hyperventilating.
    d. having a diabetic crisis.

15. Monitoring the oxygen concentration of the blood is essential when the patient has:

    a. major trauma.
    b. end-stage COPD.
    c. end-stage diabetes.
    d. an increased hematocrit.

16. How does the brain monitor the concentration of carbon dioxide in the blood?

    a. The brain does not monitor the CO_2 level.
    b. Chemoreceptors send messages to the brain.
    c. It measures the concentration in the blood in the aorta.
    d. It measures the concentration in the cerebral blood flow.

17. The gas that comprises the majority of atmospheric air is:

    a. oxygen.
    b. nitrogen.
    c. hydrogen.
    d. carbon monoxide.

18. Which of the following is unlikely to contribute to an alteration in respiratory depth?

    a. fractured ribs
    b. diabetic coma
    c. fractured radius
    d. a narcotic overdose

19. When a patient has an increased respiratory rate after a serious motorcycle collision, the EMT-I should suspect that the patient:

    a. may be in a diabetic coma.
    b. may have a serious head injury.
    c. may have been taking an opiate.
    d. is probably exhibiting hyperventilation syndrome.

20. The brain may increase the respiratory rate in response to receptors' notifying the brain that there is too much carbon dioxide in the body. This is considered:

    a. a direct result of a nerve reflex.
    b. voluntary regulation of respiration.
    c. involuntary regulation of respiration.
    d. a nonproductive feedback mechanism.

21. A patient is found in a restaurant exhibiting the signs and symptoms of an upper airway obstruction. This is most likely caused by:

    a. alcohol.
    b. talking while eating.
    c. not cutting meat small enough.
    d. a combination of the above.

22. An upper airway obstruction created by the patient's own anatomical features would most likely be caused by the:

    a. nares.
    b. tongue.
    c. vocal cords.
    d. mainstem bronchus.

23. The normal respiratory rate for a 10-year-old child is approximately _____ breaths per minute.

    a. 10–15
    b. 16–20
    c. 21–25
    d. 26–30

24. It is not uncommon for an infant to have a normal respiratory rate of approximately _____ breaths per minute.

    a. 21–25
    b. 26–30
    c. 31–35
    d. 36–40

25. The EMT-I is evaluating a patient who is in respiratory distress. Which of the following chief complaints is an unlikely cause of the distress?

    a. sternal fracture
    b. lacerated forearm
    c. acute exacerbation of COPD
    d. foreign body airway obstruction

26. Hypoxemia is a term for:

    a. reduced oxygen in the blood.
    b. increased oxygen in the blood.
    c. decreased oxygen to the coronary vessels.
    d. increased carbon dioxide levels in the lungs.

27. Hypoxia is a term for:

    a. the same condition as hypoxemia.
    b. reduced oxygen in the blood.
    c. elevated carbon monoxide in the cells.
    d. oxygen deficiency to the body sufficient to cause impaired function.

28. Which of the following is an unlikely cause of hypoxemia?
   a. increased hematocrit
   b. carbon monoxide poisoning
   c. inadequate pulmonary ventilation (e.g., COPD)
   d. low partial pressure of the atmosphere (e.g., high altitude)

29. A pulse rate that varies abnormally with the respiratory rate is referred to as:
   a. pulsus paradoxus.
   b. atrial dysrhythmia.
   c. sinus bradycardia.
   d. the pulse pressure.

30. Which of the following is not considered a modified form of respiration?
   a. agonal gasps
   b. Cheyne-Stokes
   c. Kussmaul's respirations
   d. central neurogenic hyperventilation syndrome

31. An involuntary reflex that may be absent when the patient's level of consciousness is diminished is the _____ reflex.
   a. gag
   b. blink
   c. corneal
   d. patellar

32. With regard to oxygen cylinders, which of the following activities should be avoided?
   a. Laying the tank down to keep it from falling on the regulator.
   b. Securely strapping the cylinder into the stretcher with the patient.
   c. Making sure the tank is securely fastened to a wall or cabinet.
   d. Using ferrous metal wrenches to change gauges or regulators.

33. When handling oxygen, the EMT-I should never:
   a. allow oxygen to flow near a flame source.
   b. strap the tank onto the stretcher with the patient.
   c. administer more than 8 liters per minute to the patient.
   d. line up the two pins on the regulator before tightening it.

34. The main oxygen cylinder in the ambulance usually has a _____ regulator attached to it.
   a. low-flow
   b. high-flow
   c. low-pressure
   d. high-pressure

35. When changing an oxygen cylinder, before placing the regulator on the new tank the EMT-I should:
   a. use adhesive tape to properly label the new tank.
   b. replace the washer on the regulator.
   c. crack the tank open slightly to clean any dust out of the valve.
   d. open the valve fully to prevent someone else from thinking it is empty.

36. When the EMT-I administers oxygen to a male patient who is complaining of severe chest pain, the device of choice is a _____ with a liter flow of _____ liters per minute.
   a. nasal cannula; 6
   b. nasal cannula; 10
   c. non-rebreather mask; 12
   d. partial rebreather mask; 8

37. Which of the following is a contraindication for the administration of high-concentration oxygen to a patient with mild respiratory distress?
   a. deep shock
   b. shortness of breath
   c. a history of asthma
   d. end-stage emphysema

38. When it is necessary to use supplemental oxygen for an unconscious patient who is in severe respiratory distress, the EMT-I should consider using a:
   a. nasal cannula at 6 liters per minute.
   b. bag mask to assist ventilations.
   c. non-rebreather mask at 8–10 liters per minute.
   d. none of the above.

39. Why would it be appropriate to consider using an oxygen humidifier for a patient during a lengthy inter-hospital transport?
   a. Humidified oxygen is less costly.
   b. Humidified oxygen penetrates the alveoli faster.
   c. Oxygen tends to dry out the mucous membranes.
   d. Humidified oxygen makes the patient less hypoxic.

40. The surgical opening in the neck in a patient who has had a laryngectomy is called the:
   a. stoma.
   b. larynx.
   c. tracheostomy.
   d. tracheotomy tube.

41. Why is it so important to wear a mask and eye shield when ventilating a patient?
   a. to comply with the FAA mandates
   b. to prevent breathing on a very sick patient
   c. to keep the oxygen from being absorbed into your eyes
   d. to prevent fluid droplets from entering your mouth or eyes

42. When three rescuers are available to assist on a complicated ventilation, one of the rescuers should be assigned to:
    a. compress the abdomen to relieve pressure.
    b. ensure that the ventilation rate is more than 12 per minute.
    c. provide cricoid pressure for any patient who has a tube in place.
    d. perform the Sellick maneuver on a patient who does not have an advanced airway in place.

43. When it is necessary to ventilate an adult patient using a bag mask, what should the EMT-I concentrate on providing?
    a. more than one ventilation every 5 seconds
    b. sufficient volume to achieve visible chest rise
    c. rapid ventilations to increase the SpO_2 reading
    d. rapid transport to the nearest emergency department

44. Which of the following is a complication of using a bag mask that the EMT-I should be careful to avoid?
    a. hypoventilation
    b. intact gag reflex
    c. hyperoxygenation
    d. decreased gag reflex

45. Ventilating a patient too forcefully, with too great a volume of gas, can produce:
    a. atelectasis.
    b. gastric reflux.
    c. gastric distension.
    d. inflation of the bowel.

46. When an automated transport ventilator (ATV) is available for ventilating patients; the EMT-I should avoid:
    a. using the device when the patient is hypoxic.
    b. providing excessive ventilations with the device.
    c. using the device on a patient who is not breathing on his own.
    d. using the device on a patient who has been a victim of submersion.

47. Pressure may be applied to the larynx in an attempt to gently push the airway structure back against the esophagus. This is called the:
    a. cricoid technique.
    b. Sellick maneuver.
    c. airway procedure.
    d. esophageal maneuver.

48. When the EMT-I ventilates a child, as compared to an adult, it is important to:
    a. use the pressure relief valve on the adult bag mask.
    b. increase the rate per the resuscitation standards.
    c. decrease the rate per the resuscitation standards.
    d. increase the volume to assure that the chest rises.

49. When it is necessary to ventilate a patient who has a stoma, the EMT-I should:
    a. utilize blow-by oxygen.
    b. first use a laryngoscope.
    c. always use the Sellick maneuver.
    d. try using a pediatric mask to seal around the opening.

50. A patient is no longer able to speak or cough because a large bolus of food has become lodged in her throat. This is called a:
    a. laryngospasm.
    b. crushed trachea.
    c. partial airway obstruction.
    d. complete airway obstruction.

51. When a patient has a partial airway obstruction with poor air exchange, the EMT-I should treat the patient as if he were:
    a. in need of a series of back blows.
    b. in need of immediate ventilation.
    c. experiencing a completely blocked airway.
    d. in distress, and wait a few minutes to see how he does.

52. When a patient has a partial airway obstruction with good air exchange, the EMT-I should:
    a. begin bagmask ventilations on the patient.
    b. immediately give a series of back blows.
    c. encourage the patient to cough, but not intervene just yet.
    d. treat the patient as if the patient were experiencing a completely blocked airway.

53. If the EMT-I suspects a complete airway obstruction in an adult patient who is still conscious, the EMT-I should:
    a. verify that the patient cannot speak.
    b. immediately give a series of back blows.
    c. observe and encourage the patient to cough.
    d. open the airway and verify that there is an obstruction.

54. As an advanced life support provider, the EMT-I can consider one additional step when confronted with a patient who has a completely blocked airway. What is that step?
    a. Start an IV right away.
    b. Begin chest compressions on the patient.
    c. Administer epinephrine to the patient right away.
    d. Attempt a direct laryngoscopy and remove the obstruction with forceps.

55. If a patient has fluid or blood in the upper airway, the EMT-I should begin to:
    a. expedite transportation of the patient.
    b. insert a flexible catheter into the pharynx.
    c. suction the patient with a rigid-tip suction catheter.
    d. prepare to insert an nasogastric tube into the patient.

56. Generally, a soft catheter is designed to be passed:
    a. through the nostrils.
    b. deep into the throat.
    c. into the patient's right nostril.
    d. through a tube such as an endotracheal tube.

57. Which of the following should be avoided when using a soft catheter?
    a. inserting the catheter with the suction turned off
    b. suctioning the patient as you withdraw the catheter
    c. not using a suction catheter on an unconscious patient
    d. inserting the catheter into the nose if you suspect a skull fracture

58. Which of the following suction devices is commonly used by the EMT-I on infant patients?
    a. manual unit
    b. bulb syringes
    c. oxygen-powered suction units
    d. battery-powered suction units

59. When suctioning the upper airway, it is a good practice for the EMT-I to:
    a. limit the attempts at suction to two per rescuer.
    b. ensure that the patient continues to be adequately oxygenated.
    c. maximize the amount of time the patient is being suctioned.
    d. be aware that stimulating the back of the throat may cause tachycardia.

60. When suctioning a patient, especially a child, it is important to:
    a. enter the nostril very slowly.
    b. suction as you enter the pharynx.
    c. limit the attempts at suctioning to two per rescuer.
    d. watch for a decrease in the pulse rate due to vagal stimuli.

61. "Deep suctioning" actually refers to the procedure of:
    a. passing a tube directly into the opening of a stoma.
    b. tracheobronchial suctioning in an intubated patient.
    c. passing a suction catheter far into the patient's pharynx.
    d. passing the rigid tip suction catheteror device far into the back of the patient's throat.

62. Having an advanced airway in place can mean that the patient has a/an:
    a. oropharyngeal airway (OPA) in place.
    b. nasopharyngeal airway (NPA) in place.
    c. modified jaw thrust.
    d. Combitube™ in place.

63. The EMT-I suspects that the patient had a full stomach prior to his collapse. Which advanced airway device would be least effective if the patient vomits?
    a. LMA™
    b. Combitube™
    c. endotracheal tube
    d. oropharyngeal or nasopharyngeal airway

64. If you suspect that a patient, especially a child, is becoming difficult to ventilate, it may be helpful to insert a/an:
    a. LMA™.
    b. nasogastric tube.
    c. endotracheal tube.
    d. tracheotomy tube.

65. A patient was found unconscious in bed. One of your first steps should be to:
    a. do a direct laryngoscopy.
    b. do a jaw-thrust maneuver.
    c. administer 4 quick breaths to the patient.
    d. place the pillow behind the patient's shoulder rather than behind her head.

66. When approaching an unconscious trauma victim, the EMT-I will need to open the airway. The technique to consider first is:
    a. the head-tilt chin-lift maneuver.
    b. Sellick's maneuver.
    c. the jaw-thrust maneuver.
    d. the two-person bagmask technique.

67. A nasopharyngeal airway should be used:
    a. when vomit or other secretions occlude the oropharynx.
    b. when trauma has caused broken teeth or loose dentures.
    c. if you need to access the oropharynx in a patient with clenched teeth.
    d. when bleeding from the nose cannot be controlled by other measures.

68. Previously referred to as the "gold standard" of airway care, _____ is a method of isolating the trachea to assist the patient with ventilations.
    a. the LMA™
    b. the esophageal obturator airway (EOA)
    c. the Combitube™
    d. endotracheal intubation

69. Why is it so important to listen to the lungs and epigastrium after inserting an ET tube?
    a. to verify that the tube is just above the carina
    b. to verify that the stomach is not being ventilated
    c. to verify that the tube is not in the right mainstem bronchus
    d. all of the above

70. What is a disadvantage of endotracheal intubation?
    a. It can be placed blindly by a person with very little training.
    b. It requires frequent retraining and practice to stay proficient.
    c. It requires expensive equipment that may not be available in the field.
    d. There are no disadvantages; this is the preferred method of managing the airway.

71. What is an advantage of endotracheal intubation?
    a. It can be placed blindly by a person with very little training.
    b. Once the tube is placed, it is basically maintenance-free.
    c. It helps isolate the trachea and can limit aspiration into the lungs.
    d. Providers are easily trained in this procedure and can maintain the skill with little effort.

72. You are managing the airway of a 25-year-old obese male who overdosed. After two attempts, you are still unable to pass an endotracheal tube, due to the size of the patient's neck. What should you do?
    a. Pass the Combitube and then tube around it.
    b. Call a more experienced medic to the scene to pass the tube.
    c. Place a pillow behind the patient's upper back and ventilate him with a bag mask.
    d. Continue to try to place the ET tube, as it is essential to bring him in with one in place.

73. When inserting a curved laryngoscope blade into a patient's mouth, the tip should be inserted into the:
    a. carina.
    b. vallecula.
    c. vocal cords.
    d. mainstem bronchus.

74. Once the EMT-I actually sees the endotracheal tube go through the vocal cords, it is also important to _____ as an alternate means of confirming the placement.
    a. apply an esophageal intubation detection device (EID)
    b. listen over both lung fields
    c. check the pulse oximeter and EtCO$_2$
    d. all of the above

75. The EMT-I needs to extubate a patient because he has regained consciousness and is fighting the tube. In this situation, the EMT-I should always have a/an _____ available.
    a. extra tube
    b. suction unit
    c. muscle relaxant
    d. positive pressure ventilator

76. After insertion of a Combitube™, the EMT-I should inflate the _____ pilot balloon first.
    a. red
    b. green
    c. larger
    d. smaller

77. The Combitube™ is also called a/an _____ airway.
    a. dual-lumen
    b. open-lumen
    c. laryngeal-mask
    d. esophageal obturator

78. Use of a Combitube™ is indicated in:
    a. cardiac arrest only.
    b. any patient who is unconscious.
    c. unconscious children without a gag reflex.
    d. unconscious adult patients without a gag reflex.

79. Which of the following is a contraindication for the use of a dual-lumen airway?
    a. a young patient who is less than 4 feet tall
    b. a patient who ingested a corrosive poison
    c. a patient who gags when the device is inserted
    d. all of the above

80. Which of the following is true of airway management in a pediatric patient?
    a. Use ET tubes that do not have a cuff for children.
    b. Carefully position the head, as the occiput is large.
    c. The sniffing position is not used when passing an ET tube in children.
    d. Never use a stylet to facilitate the passing of the endotracheal tube.

Chapter 5 Answer Form

	A	B	C	D		A	B	C	D
1.	❏	❏	❏	❏	26.	❏	❏	❏	❏
2.	❏	❏	❏	❏	27.	❏	❏	❏	❏
3.	❏	❏	❏	❏	28.	❏	❏	❏	❏
4.	❏	❏	❏	❏	29.	❏	❏	❏	❏
5.	❏	❏	❏	❏	30.	❏	❏	❏	❏
6.	❏	❏	❏	❏	31.	❏	❏	❏	❏
7.	❏	❏	❏	❏	32.	❏	❏	❏	❏
8.	❏	❏	❏	❏	33.	❏	❏	❏	❏
9.	❏	❏	❏	❏	34.	❏	❏	❏	❏
10.	❏	❏	❏	❏	35.	❏	❏	❏	❏
11.	❏	❏	❏	❏	36.	❏	❏	❏	❏
12.	❏	❏	❏	❏	37.	❏	❏	❏	❏
13.	❏	❏	❏	❏	38.	❏	❏	❏	❏
14.	❏	❏	❏	❏	39.	❏	❏	❏	❏
15.	❏	❏	❏	❏	40.	❏	❏	❏	❏
16.	❏	❏	❏	❏	41.	❏	❏	❏	❏
17.	❏	❏	❏	❏	42.	❏	❏	❏	❏
18.	❏	❏	❏	❏	43.	❏	❏	❏	❏
19.	❏	❏	❏	❏	44.	❏	❏	❏	❏
20.	❏	❏	❏	❏	45.	❏	❏	❏	❏
21.	❏	❏	❏	❏	46.	❏	❏	❏	❏
22.	❏	❏	❏	❏	47.	❏	❏	❏	❏
23.	❏	❏	❏	❏	48.	❏	❏	❏	❏
24.	❏	❏	❏	❏	49.	❏	❏	❏	❏
25.	❏	❏	❏	❏	50.	❏	❏	❏	❏

	A	B	C	D		A	B	C	D
51.	❑	❑	❑	❑	66.	❑	❑	❑	❑
52.	❑	❑	❑	❑	67.	❑	❑	❑	❑
53.	❑	❑	❑	❑	68.	❑	❑	❑	❑
54.	❑	❑	❑	❑	69.	❑	❑	❑	❑
55.	❑	❑	❑	❑	70.	❑	❑	❑	❑
56.	❑	❑	❑	❑	71.	❑	❑	❑	❑
57.	❑	❑	❑	❑	72.	❑	❑	❑	❑
58.	❑	❑	❑	❑	73.	❑	❑	❑	❑
59.	❑	❑	❑	❑	74.	❑	❑	❑	❑
60.	❑	❑	❑	❑	75.	❑	❑	❑	❑
61.	❑	❑	❑	❑	76.	❑	❑	❑	❑
62.	❑	❑	❑	❑	77.	❑	❑	❑	❑
63.	❑	❑	❑	❑	78.	❑	❑	❑	❑
64.	❑	❑	❑	❑	79.	❑	❑	❑	❑
65.	❑	❑	❑	❑	80.	❑	❑	❑	❑

CHAPTER

History Taking

1. Which of the following may impair the EMT-I's ability to collect medical history?
   a. positive body language
   b. ineffective listening skills
   c. a professional demeanor
   d. good eye contact with the patient

2. Which of the following is considered a diagnostic rather than a technique of history taking?
   a. measuring the $EtCO_2$
   b. establishing a rapport with the patient
   c. investigating the patient's chief complaint
   d. questioning the patient about his or her medical conditions

3. When is it important to use open-ended questions?
   a. when there is a lot of time to be filled up
   b. when it is necessary to limit the patient's response
   c. open-ended questions should not be used on emergency calls
   d. when the EMT-I would like the patient to describe his or her symptoms in detail

4. When is it important to use closed-ended questions?
   a. when there is a lot of time to be filled up
   b. whenever the patient is complaining of pain
   c. when it is necessary to speed up the information gathering
   d. closed-ended questions should not be used on emergency calls

5. Which of the following is an example of an open-ended question?
   a. asking the patient his age
   b. asking the patient if she is allergic to penicillin
   c. asking the patient to list the medications she takes daily
   d. asking the patient to describe his last incidence of chest pain

6. When the EMT-I is gathering a history from a patient, it is sometimes appropriate to ask very specific follow-up questions. This technique is known as:
   a. reflection.
   b. clarification.
   c. confrontation.
   d. empathetic response.

7. An EMT-I takes the information obtained from confrontation, combines it with suggestions from evidence gathered from the patient and scene, and tries to determine what the patient's problem might be. This process is referred to as:
   a. diagnosis.
   b. differential.
   c. clarification.
   d. interpretation.

8. The EMT-I supports and encourages the patient while the patient explains his or her problem. This technique is referred to as:
   a. facilitation.
   b. clarification.
   c. confrontation.
   d. body language.

9. Using facial expressions or statements such as, "I see" or "That must have been difficult," to display an understanding of the patient's situation is a history-taking technique known as:
   a. reflection.
   b. facilitation.
   c. clarification.
   d. empathetic response.

10. The EMT-I questions the patient to establish a relationship between the EMT-I and the patient, and to elicit pertinent information about the patient's medical history. This is commonly done in the:
    a. health history.
    b. initial assessment.
    c. rapid trauma exam.
    d. ongoing assessment.

11. The history of an adult patient should include each of the following, except:

a. current health status.
b. preliminary data, such as age and sex.
c. which hospital the patient would like to be taken to today.
d. a review of the body systems and general physical exam.

12. The review of body systems should include an assessment of:

a. the skin and gastrointestinal tract.
b. the patient's current and past health history.
c. preliminary data, such as age and sex.
d. a complete list of prescription and over-the-counter medications.

13. Which of the following is an example of a special challenge to the EMT-I who is obtaining a history?

a. the silent patient
b. the intoxicated patient
c. a patient needing reassurance
d. all of the above

14. During your assessment and history taking, you begin to suspect that the patient may have a hearing problem. It would be appropriate to avoid which of the following actions?

a. speaking slowly in a low-pitched voice
b. shouting at the patient so she can hear you clearly
c. speaking to the patient's best ear if one is better than the other
d. positioning yourself in front of the patient so he can see your lips

15. If your patient is in pain and crying, the best approach for the EMT-I is to:

a. ask the patient to try to quiet down.
b. tell him that it does not really hurt that bad.
c. just ignore the crying, as it will eventually stop.
d. be patient and accept the crying as a natural venting of emotions.

Chapter 6 Answer Form

	A	B	C	D
1.	❏	❏	❏	❏
2.	❏	❏	❏	❏
3.	❏	❏	❏	❏
4.	❏	❏	❏	❏
5.	❏	❏	❏	❏
6.	❏	❏	❏	❏
7.	❏	❏	❏	❏
8.	❏	❏	❏	❏

	A	B	C	D
9.	❏	❏	❏	❏
10.	❏	❏	❏	❏
11.	❏	❏	❏	❏
12.	❏	❏	❏	❏
13.	❏	❏	❏	❏
14.	❏	❏	❏	❏
15.	❏	❏	❏	❏

Patient Assessment

CHAPTER 7

Techniques of Physical Examination

1. When the EMT-I feels each of the four quadrants of the abdomen for tenderness or rigidity, which technique of physical examination is she using?
   a. palpation
   b. inspection
   c. percussion
   d. auscultation

2. Listening to the sound of an internal organ with a stethoscope is referred to as:
   a. palpation.
   b. inspection.
   c. percussion.
   d. auscultation.

3. Tapping on the outer surface of the body, in an attempt to determine if there is a solid mass or hollow area beneath, is called:
   a. palpation.
   b. inspection.
   c. percussion.
   d. auscultation.

4. The EMT-I compares the right extremity to the left extremity while looking for swelling of the knee. This physical examination technique is referred to as:
   a. inspection.
   b. lateralizing.
   c. pitting edema.
   d. range of motion.

5. How can the EMT-I obtain an accurate respiratory rate while the patient is watching the EMT-I take her vital signs?
   a. Use the pulse oximeter to estimate the rate.
   b. The respiratory rate is only an estimate most of the time.
   c. Hold the wrist and count first the pulse, then breaths, for 15 seconds each.
   d. Tell the patient to stop talking because you are counting her respirations.

6. In noisy situations, such as in the back of a moving ambulance, the EMT-I may take the patient's blood pressure using the _____ method.
   a. palpation
   b. reflection
   c. estimation
   d. auscultation

7. While obtaining the patient's vital signs, the EMT-I notes that the adult patient has a BP of 150/100 mm Hg. This is usually considered:
   a. tachycardia.
   b. hypotensive.
   c. hypertensive.
   d. normal for an adult.

8. When an adult patient has a sustained pulse rate of _____, this is considered _____.
   a. 50 or less; hypotension
   b. 60 or more; bradycardia
   c. 100 or more; tachycardia
   d. 100 or more; hypertension

9. You arrive at the scene of a car/tree collision. A first responder with the patient reports that the patient is conscious, but confused. Given all that you know so far, what is the patient's mental status?
   a. alert
   b. verbal
   c. painful
   d. unresponsive

10. Why is it so important to determine the patient's mental status?
    a. It is needed for the PCR.
    b. It is not important to monitor the patient's mental status.
    c. You should not take seriously patients who are not alert.
    d. A patient who is not alert may have a serious head injury.

11. Why is it important to consider doing a generalized survey when there is time?
   a. It will help the EMT-I prioritize the life threats.
   b. It will help the EMT-I focus on the patient's vital signs.
   c. It will help to identify life threats that must be managed right away.
   d. The generalized survey can yield subtle findings that may relate to the chief complaint.

12. When examining a patient's skin, the EMT-I should note the:
   a. vasculature.
   b. color and condition.
   c. possible sites for establishing an IV.
   d. all of the above.

13. What is the relevance of skin tenting in a patient?
   a. The patient usually has the flu.
   b. The patient may be dehydrated.
   c. The patient usually has hypertension.
   d. There is no clinical relevance to this sign.

14. A patient has large nails that appeared squared. This is referred to as _____ and is often found in _____.
   a. clubbing; smokers
   b. clipping; obese males
   c. clipping; mature adults
   d. clubbing; skinny females

15. When a patient is dehydrated, the EMT-I may make a physical examination finding called:
   a. tenting.
   b. clubbing.
   c. Battle's sign.
   d. evaporation.

16. The EMT-I examines the skin of a child who has a fever and locates swollen, pus-filled growths all over the skin. The EMT-I should:
   a. be careful not to pop any of the growths.
   b. use the appropriate form of BSI precautions.
   c. not allow a pregnant EMT near the patient.
   d. all of the above.

17. While assessing a patient's head, the EMT-I notices swelling and discoloration over the mastoid process behind the ear. What is this finding called?
   a. tenting
   b. Battle's sign
   c. Cushing's sign
   d. periorbital edema

18. As you examine the face of a patient who was involved in a bar fight, you notice that there is blood in his nostrils. What is this finding most likely from?
   a. epistaxis
   b. a CSF leak
   c. raccoon eyes
   d. frothy pulmonary edema

19. During an examination of the eyes, the EMT-I will ask the patient to hold his head still and, with his eyes only, follow the EMT-I's finger in a/an _____ motion.
   a. "H"
   b. "J"
   c. figure-eight
   d. circular

20. When examining a patient's eyes, the EMT-I should avoid:
   a. stimulating a reaction to light.
   b. stimulating extraocular movement.
   c. stimulating a change in the size of each pupil.
   d. shining a light into both eyes at the same time.

21. What is the significance of a constricted pupil?
   a. The patient is suffering from hypoxia.
   b. The patient may have a brain stem injury.
   c. The patient has severe swelling inside the head.
   d. There is no significance if the patient is looking into the sunlight.

22. When assessing a patient's eyes, what is an important question to ask?
   a. What color are your eyes?
   b. Do you normally wear sunglasses?
   c. Do you have the ability to make tears?
   d. Do you have contact lenses in at the moment?

23. While examining the ears of a patient who has a suspected head injury, the EMT-I notices blood and some clear fluid leaking from the ear. What could this mean?
   a. The patient has a lymphatic gland leak.
   b. The patient has not cleaned his ear today.
   c. The patient may have a basilar skull fracture.
   d. The patient may have been swimming earlier in the day.

24. (Continuing with the preceding question) What type of fluid is most likely leaking from the patient's ears?
   a. liquid wax
   b. cervical fluid
   c. lymphatic fluid
   d. cerebrospinal fluid

25. You are treating a patient whom you suspect may have sustained a ruptured eardrum. What is a likely cause of this type of injury?
    a. a fall from a height
    b. a motor vehicle crash
    c. exposure to a toxic environment
    d. an explosion within a confined space

26. While examining a patient's nose, the EMT-I notices that the hairs are singed; the patient also has a productive cough with dark sputum. What likely caused these findings?
    a. The patient has acute pulmonary edema.
    b. The patient is having an allergic reaction to shellfish.
    c. The patient may have inhaled superheated fumes at a fire scene.
    d. The patient has had an upper respiratory infection for the past few days.

27. During the interview, your patient tells you he has a deviated septum. What value does this piece of history have to the field management of this patient?
    a. The patient is probably a cocaine abuser.
    b. The patient is prone to frequent nosebleeds.
    c. The patient will not be able to take an NG tube.
    d. A nasal airway may not slide easily into one of the nostrils.

28. When assessing a patient with facial injuries who was involved in a fist fight, it is important for the EMT-I to examine the:
    a. right side and then the left side.
    b. scalp before any other parts of the body.
    c. patient before allowing him to walk around.
    d. patient's mouth for broken teeth and bleeding.

29. When examining a patient's neck, it is helpful to try to determine the:
    a. size of the larynx.
    b. duration of each breath.
    c. relationship of the structures to the midline.
    d. length of endotracheal tube that may be needed.

30. When interviewing your patient, you find out that she was in a car crash and struck her neck against the steering wheel. She has a very raspy voice with low volume. What should you suspect?
    a. She has the symptoms of a cold.
    b. She is having an allergic reaction.
    c. She may have a complete cervical spine dislocation.
    d. She may have fractured her larynx.

31. Your conscious patient fell off a ladder and struck the back of his neck on the corner of a desk. If you suspect that a patient, like this one, may have a cervical spine injury, it is important to:
    a. apply a rigid collar.
    b. open the airway with a jaw thrust.
    c. fully immobilize the entire spine on a backboard.
    d. all of the above.

32. You are conducting a physical examination on a patient who sustained a crushing injury to the chest. Upon inspection, you note a section of ribs that seems to move out as the rest of the chest moves in. What would you expect to feel during palpation of this patient?
    a. a large hole in the side of the chest wall
    b. a similar motion on both sides of the chest wall
    c. the sensation of a pneumothorax under the skin
    d. a segment of ribs that is unstable, with a feeling of crepitus

33. If you percussed the chest wall of a patient who has pneumonia or a tumor in the lung, what would you expect to hear over the affected area?
    a. a very tympanic sound
    b. a dull sound compared to the rest of the lung fields
    c. percussion is done on the abdomen, not the chest wall
    d. it is not possible to hear the difference from one area of the lung to another

34. Which of the following is *not* a reason why a patient may have decreased ventilation volume?
    a. overdose of a narcotic or opiate
    b. Kussmaul's respirations in the diabetic patient
    c. flail chest has occurred from a forceful blow to the chest wall
    d. pneumothorax from a gunshot wound to the chest

35. When conducting a physical exam on a trauma patient, the EMT-I should look for:
    a. life-threatening injuries only.
    b. a list of medications in the patient's belongings.
    c. a driver's license or other form of identification.
    d. injuries to both the anterior and posterior chest.

36. When the EMT-I percusses the posterior chest wall of a patient, it is important to assess for:
    a. deformity of the spine.
    b. osteoporosis of the spine.
    c. perforation of the diaphragm.
    d. excursion or movement of the diaphragm.

37. Breath sounds that may be heard in the bases of the lungs, and are caused by a small amount of moisture or fluid in the lungs, are called:

 a. rales.
 b. rhonchi.
 c. wheezes.
 d. pleural rub.

38. The musical tones that can be heard in a patient's chest when the bronchioles are constricted are called:

 a. rales.
 b. rhonchi.
 c. a wheeze.
 d. pleural rub.

39. The sound heard when there is a lack of fluid or in-flammation of the membranes that surround the lung is called:

 a. rales.
 b. rhonchi.
 c. a wheeze.
 d. pleural rub.

40. When palpating peripheral pulses, it is important to assess the:

 a. depth and quality.
 b. time, depth, and pattern.
 c. temperature and condition.
 d. rate, regularity, and strength.

41. To properly assess the jugular vein for distention, the patient should be in the _____ position.

 a. prone
 b. supine
 c. Fowler's
 d. semi-Fowler's

42. A patient has a crush injury to the chest that is limiting the flow of blood into the right atrium. The EMT-I should expect to see:

 a. distended neck veins.
 b. depressed neck veins.
 c. distended carotid arteries.
 d. depressed carotid arteries.

43. When examining the heart, the EMT-I should note the _____, which may be seen or felt as a pulsation on the chest wall.

 a. distal aorta
 b. right atrium
 c. right ventricle
 d. point of maximal impulse (PMI)

44. The "lub" and "dub" sounds heard upon auscultation of the heart are actually caused by the:

 a. movement of the aorta.
 b. movement of the valves.
 c. pulsation of the ventricle.
 d. rubbing of the membrane that surrounds the heart.

45. You are listening for heart sounds and hear a galloping sound. This is considered:

 a. normal in an enlarged heart.
 b. abnormal, and may indicate a problem.
 c. normal, and is expected in most patients.
 d. abnormal, and the cause of a slow heart rhythm.

46. You can hear a rubbing sound upon auscultation of a patient's lungs. This is called:

 a. pleural rub if it can be heard all the time.
 b. pericardial rub if it can be heard upon inhalation.
 c. pericardial rub if it can be heard upon exhalation.
 d. pleural rub if it can be heard upon inhalation or exhalation.

47. When examining a patient's abdomen, the EMT-I should always remember to assess:

 a. all four quadrants.
 b. with deep palpation.
 c. the painful section first.
 d. for rebound tenderness.

48. A patient is found to have a soft and supple abdomen. This is considered a _____ finding.

 a. normal
 b. abnormal
 c. pathological
 d. inappropriate

49. In which circumstance would the EMT-I need to examine the female external genitalia?

 a. the patient is a victim of sexual abuse
 b. as a routine part of the physical examination
 c. if the EMT-I suspects that labor is causing crowning
 d. the EMT-I should not examine this location; it can wait until arrival at the ED

50. Which of the following is an example of a situation in which it may be necessary to examine the male external genitalia?

 a. the patient was kicked in the groin
 b. the patient caught his scrotum in his zipper
 c. the patient sustained a serious soft tissue injury
 d. all of the above

51. When examining a patient whom you suspect has an extremity fracture, which of the following should you avoid assessing?

 a. distal pulses
 b. distal sensation
 c. full range of motion
 d. distal motor function

52. When examining a patient's extremities for strength, it is appropriate to check:

 a. the leg from top to bottom.
 b. the leg from distal to proximal.
 c. each arm for grip strength, one at a time.
 d. both arms for equal strength, at the same time.

53. What is the difference between light and deep palpation?
    a. Light palpation is used with patients who weigh less than 150 pounds.
    b. Deep palpation is reserved use with patients who weigh more than 150 pounds.
    c. Light palpation is reserved for the in-hospital environment.
    d. Deep palpation is usually done on the abdomen of a patient who is in the hospital.

54. What is skin turgor?
    a. the color of the skin
    b. the depth of the skin
    c. the strength or the skin
    d. the elasticity of the skin

55. Phlebitis is a condition that affects the:
    a. pulmonic system.
    b. coronary circulation.
    c. central nervous system.
    d. peripheral vascular system.

56. Examination of the nervous system should include:
    a. assessment of capillary refill time.
    b. assessment of the cranial nerves.
    c. a check of the distal pulse in the extremities.
    d. reassessment of the blood pressure and pulse oximetry.

57. The sounds heard with a stethoscope while taking a BP are called:
    a. Levine's sign.
    b. Turner's sounds.
    c. Babinski's sign.
    d. Korotkoff's sounds.

58. Elderly patients commonly have:
    a. extreme sensitivity to light.
    b. faster reflexes than younger patients.
    c. pitting edema whenever they are supine.
    d. poor skin turgor, due to deterioration of connective tissue.

59. Where is the apical pulse heard or felt?
    a. in the wrist of either arm
    b. in the midaxillary line at the second intercostal space
    c. in the midaxillary line at the fifth intercostal space
    d. in the midaxillary line at the fourth to sixth intercostal spaces.

60. After conducting a physical examination, the EMT-I should be careful to:
    a. redo the exam every 15 minutes.
    b. properly document the findings on the PCR.
    c. avoid any complicated questions from the patient.
    d. explain all the pertinent negative findings to the patient.

Chapter 7 Answer Form

	A	B	C	D		A	B	C	D
1.	❏	❏	❏	❏	26.	❏	❏	❏	❏
2.	❏	❏	❏	❏	27.	❏	❏	❏	❏
3.	❏	❏	❏	❏	28.	❏	❏	❏	❏
4.	❏	❏	❏	❏	29.	❏	❏	❏	❏
5.	❏	❏	❏	❏	30.	❏	❏	❏	❏
6.	❏	❏	❏	❏	31.	❏	❏	❏	❏
7.	❏	❏	❏	❏	32.	❏	❏	❏	❏
8.	❏	❏	❏	❏	33.	❏	❏	❏	❏
9.	❏	❏	❏	❏	34.	❏	❏	❏	❏
10.	❏	❏	❏	❏	35.	❏	❏	❏	❏
11.	❏	❏	❏	❏	36.	❏	❏	❏	❏
12.	❏	❏	❏	❏	37.	❏	❏	❏	❏
13.	❏	❏	❏	❏	38.	❏	❏	❏	❏
14.	❏	❏	❏	❏	39.	❏	❏	❏	❏
15.	❏	❏	❏	❏	40.	❏	❏	❏	❏
16.	❏	❏	❏	❏	41.	❏	❏	❏	❏
17.	❏	❏	❏	❏	42.	❏	❏	❏	❏
18.	❏	❏	❏	❏	43.	❏	❏	❏	❏
19.	❏	❏	❏	❏	44.	❏	❏	❏	❏
20.	❏	❏	❏	❏	45.	❏	❏	❏	❏
21.	❏	❏	❏	❏	46.	❏	❏	❏	❏
22.	❏	❏	❏	❏	47.	❏	❏	❏	❏
23.	❏	❏	❏	❏	48.	❏	❏	❏	❏
24.	❏	❏	❏	❏	49.	❏	❏	❏	❏
25.	❏	❏	❏	❏	50.	❏	❏	❏	❏

	A	B	C	D			A	B	C	D
51.	❑	❑	❑	❑		56.	❑	❑	❑	❑
52.	❑	❑	❑	❑		57.	❑	❑	❑	❑
53.	❑	❑	❑	❑		58.	❑	❑	❑	❑
54.	❑	❑	❑	❑		59.	❑	❑	❑	❑
55.	❑	❑	❑	❑		60.	❑	❑	❑	❑

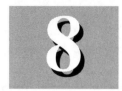

Patient Assessment

1. When dispatched to a home for an elderly woman who is having breathing difficulties, the EMT-I should suspect a potential hazard if:
   a. the front door is unlocked.
   b. there is no noise coming from the house.
   c. it is night time and the porch light has not been turned on.
   d. a relative of the patient is waiting at the front door.

2. Which of the following is an example of a potential hazard to the EMT-I who is caring for a patient in a typical living room or family room?
   a. a set of ski poles
   b. a set of carving knives
   c. a 12-inch-high marble statue
   d. a hammer or other hand tools

3. Which of the following is most likely to pose the greatest hazard to the EMT-I?
   a. an unregistered exotic pet
   b. a beer bottle on the end table in the living room
   c. an improperly vented fireplace that is leaking carbon monoxide
   d. a decorative sword on the wall of the family room.

4. You enter a home and suspect that it is actually a clandestine lab. The best approach to take is to:
   a. turn off all the burners.
   b. tell the occupants that they are under arrest.
   c. discreetly notify the police and do not touch anything.
   d. tell the occupants that the house is surrounded and they must all leave.

5. When treating a patient whom you suspect may be a gang member, always:
   a. ask before you cut off any clothing.
   b. be respectful of the patient and his or her belongings.
   c. consider that minors often carry weapons.
   d. all of the above.

6. At the scene of a motor vehicle collision, the greatest hazard to the EMT-I is likely to be:
   a. angry patients or bystanders.
   b. a car that could burst into flame.
   c. biohazards contained in the vehicles.
   d. the traffic flow.

7. You are responding to a call for a three-car collision with multiple citizen reports of injuries on the scene. In this situation, it is common for dispatch to:
   a. send police to the scene for traffic control and investigation.
   b. send the fire department to stand by with a charged line and wash down the area as needed.
   c. wait to send a second ambulance until the existence of multiple patients is confirmed.
   d. withhold EMS response until police send an update from the scene.

8. A patient who was involved in a frontal collision has injuries to his head and neck. This type of collision is often described as the _____ mechanism of injury.
   a. up-and-over
   b. axial-loading
   c. down-and-under
   d. restrained-patient

9. A patient has called the ambulance because of respiratory distress. He states that he has a long history of emphysema and is usually on home oxygen. The most likely nature of illness (NOI) is a/an:
   a. serious car crash.
   b. allergy to a bee sting.
   c. recent upper respiratory infection.
   d. exposure to an infectious disease.

10. Why is it important for the EMT-I to recognize and appreciate the MOI?
    a. It can help predict injury patterns.
    b. It will let the EMT-I make a field diagnosis.
    c. It will help determine the hazards on the scene.
    d. It helps the EMT-I understand the patient's medical history.

11. As early as possible after arriving at the scene of an emergency, the EMT-I should:

    a. prepare to transport the patient.

    b. conduct a detailed assessment of each patient found on the scene.

    c. identify the total number of patients and call for any additional needed help.

    d. all of the above.

12. Which of the following steps is performed after the scene size-up rather than during it?

    a. taking BSI precautions

    b. conducting an initial assessment of the patient

    c. determining if there are any hazards to you and your crew

    d. ensuring that you have appropriate help en route to the scene

13. Why is it important to identify the need for additional help or assistance as soon as possible on EMS calls?

    a. it may take time for additional helpers to respond

    b. you may need their help so that you are free to do patient care

    c. their services may be required to make the scene safe for you

    d. all of the above

14. Which of the following is part of the initial assessment rather than the general impression of the patient?

    a. patient priority

    b. the patient's sex

    c. the patient's approximate age

    d. the patient's degree of distress

15. A patient was involved in a fall and may have struck his head. When you arrive, he seems confused and is not clear about who you are or who he is. What would you classify his mental status as?

    a. alert

    b. obtunded

    c. semi-conscious

    d. verbally responsive

16. (Continuing with the preceding question) After about five minutes, the patient begins to answer all your questions correctly. What would you classify his mental status as now?

    a. alert

    b. obtunded

    c. semi-conscious

    d. verbally responsive

17. (Continuing with the preceding questions) The patient arrived at the ED after 30 minutes with the mental status you selected as an answer to question #16. What would be important to note in your oral report and on the PCR?

    a. how the patient smelled and what he was wearing

    b. the patient's baseline mental status as discovered on the scene

    c. only the patient's best mental status is of significance for reporting

    d. how cooperative the patient was with assessment and how well you were received by the ED

18. You are managing a patient who collapsed in a restaurant. Witnesses state that she was not eating at the time, but did seem to have a convulsion as she fell out of her chair. At this point the patient is unconscious and does not respond to painful stimuli. What is her mental status?

    a. alert

    b. verbal

    c. painful

    d. unresponsive

19. A painful stimulus is applied to a patient to determine his mental status. An appropriate response from the patient is to:

    a. withdraw from the pain source.

    b. give no obvious response to the pain.

    c. demonstrate decorticate posturing.

    d. demonstrate decerebrate posturing.

20. When assessing the airway of an unconscious patient, it is important to:

    a. stimulate a gag reflex.

    b. immediately suction out the airway.

    c. open the mouth and perform a finger sweep for foreign matter.

    d. maintain manual head/neck stabilization if you suspect trauma.

21. When a patient does not have a gag reflex, it is important for the EMT-I to:

    a. immediately suction out the airway.

    b. ventilate the patient with a bag mask.

    c. administer oxygen with a nasal cannula.

    d. attempt insertion of an oropharyngeal airway.

22. You are managing the airway of an unconscious patient who may have struck his head when he fell to the ground. In this situation, it is appropriate to use the:

    a. jaw thrust with head tilt.

    b. chin-lift, neck-lift maneuver.

    c. head-tilt, chin-lift maneuver.

    d. jaw thrust with head stabilization.

23. When assessing a scene, you should first determine if _____ needed as soon as you approach the patient.
    a. an ALS unit is
    b. a Sager splint is
    c. spinal precautions are
    d. bag-mask ventilation is

24. Once it is determined that the patient's airway is open, the EMT-I should next:
    a. check the radial pulse.
    b. reassess the patient's mental status.
    c. check the patient for breathing.
    d. begin the initial assessment of the patient.

25. When a patient has sustained multiple rib fractures from a blunt injury to the chest, the EMT-I should suspect that the:
    a. patient will be very cold.
    b. pulse will not be present.
    c. mental status will be altered.
    d. breathing may not be adequate.

26. When assessing the patient for breathing, always:
    a. look for chest rise.
    b. obtain a pulse oximetry reading.
    c. determine the exact tidal volume.
    d. listen to the lungs with a stethoscope, but only if the patient is in distress.

27. When a patient has decreased respiratory excursion because of an injury to the chest wall, you can expect that the patient will involuntarily _____ in an effort to maintain an adequate minute volume.
    a. stop the respirations
    b. increase the respiratory rate
    c. decrease the respiratory rate
    d. increase the ventilation volume

28. A patient has an open airway, is breathing adequately, and has an adequate pulse. In the examination of this patient, the EMT-I should next:
    a. rule out a neck injury.
    b. assign a priority to the patient.
    c. quickly check for external bleeding.
    d. determine if any fractures are present.

29. A trauma patient has numerous cuts and abrasions, as well as one seriously bleeding injury in the right arm. The EMT-I should:
    a. prioritize the patient as high and transport immediately.
    b. skip over the bleeding injuries, as they are not life-threatening.
    c. place a tourniquet on the upper arm and continue the assessment.
    d. control the bleeding in the arm and proceed with the initial assessment.

30. When initially assessing a patient's skin, the EMT-I should check for:
    a. hygiene.
    b. pigmentation.
    c. loss of skin turgor.
    d. color, temperature, and condition.

31. While assessing a patient, the EMT-I notes that the patient has blue coloring around the lips. This is called _____ and is likely caused by _____.
    a. cyanosis; hypoxia
    b. pallor; CO poisoning
    c. mottled; poisoning
    d. flushed; hypertension

32. A patient is shivering and has warm skin compared to the skin temperature on the back of your hand. This is likely due to:
    a. asthma.
    b. hypothermia.
    c. hypoglycemia.
    d. a fever or infection.

33. You feel that a patient's skin is cold and dry compared to the skin temperature on the back of your hand. As an EMT-I, you know that this finding:
    a. is probably because the patient is elderly.
    b. means that the patient is taking many medications.
    c. means that the patient needs supplementary oxygen.
    d. indicates that you should actually measure the body temperature with a thermometer.

34. Skin tenting may be found in patients who are:
    a. young.
    b. dehydrated.
    c. very hot to the touch.
    d. normally allergic to bees.

35. Upon completing the steps of the initial assessment, the EMT-I should have:
    a. made a decision as to transport priority.
    b. discovered if the patient has a health care proxy.
    c. obtained a complete list of all the patient's medications.
    d. contacted medical control for approval of transport destination.

36. Which of the following patients would not normally be considered a high priority for immediate transport?
    a. a patient who has cardiac chest pain and is hypotensive
    b. a patient who has respiratory depression from a drug overdose
    c. a patient who may have sustained an injury to the lower back from a fall
    d. a woman who is experiencing a complicated out-of-hospital delivery with an arm presentation

37. If you have adequate resources to provide the appropriate treatment on the scene, which patient is the highest priority for transport?

   a. a 37-year-old female with a suspected ectopic pregnancy

   b. a 45-year-old male with a open fracture of the right fibula and tibia

   c. a 98-year-old male who has been in cardiac arrest for an unknown period of time

   d. a 59-year-old female who is dizzy and nauseated when she stands up

38. When should the orthostatic vital signs of a trauma victim be assessed?

   a. immediately after the initial assessment

   b. whenever the patient complains of dizziness

   c. a set of orthostatic vitals should be taken on all patients

   d. only if you have to convince the patient to go to the hospital

39. When conducting a physical examination on a medical patient who is responsive, the EMT-I provides a/an _____ exam.

   a. initial

   b. detailed

   c. focused

   d. complete

40. If the patient with a medical complaint has an altered mental status, the physical exam that is conducted is very similar to a/an:

   a. rapid trauma exam.

   b. comprehensive exam.

   c. detailed physical exam.

   d. initial assessment and interview.

41. If the patient is complaining of weakness on the left side and has slurred speech, the EMT-I should:

   a. do a focused neuro exam.

   b. conduct a rapid trauma exam.

   c. do a detailed physical exam right away.

   d. skip further assessment and rush the patient to the ED.

42. Why should the MOI be reconsidered in the focused history (FH) and physical exam (PE) of a trauma patient?

   a. to definitely rule out any spine injury

   b. all patients should undergo a rapid trauma exam

   c. the patient most likely has trauma to the back

   d. you want to be sure that no significant trauma was involved

43. Which patient will not routinely get a rapid trauma exam?

   a. the critical trauma patient

   b. all patients must undergo a rapid trauma exam

   c. the patient who has fractures to the lower extremities

   d. the patient who has a minor laceration or sprained ankle

44. The rapid trauma exam includes an examination of each of the following body regions, except the:

   a. head.

   b. pelvis.

   c. mouth.

   d. posterior.

45. During your rapid trauma assessment, you locate a flail chest that you did not previously find. You should:

   a. skip over it, as it is usually not that serious.

   b. wait until the detailed physical exam to manage the injury.

   c. mark it down on the PCR and continue with the evaluation.

   d. treat it as if found during the initial assessment and begin to stabilize.

46. The ongoing assessment includes:

   a. reassessing any interventions.

   b. performing serial vital signs.

   c. redoing the initial assessment as needed.

   d. all of the above.

47. Following the assessment algorithm, which patient should undergo a detailed physical exam en route to the ED?

   a. the unconscious cardiac patient

   b. the hypoglycemic diabetic patient

   c. the patient who is just coming out of a seizure

   d. the patient who is unconscious from serious head trauma

48. Why is the initial assessment repeated during the ongoing assessment?

   a. in case the EMT-I forgot to do one previously

   b. to reassess life threats and treat them quickly

   c. to fill the time during travel to the ED

   d. to make sure that even medical patients receive an initial assessment

49. Compared to the rapid trauma exam, the detailed physical exam is:

   a. basically the same.

   b. excludes auscultation.

   c. excludes DCAP-BTLS.

   d. a much more detailed look at the head.

50. During the detailed physical exam, the EMT-I should examine the ears for:
   a. wax accumulation.
   b. chronic hearing loss.
   c. blood or leaking fluid.
   d. color, temperature, and condition.

51. When a medical patient is not responsive, the EMT-I can obtain clues about the patient's medical history from:
   a. an interview.
   b. a physical examination.
   c. the presence of a Medic Alert® bracelet.
   d. a call to the patient's primary care physician.

52. Why is it important to trend vital signs?
   a. It is not important to determine if there are trends.
   b. The PCR has numerous spots for vitals to be listed.
   c. Trending can help the EMT-I determine if the patient's condition is changing.
   d. none of the above

53. Which of the following is a component of the ongoing assessment?
   a. OPQRST
   b. DCAP-BTLS
   c. SAMPLE history
   d. reassessment of the vital signs

54. What does the "S" in OPQRST stand for?
   a. signs
   b. stable
   c. severity
   d. symptoms

55. What does the "A" in DCAP-BTLS stand for?
   a. alert
   b. abrasions
   c. ambulatory
   d. assessment

Chapter 8 Answer Form

	A	B	C	D		A	B	C	D
1.	❑	❑	❑	❑	25.	❑	❑	❑	❑
2.	❑	❑	❑	❑	26.	❑	❑	❑	❑
3.	❑	❑	❑	❑	27.	❑	❑	❑	❑
4.	❑	❑	❑	❑	28.	❑	❑	❑	❑
5.	❑	❑	❑	❑	29.	❑	❑	❑	❑
6.	❑	❑	❑	❑	30.	❑	❑	❑	❑
7.	❑	❑	❑	❑	31.	❑	❑	❑	❑
8.	❑	❑	❑	❑	32.	❑	❑	❑	❑
9.	❑	❑	❑	❑	33.	❑	❑	❑	❑
10.	❑	❑	❑	❑	34.	❑	❑	❑	❑
11.	❑	❑	❑	❑	35.	❑	❑	❑	❑
12.	❑	❑	❑	❑	36.	❑	❑	❑	❑
13.	❑	❑	❑	❑	37.	❑	❑	❑	❑
14.	❑	❑	❑	❑	38.	❑	❑	❑	❑
15.	❑	❑	❑	❑	39.	❑	❑	❑	❑
16.	❑	❑	❑	❑	40.	❑	❑	❑	❑
17.	❑	❑	❑	❑	41.	❑	❑	❑	❑
18.	❑	❑	❑	❑	42.	❑	❑	❑	❑
19.	❑	❑	❑	❑	43.	❑	❑	❑	❑
20.	❑	❑	❑	❑	44.	❑	❑	❑	❑
21.	❑	❑	❑	❑	45.	❑	❑	❑	❑
22.	❑	❑	❑	❑	46.	❑	❑	❑	❑
23.	❑	❑	❑	❑	47.	❑	❑	❑	❑
24.	❑	❑	❑	❑	48.	❑	❑	❑	❑

	A	B	C	D			A	B	C	D
49.	❏	❏	❏	❏		53.	❏	❏	❏	❏
50.	❏	❏	❏	❏		54.	❏	❏	❏	❏
51.	❏	❏	❏	❏		55.	❏	❏	❏	❏
52.	❏	❏	❏	❏						

CHAPTER

Clinical Decision Making

1. The most obvious difference between emergency care in the out-of-hospital setting and the in-hospital setting is:
    a. a relatively controlled environment in the hospital.
    b. the approach to patient assessment.
    c. that the patients in the hospital are sicker.
    d. a more diverse range of patient care in the field.

2. A patient with an isolated extremity injury without neurovascular compromise is an example of a situation that is:
    a. not life-threatening.
    b. critically life-threatening.
    c. potentially life-threatening.
    d. a major single-system trauma.

3. Which of the following is a disadvantage of using protocols and standing orders?
    a. Standing orders define performance parameters.
    b. Protocols often omit patients with multisystem failure.
    c. Protocols promote a standard approach to patient care.
    d. Standing orders speed the application of critical-care interventions.

4. Which of the following is an advantage of using protocols and standing orders?
    a. Protocols provide structure for the EMT-I provider.
    b. Standing orders are helpful for patients with non-specific complaints.
    c. Standing orders and protocols only fit patients with "textbook" injuries or illnesses.
    d. Protocols offer the EMT-I help when caring for a patient who has concurrent disease processes.

5. The foundation of being an effective EMT-I is having the ability to think and work under pressure. This includes:
    a. implementing appropriate patient management.
    b. gathering, evaluating, and processing information.
    c. articulating and documenting reasons for the decisions made.
    d. all of the above.

6. The hormonal fight-or-flight response to stress can affect the EMT-I's decision-making ability:
    a. positively.
    b. negatively.
    c. both positively and negatively.
    d. by causing him or her to take a deep breath.

7. Which of the following is *not* a strategy for effective thinking that the EMT-I may use on the job?
    a. staying calm
    b. planning for the worst
    c. reassessing frequently
    d. using a radical plan of action

8. The "six Rs" of putting it all together, as described by the DOT National Standard Curriculum for the EMT-I, include: read the patient, read the scene, react, reevaluate, revise, and:
    a. regain.
    b. review.
    c. recover.
    d. reassess.

9. When the EMT-I is reading the scene of an incident, she is considering which of the following?
    a. mechanism of injury
    b. transportation considerations
    c. staying calm to avoid panicking
    d. the initial assessment

10. During a call in which you are treating a patient who has crushing chest pain, you suddenly realize that you have forgotten the new standing-order dose of nitroglycerin. Which of the following is the most appropriate action?
    a. Use the old standing-order dose.
    b. Look up the correct dose in your protocol reference.
    c. Guess at the dose, because it is too embarrassing to ask medical control.
    d. Administer one dose right away, and then call your supervisor for the newest dose.

11. Which of the following is *not* a fundamental element of critical thinking for the EMT-I?

a. documenting medical ambiguity

b. analyzing and comparing similar situations

c. differentiating between relevant and irrelevant data

d. focusing on specific, as well as multiple, elements of data

12. The EMT-I's critical thinking incorporates the patient's active participation in the process. Which of the following is a way to encourage the patient to participate?

a. Ask the patient questions.

b. Have the patient sign the billing form.

c. Direct the patient to state the chief complaint.

d. Reassess the patient's response to treatment interventions.

13. Behaviors that can help the EMT-I think effectively while working under pressure include:

a. maintaining a systematic assessment pattern.

b. being optimistic and hoping for the best outcome.

c. assuming the best possible outcome and planning for it.

d. walking away, taking a few moments to regroup, and beginning again.

14. The first component in the sequence of critical thinking for the EMT-I is:

a. managing the patient using protocols.

b. interpretation and processing of information.

c. collecting information and formulating concepts.

d. the application of treatment using differential assessment.

15. You have just finished obtaining baseline vital signs on a patient who incurred an isolated ankle injury after tripping and falling. The blood pressure was 290/170 mm Hg. What is most appropriate action to take next?

a. Ask the patient if this reading is normal for her.

b. Ask your partner to reassess the blood pressure.

c. Call medical control and request permission to treat the hypertension.

d. Follow standing orders or local protocols for treatment of hypertensive crisis.

Chapter 9 Answer Form

	A	B	C	D		A	B	C	D
1.	❑	❑	❑	❑	9.	❑	❑	❑	❑
2.	❑	❑	❑	❑	10.	❑	❑	❑	❑
3.	❑	❑	❑	❑	11.	❑	❑	❑	❑
4.	❑	❑	❑	❑	12.	❑	❑	❑	❑
5.	❑	❑	❑	❑	13.	❑	❑	❑	❑
6.	❑	❑	❑	❑	14.	❑	❑	❑	❑
7.	❑	❑	❑	❑	15.	❑	❑	❑	❑
8.	❑	❑	❑	❑					

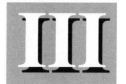

Trauma

CHAPTER 10

Communications

1. The EMT-I must be able to effectively communicate patient assessment and management information to the ED physician, so that:
   a. the EMT-I can act as the patient's advocate.
   b. the physician can assist the EMT-I with treatment orders.
   c. the patient can get definitive care as soon as possible.
   d. registration staff can prepare for the patient's arrival.

2. The EMT-I is expected to be effective in which mode(s) of communication?
   a. research
   b. interrogation
   c. prearrival instructions
   d. verbal, written, and electronic

3. Which of the following is an example of the notification phase of communication?
   a. The EMT-I communicates with medical control about treatment of the patient.
   b. The EMT-I notifies the dispatcher where the ambulance is transporting the patient.
   c. Emergency medical dispatch (EMD) receives a call for help and dispatches an ambulance.
   d. The EMT-I notifies the dispatcher that the ambulance is back in service, after clearing the hospital.

4. Many EMS services have stopped using special codes (e.g., 10-codes) and have changed to plain English because:
   a. special codes prevent confusion.
   b. that is the way it is done on television.
   c. many providers were making up their own phrases.
   d. special codes increase the possibility of multiple interpretations.

5. During which of the following EMS events is the use of special codes preferred over plain English?
   a. multiple-casualty incident
   b. training and practice drills
   c. hazardous materials incident
   d. television shows about EMS

6. Which of the following can impede verbal communication between the EMT-I and a patient?
   a. speaking clearly
   b. providing feedback
   c. using technical terminology
   d. interacting with the patient's family

7. Which of the following can enhance verbal communication by the EMT-I?
   a. Only use technical terms when talking on the radio.
   b. Use terms that are easy to understand and avoid mumbling.
   c. Decode the message from the sender and then acknowledge.
   d. Use a monotone voice when speaking into a radio microphone.

8. The documentation that is written for prehospital care is important because:
   a. it is the written and legal record of the incident.
   b. it is directly related to the continuity of patient care.
   c. it protects the patient's confidentiality regarding emergency care.
   d. all decisions about the patient's care will be made based on the PCR.

9. Which of the following impedes effective written communication?
   a. documenting opinionated information
   b. failing to document subjective information
   c. failing to add your interpretation of why the patient acted a certain way
   d. providing a complete and accurate portrait of the care provided to the patient

10. Which of the following approaches can improve written communication by the EMT-I?
    a. Whenever possible, avoid using abbreviations.
    b. Document patient statements on a PCR using exact quotations.
    c. Use abbreviations from a comprehensive medical list.
    d. Whenever possible, include subjective patient information on the PCR.

11. Which statement is most accurate? The release of patient information:

    a. to a third party for billing purposes is legal.
    b. requires written permission from the patient in all cases.
    c. is not illegal if it is not true or accurate information.
    d. to another health care provider requires the patient's written consent.

12. Verbal communication can be face-to-face or over the telephone or radio. In which of the following situations would verbal communication be of least significance?

    a. interacting with bystanders
    b. interpreting body language
    c. communicating with the triage nurse
    d. receiving call information from dispatch

13. To gain legal access to medical information exchanged electronically, an individual must:

    a. have e-mail capabilities.
    b. know how to turn on a computer.
    c. obtain a court order or search warrant.
    d. transmit the request on the computer.

14. Which of the following is most accurate about radio transmissions?

    a. Radio transmissions are public and open for all to hear.
    b. Only specific channels are public and open for all to hear.
    c. Radio transmission interference can override system signals.
    d. It is acceptable to use a patient's first name in a radio transmission.

15. When a radio transmits and receives at the same time, it is called:

    a. analog transmission.
    b. duplex communication.
    c. trunked communication.
    d. multiplex communication.

16. _____ is/are the means of alerting EMS, fire, and police agencies in each community.

    a. Prearrival instructions
    b. The system dispatcher
    c. A public safety access point
    d. The emergency medical dispatcher

17. The Federal Communications Commission (FCC) is responsible for:

    a. modifying computer-aided dispatch.
    b. regulating all aspects of the communication industry.
    c. diminishing competition in all communication markets.
    d. enforcing the use of special codes within specific agencies.

18. The emergency medical dispatcher (EMD) is an integral part of the EMS team and in some cases can save lives by:

    a. providing prearrival instructions.
    b. dispatching the police together with EMS.
    c. retrieving information on the history of a residence.
    d. dispatching the fire department together with EMS.

19. The EMD is trained to determine the answer to four key questions from the caller's responses. Which of the following may the EMD get information about after asking the four key questions?

    a. Is the patient breathing?
    b. Is the patient conscious?
    c. What is the patient's chief complaint?
    d. What is the patient's past medical history?

20. During which time interval does the dispatcher determine the type of call, the most appropriate units to dispatch, and their level of response?

    a. queue
    b. scene
    c. response
    d. transport

21. When the EMD interrogates someone who is in direct contact with the patient, but is not the actual patient, she is speaking to a _____-party caller.

    a. first
    b. second
    c. third
    d. fourth

22. The procedure of providing verbal communication of patient information to the hospital is:

    a. the same in every community.
    b. the same for BLS and ALS reports.
    c. based on a format that is standard, but varies slightly in each community.
    d. designed to reduce the length of radio transmissions and convey a precise message.

23. The primary purpose of a verbal report over the radio to the ED is to:

    a. relay the patient's vital signs.
    b. get the report recorded for future reference.
    c. give the staff time to prepare for the patient.
    d. let the patient know that a room has been reserved.

24. After receiving medical orders, the EMT-I repeats the order back to the physician. This is called *echoing,* and it should always done to:

    a. permit time to properly document the order.
    b. ensure that the order is recorded for quality purposes.
    c. allow the patient to hear and understand the order.
    d. ensure that the message was received and understood correctly.

25. Which of the following steps is *not* part of the basic model of communication?
    a. sender sends the message
    b. sender decodes the message
    c. receiver decodes the message
    d. receiver gives feedback to the sender

26. The ability to transmit physiological patient information (e.g., heart rate) over the airwaves or cellular band is called:
    a. simplex.
    b. telemetry.
    c. frequency modulation.
    d. amplitude modulation.

27. Which of the following is the radio frequency that ranges between 30 and 300 MHz?
    a. trunked
    b. very high
    c. ultra high
    d. mega high

28. Which of the following can cause radio interference on the scene of an EMS call?
    a. computer
    b. electric motor
    c. fluorescent light fixture
    d. all of the above

29. Another term for voice transmission is:
    a. analog.
    b. duplex.
    c. simplex.
    d. repeater.

30. Computer-aided dispatch is used to help the EMD:
    a. provide prearrival instructions.
    b. determine which unit to send to a call.
    c. keep the caller calm until an EMS unit arrives.
    d. keep all the necessary frequencies open and available.

Chapter 10 Answer Form

	A	B	C	D		A	B	C	D
1.	❏	❏	❏	❏	16.	❏	❏	❏	❏
2.	❏	❏	❏	❏	17.	❏	❏	❏	❏
3.	❏	❏	❏	❏	18.	❏	❏	❏	❏
4.	❏	❏	❏	❏	19.	❏	❏	❏	❏
5.	❏	❏	❏	❏	20.	❏	❏	❏	❏
6.	❏	❏	❏	❏	21.	❏	❏	❏	❏
7.	❏	❏	❏	❏	22.	❏	❏	❏	❏
8.	❏	❏	❏	❏	23.	❏	❏	❏	❏
9.	❏	❏	❏	❏	24.	❏	❏	❏	❏
10.	❏	❏	❏	❏	25.	❏	❏	❏	❏
11.	❏	❏	❏	❏	26.	❏	❏	❏	❏
12.	❏	❏	❏	❏	27.	❏	❏	❏	❏
13.	❏	❏	❏	❏	28.	❏	❏	❏	❏
14.	❏	❏	❏	❏	29.	❏	❏	❏	❏
15.	❏	❏	❏	❏	30.	❏	❏	❏	❏

Documentation

1. Which statement regarding the importance of EMS documentation is most accurate?
   a. Poor documentation is an indication of a poor assessment.
   b. The most experienced crew member should review every prehospital care report (PCR).
   c. The EMT-I's omission of any run data on EMS documentation is subject to disciplinary action.
   d. If a patient confesses to a crime during transport, the statement should not be documented.

2. When documenting, the EMT-I should choose the proper terminology. Which of the following is the correct term for an area of necrosis in a tissue or organ resulting from obstruction of the local circulation by a thrombus or embolus?
   a. injury
   b. infarct
   c. infection
   d. ischemia

3. The abbreviation SpO_2 stands for:
   a. sensitivity of pressurized oxygen.
   b. specificity of the pressure of oxygen.
   c. saturation of the pressure of oxygen.
   d. saturation of partial pressure of oxygen.

4. Which of the following is administrative information that is recorded on a PCR?
   a. run times
   b. vital signs
   c. chief complaint
   d. mechanism of injury

5. Which of the following medical terms is misspelled?
   a. cefalad
   b. mediad
   c. retraction
   d. adduction

6. Many patients have some form of insurance that requires specific information about the patient and the call before the insurer will pay the bill. The EMS agency must provide this specific information to the _____ to receive payment.
   a. patient
   b. first-party payer
   c. second-party payer
   d. third-party payer

7. Which of the following is an example of pertinent information that should be included on a PCR?
   a. These people are usually so nice.
   b. That patient really had it coming to him.
   c. This is the patient's fourth taxi ride this month.
   d. The patient was calm and cooperative during the transport.

8. Which of the following is an example of objective language?
   a. The patient smelled of cigarettes and beer.
   b. The patient's home was filthy and disorganized.
   c. The patient was crying because she was depressed.
   d. The patient stated that he vomited twice this morning.

9. When documenting a medication administration, what information must the EMT-I include on the PCR?
   a. expiration date of the drug
   b. how the drug is metabolized
   c. the patient's response to the drug
   d. the type of drug-packaging device

10. Which of the following is the correct abbreviation for the term "millimeters of mercury"?
    a. Torr
    b. MMR
    c. mmM
    d. mm Hg

11. Which of the following is most correct regarding a patient's right to have medical conditions held in confidence?
    a. Triage tags should not include any patient-specific identifying information.
    b. To avoid breaching the patient's confidentiality rights, PCRs should not be used for educational purposes.
    c. To avoid breaching the patient's confidentiality rights, PCRs should not be used for quality improvement.
    d. PCRs that are used for quality improvement or educational purposes should not include the patient's name.

12. Incomplete, inaccurate, or illegible information on a PCR:
    a. always creates the opportunity for a lawsuit.
    b. is the ultimate responsibility of an EMS agency's supervisor.
    c. may indicate that the EMT-I did not provide proper patient care.
    d. is the ultimate responsibility of an EMS agency's medical director.

13. In many EMS agencies, the first form of documentation used for patient information at the scene of a multiple-casualty incident (MCI) is:
    a. triage tags.
    b. sector labels.
    c. identification vests.
    d. an operation flowsheet.

14. The section of the PCR that describes the call in a written report is the:
    a. outline.
    b. narrative.
    c. addendum.
    d. administrative portion.

15. Which of the following are two types of written formats EMT-Is use in documenting patient information on PCRs?
    a. AVPU and GCS
    b. SAMPLE and GCS
    c. OPQRST and APGAR
    d. SOAP and CHEATED

16. Which of the following is prehospital patient documentation prepared by the EMT-I?
    a. standing orders
    b. advance directive
    c. do not attempt resuscitation
    d. refusal of medical attention

17. Documentation of which of the following findings is vital in defending your care of a patient you intubated in the prehospital setting?
    a. the pulse oximetry reading
    b. the size of the endotracheal tube
    c. auscultation of bilateral breath sounds
    d. the patient's mental status prior to intubation

18. What is meant by the phrase "the documentation should stand on its own"?
    a. The PCR contains no pertinent negatives.
    b. The PCR does not contain any extraneous language.
    c. The PCR contains no statements to questions that do not appear in a check box.
    d. The PCR contains complete and accurate information regarding the patient's needs and the care provided.

19. A 55-year-old male is complaining of substernal chest pain that began 30 minutes ago. He feels nauseated, is sweating, and denies shortness of breath. The patient has had this type of pain before, but today is the worst ever. Which of the following is a pertinent negative finding with this patient?
    a. no shortness of breath
    b. never had pain this bad
    c. less than 60 years of age
    d. pain began less than an hour ago

20. Near the end of your shift, you realize that you forgot to document an important item on a PCR written earlier in the shift. The PCR copies have already been distributed. What is the appropriate method for making corrections or additions to the PCR?
    a. Add the pertinent information to the copy you have.
    b. Advise the EMS supervisor of the omission and leave it at that.
    c. Document the information on an addendum and distribute copies of the addendum.
    d. Do nothing unless the matter comes up in the quality assurance (QA) review.

21. The EMT-I who makes changes to a PCR before distributing the copies is:
    a. guilty of record tampering.
    b. knowingly filing a false instrument.
    c. doing the right thing and cannot be sued.
    d. doing the right thing if she initials the changes.

22. Which of the following is an example of an unusual situation that would be documented on a special incident report rather than a PCR?
    a. a hostile or abusive patient
    b. a patient who required physical restraint
    c. an emergency vehicle collision en route to a call
    d. radio failure that delayed direct medical control

23. Which of the following is most correct regarding the use of abbreviations in the PCR?
    a. Abbreviations are typically considered extraneous.
    b. Abbreviations are confusing and should be avoided.
    c. The use of abbreviations is acceptable if you use your own.
    d. The use of standard abbreviations is acceptable in many EMS systems.

24. When writing a PCR, the EMT-I must remember that it is a legal document and ensure that the terms and expressions used are:
    a. biased.
    b. subjective.
    c. standardized.
    d. discriminatory.

25. During a patient interview, the patient disclosed information to questions that do not appear in the check boxes on the PCR. The EMT-I should document that information by:
    a. using a special incident form in addition to the PCR.
    b. document the patient's statements in the narrative using quotation marks.
    c. paraphrase the patient's statement into the administrative section.
    d. writing in additional check boxes that correspond with the information.

Chapter 11 Answer Form

	A	B	C	D		A	B	C	D
1.	❏	❏	❏	❏	14.	❏	❏	❏	❏
2.	❏	❏	❏	❏	15.	❏	❏	❏	❏
3.	❏	❏	❏	❏	16.	❏	❏	❏	❏
4.	❏	❏	❏	❏	17.	❏	❏	❏	❏
5.	❏	❏	❏	❏	18.	❏	❏	❏	❏
6.	❏	❏	❏	❏	19.	❏	❏	❏	❏
7.	❏	❏	❏	❏	20.	❏	❏	❏	❏
8.	❏	❏	❏	❏	21.	❏	❏	❏	❏
9.	❏	❏	❏	❏	22.	❏	❏	❏	❏
10.	❏	❏	❏	❏	23.	❏	❏	❏	❏
11.	❏	❏	❏	❏	24.	❏	❏	❏	❏
12.	❏	❏	❏	❏	25.	❏	❏	❏	❏
13.	❏	❏	❏	❏					

CHAPTER 12

Trauma Systems and Mechanism of Injury

1. The components of a comprehensive trauma system include each of the following, except:
   a. hospice care.
   b. definitive care.
   c. critical trauma care.
   d. injury prevention programs.

2. Trauma centers are classified into four levels based on the:
   a. number of employees working at the facility.
   b. resources and programs available at the facility.
   c. ability of a facility to receive patients by Medevac.
   d. statistics of high frequency of traumatic injuries in the geographic area.

3. You want to know the criteria for transporting a trauma patient to a Level I trauma center in your community. You can typically find this information:
   a. in your local protocols.
   b. listed in the NAEMT website.
   c. by contacting medical control.
   d. in the EMT-Intermediate training text.

4. Which of the following is a criterion for air-medical transport?
   a. critical burn patient
   b. morbidly obese patient
   c. traumatic cardiac arrest
   d. patient with barotrauma

5. The strength, direction, and nature of energy forces that cause injury are referred to as:
   a. inertia.
   b. kinetic energy.
   c. mechanism of injury.
   d. conservation of energy.

6. Kinetic energy, as it relates to mechanism of injury, means that the:
   a. speed the object was traveling is significant.
   b. less speed there is, the more energy there is.
   c. lighter the weight of the patient, the more energy there is.
   d. heavier the weight of the patient, the more energy there is.

7. When a bullet is fired into the body, the energy forces from the bullet are transferred to the tissues, causing the tissues to move away from the track of the projectile. This is referred to as:
   a. velocity.
   b. cavitation.
   c. an index of suspicion.
   d. conservation of energy.

8. The driver of a vehicle involved in a motor vehicle collision (MVC) strikes the left side of his head on the window. The injury that causes the brain to be damaged on the same side as the impact is called a _____ injury.
   a. coup
   b. parietal
   c. temporal
   d. contrecoup

9. A 65-year-old male who was involved in a rear-end collision, with a significant MOI, had a brief loss of consciousness as reported by a passenger in the vehicle. Your assessment reveals that he is alert, complaining of pain, and denies tenderness of the cervical spine or back. Which of the following factors make the patient unreliable and should cause you to consider immobilizing the patient to a long backboard?
   a. no complaint of pain
   b. the age of the patient
   c. the loss of consciousness
   d. the patient is alert during the assessment

10. A 24-year-old male was riding his motorcycle through an intersection when he was struck from the right side at approximately 20 mph. The collision caused him to hit the ground and the bike to fall on him. Which of the following directions of force can you suspect his cervical spine most likely sustained?

a. rotation
b. distraction
c. hyperextension
d. vertical compression

11. Sternal contusions, facial abrasions, soft tissue injuries to the nose, and burns or abrasion to the forearms are injuries associated with which MOI?

a. rapid acceleration
b. seatbelt activation
c. airbag deployment
d. penetrating trauma

12. In the kinetic energy formula, the variable that contributes the most to significant injury is:

a. mass.
b. force.
c. inertia.
d. velocity.

13. Which of the following is most correct about penetrating and blunt trauma injuries?

a. Both types of injuries can be lethal.
b. Only blunt injuries create a temporary cavity.
c. Only penetrating injuries penetrate body tissues.
d. Blunt trauma is easier to recognize than penetrating trauma.

14. Each phase of a blast has a different energy pattern and potential for injury. When the energy pattern causes a victim to become a flying object that strikes other objects, the resulting injuries are recognized as occurring in the _____ phase.

a. primary
b. secondary
c. tertiary
d. fourth

15. Some bullets are designed to tumble when they are fired, because a tumbling bullet will:

a. travel faster and further.
b. create a cavity that leaves a permanent hole.
c. create a smaller entry point with a larger exit point.
d. create a large entry point and more tissue damage.

Chapter 12 Answer Form

	A	B	C	D
1.	❏	❏	❏	❏
2.	❏	❏	❏	❏
3.	❏	❏	❏	❏
4.	❏	❏	❏	❏
5.	❏	❏	❏	❏
6.	❏	❏	❏	❏
7.	❏	❏	❏	❏
8.	❏	❏	❏	❏

	A	B	C	D
9.	❏	❏	❏	❏
10.	❏	❏	❏	❏
11.	❏	❏	❏	❏
12.	❏	❏	❏	❏
13.	❏	❏	❏	❏
14.	❏	❏	❏	❏
15.	❏	❏	❏	❏

CHAPTER 13

Hemorrhage and Shock

1. The outcome for a patient who is hemorrhaging and has signs of shock will be affected most by:
   a. severity of bleeding.
   b. whether or not the patient is a smoker.
   c. the medications the patient is prescribed.
   d. how aggressive local treatment protocols are.

2. During which stage of shock does the body shunt blood from less vital organs and redirect it to the heart, brain, and lungs?
   a. irreversible
   b. compensatory
   c. decompensatory
   d. all of the above

3. When a patient has signs and symptoms of hypo-volemic shock and no external bleeding is apparent, the EMT-I should:
   a. rule out dehydration as the cause.
   b. consider head injury as the cause.
   c. rule out inferior-wall myocardial infarction.
   d. consider occult gastrointestinal (GI) bleeding as the cause.

4. A patient tells you that he has been passing bloody stools. The term for this condition is:
   a. hemoptysis.
   b. hematemesis.
   c. hematochezia.
   d. occult bleeding.

5. A 14-year-old male fell while skateboarding and incurred an isolated injury to the lower leg. There is an open injury with deformity, and you suspect a possible fracture of the tibia and the fibula. There is significant bleeding, and the bone and fascia are exposed. The first step in the care of this injury is to:
   a. obtain a blood pressure.
   b. apply direct pressure and elevation.
   c. apply pressure on the proximal pressure point.
   d. splint the lower leg before attempting any bleeding control.

6. How does the application of a cold pack or ice help to control bleeding?
   a. Cooling helps to reduce swelling.
   b. Cooling promotes vasoconstriction.
   c. Cooling facilitates the clotting process.
   d. All of the above.

7. Your patient has arterial bleeding in the lower leg. Direct pressure and elevation have not slowed the bleeding. What action should you take next to stop the bleeding?
   a. Apply a tourniquet just below the knee.
   b. Apply a tourniquet just above the knee.
   c. Apply direct pressure on the popliteal artery.
   d. Start two large-bore IVs and administer a fluid challenge.

8. When treating a patient who has a gunshot wound to the upper thigh, you can consider bleeding to be controlled when:
   a. no blood is seeping through the bandage.
   b. the heart rate stays under 100 beats per minute.
   c. the patient's blood pressure remains normotensive.
   d. none of the above.

9. The role of IV fluid administration for the patient who is in hypovolemic shock is:
   a. autoregulation.
   b. vasoconstriction.
   c. volume expansion.
   d. hemorrhage control.

10. When the body senses a decrease in systolic blood pressure to less than 80 mm Hg, the vasomotor center is stimulated to:
    a. increase the arterial pressure.
    b. increase the release of insulin.
    c. inhibit the release of epinephrine.
    d. inhibit the release of norepinephrine.

11. Your patient was the driver of a vehicle that was involved in a serious crash. From your baseline assessment and serial assessment findings, you have observed that the patient has a narrowing pulse pressure. This finding indicates that the patient:
    a. is experiencing decompensating shock.
    b. is experiencing early hypovolemic shock.
    c. has a head injury in addition to internal hemorrhage.
    d. has a head injury that is causing hypovolemic shock.

12. How does the body sense blood loss?
    a. Baroreceptors sense decreased arterial blood flow.
    b. Baroreceptors sense decreased venous blood flow.
    c. Chemoreceptors sense decreased arterial blood flow.
    d. Chemoreceptors sense decreased venous blood flow.

13. What causes the capillaries to switch from aerobic to anaerobic metabolism?
    a. metabolic acidosis
    b. minimal blood flow to the capillaries
    c. increased production of lactic acid
    d. increased production of carbon dioxide

14. During a decreased state of perfusion, the cells go through a series of changes. In the first phase,
    a. the result is metabolic acidosis.
    b. plasma leaks from the capillaries.
    c. the capillaries become engorged with fluid.
    d. the cells switch from aerobic to anaerobic metabolism.

15. Which of the following is the correct sequence of phases the cells go through during a decreased state of perfusion?
    a. ischemic, stagnation, and washout
    b. stagnation, ischemic, and washout
    c. washout, ischemic, and stagnation
    d. stagnation, washout, and ischemic

16. The series of changes that the cells go through during decreased states of perfusion ultimately lead to _____ shock.
    a. metabolic
    b. obstructive
    c. cardiogenic
    d. hypovolemic

17. Stroke volume is defined as:
    a. adequate perfusion to tissues.
    b. the clinical signs of shock or inadequate perfusion.
    c. the heart rate divided by the amount of cardiac output in one hour.
    d. the amount of blood ejected from the left ventricle with each contraction.

18. Adequate perfusion depends on there being no interference with cardiac output, systemic vascular resistance, and:
    a. normal urine output.
    b. the transport of blood.
    c. normal insulin production.
    d. release of norepinephrine.

19. When a person donates a pint of blood, she can go into which stage or phase of shock?
    a. one
    b. two
    c. three
    d. four

20. What type of IV fluid is the accepted choice for EMT-Is to administer to patients with hypovolemia from trauma?
    a. blood substitutes
    b. isotonic solutions
    c. hypotonic solutions
    d. hypertonic solutions

21. Which of the following bleeding wounds would it be appropriate to pack with a large sterile dressing?
    a. uncontrolled bleeding from the ear
    b. bright red bleeding from the rectum
    c. a large gaping wound in the upper arm
    d. severe postpartum vaginal hemorrhage

22. A patient is vomiting bright red blood. This finding suggests that the:
    a. bleeding is coming from the lungs or upper GI.
    b. patient has lower GI bleeding.
    c. patient will also have bleeding from the rectum.
    d. patient will have orthostatic vital sign changes.

23. Which finding is associated with decompensated (rather than compensated) hypovolemic shock?
    a. anxiety
    b. abdominal pain
    c. normal blood pressure
    d. decreased mental status

24. You respond to an emergency call to the local nursing home for a patient in respiratory distress. She is responsive to pain, is gasping for air, and appears to be in shock. Her vital signs are: respiratory rate, 40/labored; pulse rate, 48/irregular; BP, 70/50. The staff reports that she was well until about one hour ago, when she suddenly developed shortness of breath and chest pain. What type of shock do you suspect the patient is experiencing?
    a. distributive
    b. obstructive
    c. cardiogenic
    d. hypovolemic

25. Your patient, who is coming out of a health care facility, is being taken to the ED for a simple pneumothorax. During the transport the patient suddenly deteriorates. He develops severe respiratory distress, jugular vein distention, and absent breath sounds on the affected side. He is now hypotensive, pale, and clammy. You suspect that he has a tension pneumothorax. What type of shock is he experiencing?
    a. distributive
    b. obstructive
    c. cardiogenic
    d. hypovolemic

26. A 12-year-old female with a known allergy to nuts is experiencing a severe allergic reaction. She is pale, diaphoretic, and moist. Her breath sounds are diminished bilaterally, and she has a weak and rapid distal pulse. What type of shock is she exhibiting?
    a. distributive
    b. obstructive
    c. cardiogenic
    d. hypovolemic

27. You are dispatched for an unresponsive patient. When you arrive, you find a 66-year-old female sitting on the floor conscious and alert. Witnesses report a 30-second loss of conscious with no injuries sustained during the collapse. The patient's only complaint is dizziness. What is the first action to take with this patient?
    a. lay her down
    b. obtain a blood pressure
    c. administer high-concentration oxygen
    d. start an IV and administer a fluid bolus

28. The presence of orthostatic changes in a patient's vital signs suggests:
    a. inner ear infection.
    b. epidural hematoma.
    c. subdural hematoma.
    d. intravascular volume depletion.

29. Coffee-ground-like vomitus is associated with:
    a. colon cancer.
    b. ingesting tomatoes.
    c. bleeding from the stomach.
    d. bleeding from the lower GI tract.

30. Bright red bleeding from the rectum can result from many causes and is typically considered:
    a. a serious condition.
    b. non-life-threatening.
    c. as minor as a nosebleed.
    d. to be from hemorrhoids.

31. What mechanism of shock is associated with an isolated spinal or head injury?
    a. distributive
    b. obstructive
    c. cardiogenic
    d. hypovolemic

32. Decreased perfusion that leads to decompensated shock or irreversible shock can be caused by significant blood loss, by kinking of the great vessels (as in tension pneumothorax), or by:
    a. an allergic reaction.
    b. loss of vasomotor tone.
    c. a failure in the buffer system.
    d. loss of capillary hydrostatic pressure.

33. The grade or stage of shock that involves 15 to 25 percent intravascular loss is:
    a. one.
    b. two.
    c. three.
    d. four.

34. The suggested effect from the use of a pneumatic anti-shock garment (PASG) is that inflation of the PASG leads to:
    a. dilation of blood vessels.
    b. increased heart rate and respiratory rate.
    c. increased force of contraction of the heart.
    d. increased blood pressure and organ perfusion.

35. The indication for the use of a PASG is hypovolemia associated with:
    a. chest trauma.
    b. pelvic fractures.
    c. cardiogenic shock.
    d. pulmonary edema.

36. _____ shock occurs when toxins in the body cause blood vessels to dilate, allowing blood to pool in the extremities and fluid to leak into the surrounding tissues.
    a. Septic
    b. Vasogenic
    c. Cardiogenic
    d. Anaphylactic

37. Your patient is a 30-year-old female who is complaining of vaginal bleeding. She tells you that she feels dizzy, weak, and has cramping. What is the most serious complication of her chief complaint?
    a. anemia
    b. pregnancy
    c. hypovolemic shock
    d. compensated shock

38. You are administering IV fluids to a patient in decompensated shock. You should recall that only about one-third of the IV fluid infused stays in the:

a. interstitial fluid.
b. intracellular space.
c. extracellular space.
d. intravascular space.

39. Within an hour of infusion of a crystalloid IV fluid, such as normal saline, approximately two-thirds of the fluids infused will move into the:

a. cells.
b. lungs.
c. kidneys.
d. interstitial space.

40. You are starting an IV on a patient with an isolated extremity injury. When the patient sees his own blood in the IV catheter, he rolls his eyes and faints. What type of shock is this?

a. cardiogenic
b. neurogenic
c. psychogenic
d. hypovolemic

Chapter 13 Answer Form

	A	B	C	D			A	B	C	D
1.	❏	❏	❏	❏		21.	❏	❏	❏	❏
2.	❏	❏	❏	❏		22.	❏	❏	❏	❏
3.	❏	❏	❏	❏		23.	❏	❏	❏	❏
4.	❏	❏	❏	❏		24.	❏	❏	❏	❏
5.	❏	❏	❏	❏		25.	❏	❏	❏	❏
6.	❏	❏	❏	❏		26.	❏	❏	❏	❏
7.	❏	❏	❏	❏		27.	❏	❏	❏	❏
8.	❏	❏	❏	❏		28.	❏	❏	❏	❏
9.	❏	❏	❏	❏		29.	❏	❏	❏	❏
10.	❏	❏	❏	❏		30.	❏	❏	❏	❏
11.	❏	❏	❏	❏		31.	❏	❏	❏	❏
12.	❏	❏	❏	❏		32.	❏	❏	❏	❏
13.	❏	❏	❏	❏		33.	❏	❏	❏	❏
14.	❏	❏	❏	❏		34.	❏	❏	❏	❏
15.	❏	❏	❏	❏		35.	❏	❏	❏	❏
16.	❏	❏	❏	❏		36.	❏	❏	❏	❏
17.	❏	❏	❏	❏		37.	❏	❏	❏	❏
18.	❏	❏	❏	❏		38.	❏	❏	❏	❏
19.	❏	❏	❏	❏		39.	❏	❏	❏	❏
20.	❏	❏	❏	❏		40.	❏	❏	❏	❏

CHAPTER

Burns

1. The immediate scar that forms on the skin following a burn is:
   a. an eschar formation.
   b. in no way life-threatening.
   c. only associated with radiation burns.
   d. only associated with electrical burns.

2. Which of the following time periods presents the greatest risk of sunburn?
   a. 10:00 a.m. to 2:00 p.m.
   b. 11:00 a.m. to 3:00 p.m.
   c. 12:00 p.m. to 4:00 p.m.
   d. 1:00 p.m. to 5:00 p.m.

3. Preexisting medical problems associated with _____ can make it difficult for the patient to handle the significant movement of body fluids that occurs with a burn injury.
   a. the skin
   b. the heart
   c. hyperlipidemia
   d. behavioral disorders

4. Direct contract with harsh solvents, dry ice, and drain cleaners is primarily associated with what type of burn?
   a. thermal
   b. ionizing
   c. chemical
   d. inhalation

5. A burn that extends to the fascia is classified as:
   a. superficial.
   b. deep fascia.
   c. full-thickness.
   d. partial-thickness.

6. One method of estimating the body surface area (BSA) affected by a burn on an infant is to:
   a. use the Broselow tape.
   b. apply the Parkland formula.
   c. use the surface area of the EMT-I's palm to correspond to 1 percent of the patient's BSA.
   d. use the surface area of the patient's palm to correspond to 1 percent of the patient's BSA.

7. An infant's head accounts for what percentage of body surface area, according to the rule of nines?
   a. 9 percent
   b. 13.5 percent
   c. 18 percent
   d. 21.5 percent

8. Which of the following is most accurate about determining the severity of a burn injury?
   a. The rule of nines applies equally to adults and children.
   b. The severity of a burn for a child involves less BSA than for an adult.
   c. The severity of a burn for an adult patient involves less BSA than for a child.
   d. The severity of a burn for adults and children is the same when the same amount of BSA is affected.

9. Sunburns sustained during childhood can lead to what dangerous condition in adulthood?
   a. cellulite
   b. contact dermatitis
   c. necrotizing fasciitis
   d. malignant melanoma

10. The patient's _____ is an important factor in how well his or her body can handle a burn injury.
    a. age
    b. gender
    c. height
    d. weight

11. Which of the following typically produces the most severe burn?
    a. hot tar
    b. hot coffee
    c. hot grease
    d. pepper spray

12. The EMT-I should suspect _____ in an unconscious victim who was rescued from a fully involved house fire.

   a. massive internal injuries
   b. hearing impairment and vision loss
   c. soft tissue and musculoskeletal injuries
   d. airway compromise from inhaling superheated gases

13. A burn victim has singed nasal hairs and is spitting up black soot. In addition to provision of high-concentration oxygen, the primary treatment for this patient is:

   a. hyperbaric therapy.
   b. airway maintenance.
   c. fluid volume replacement.
   d. flushing of the nose and mouth.

14. The organ(s) most commonly injured by burns is/are the:

   a. skin.
   b. eyes.
   c. lungs.
   d. heart.

15. How does a circumferential burn of the chest contribute to respiratory compromise?

   a. The eschar does not allow the chest to expand for ventilation.
   b. The eschar produces sloughing in and swelling of the lower airways.
   c. The burn stimulates the release of catecholamines, which produce pulmonary edema.
   d. The eschar stimulates a fluid shift from the intravascular space, leading to hypoxia.

16. When a large area of skin is damaged by a thermal burn, the patient is at risk of quickly developing:

   a. anemia.
   b. hypothermia.
   c. dysrhythmias.
   d. hypoglycemia.

17. A partial-thickness burn affects what structures?

   a. fascia
   b. muscles
   c. sweat ducts
   d. mucous membranes

18. The first step in the care of a patient with a thermal burn is to:

   a. protect the airway.
   b. stop the burning.
   c. estimate the BSA affected.
   d. administer high-concentration oxygen.

19. A 16-year-old female has a superficial burn over her entire back. Care for this burn includes:

   a. applying a burn ointment.
   b. transport to a burn center.
   c. applying a moist, sterile burn dressing.
   d. covering the burn area with a dry burn dressing.

20. A 23-year-old male has reddening, blisters, and peeling skin on his left cheek and neck from brief exposure to a flame. What type of burn does he have?

   a. radiation
   b. superficial
   c. chemical
   d. partial-thickness

21. Which of the following is not likely to result in a thermal burn?

   a. steam
   b. flames
   c. sunburn
   d. microwave

22. Hyperbaric therapy is useful in what type of inhalation burn injury?

   a. smoke
   b. phenols
   c. carbon monoxide
   d. any chemical inhalation

23. Inhalation injuries are most commonly associated with _____ burns.

   a. thermal
   b. radiation
   c. chemical
   d. electrical

24. Which of the following signs or symptoms indicates that a patient has experienced an inhalation injury?

   a. stridor
   b. chest pain
   c. singed facial hairs
   d. black soot on the face

25. After supporting the airway, breathing, and circulation, what is the appropriate treatment for the patient with suspected cyanide inhalation?

   a. high-dose atropine
   b. hyperbaric therapy
   c. aggressive fluid challenge
   d. amyl nitrate and thiosulfate

26. Your patient was removed from his workplace, where he was exposed to superheated gases. He has respiratory distress, wheezing, and difficulty swallowing, and is cyanotic. What can you do to keep his airway from swelling any further?

   a. There is nothing you can do.
   b. Administer humidified oxygen.
   c. Endotracheally intubate the patient.
   d. Administer high-concentration oxygen.

27. Which phase of a blast injury has the greatest potential for injury to the lower airways?
    a. primary
    b. secondary
    c. tertiary
    d. quaternary or fourth

28. Which of the following is typically associated with inhalation injury?
    a. steam
    b. flash burn
    c. pepper spray
    d. all of the above

29. Which of the following is most correct about inhalation burn injuries?
    a. Ionizing radiation can cause injury by inhalation.
    b. Ionizing radiation does not cause inhalation burn injuries.
    c. Nonionizing radiation does not cause inhalation burn injuries.
    d. Only alpha and beta particles can be inhaled and cause tissue injury.

30. When a patient has an eye injury from a chemical agent, what should you do if the patient is wearing contact lenses?
    a. Irrigate the eyes with the lenses in place.
    b. Remove the lenses or assist the patient to remove them.
    c. Irrigate the eyes for 10 minutes and then remove the lenses.
    d. Place Morgan lenses over the contact lenses, then irrigate the eyes.

31. Most chemical burn injuries occur in:
    a. the home.
    b. house fires.
    c. an industrial setting.
    d. photo developing labs.

32. Your patient has wet pepper spray on the face, hands, and arms. What is the most effective way to remove it?
    a. Rinse it with a lot of water.
    b. Do not touch it while it is wet.
    c. Sponge it off with a dry towel.
    d. Provide continuous irrigation.

33. Which of the following chemicals should be diluted with alcohol, if available, prior to being irrigated with water?
    a. lye
    b. phenol
    c. dry lime
    d. drain cleaner

34. Which of the following is most accurate about chemical burns to the eyes?
    a. Morgan lenses are not indicated for chemical burns to the eyes.
    b. Inhalation injuries are often associated with chemical burns to the eyes.
    c. Vinegar is an excellent neutralizer for many chemical burns affecting the eyes.
    d. Chemical burns to the eyes cause a release of catecholamines, which can cause seizures.

35. What is the first action to take in treating a chemical burn?
    a. Flush the affected area with a lot of water.
    b. Wipe off as much chemical product as possible.
    c. Instruct the patient to close the eyes and mouth.
    d. Move the patient outside and downwind of the ambulance.

36. A truck driver was splashed with diesel fuel while filling his vehicle. Before you arrived, coworkers helped him rinse his face and eyes. As you approach, you can smell that he is covered with fuel. He is alert and complains of burning in both eyes. What is the first action you take?
    a. Assist the patient to a well-ventilated area.
    b. Request the fire department to help with a washdown.
    c. Continue to flush his eyes and instruct the patient to rinse his mouth.
    d. Instruct the patient to remove all his clothing; assist him if necessary.

37. (Continuing with the preceding question) The patient tells you that the fill pipe overflowed, causing the diesel fuel to splash into his face and onto his body. He denies difficulty breathing, but says he can still taste the fuel. You examine his mouth and see no burns. His lung sounds are clear. His face and neck are reddened, his eyes are bloodshot, and his vision is blurred in one eye. His vital signs are: respiratory rate, 20/regular; pulse rate, 88/regular; BP, 134/80. What is your primary focus in further treatment of this patient?
    a. continued irrigation of both eyes
    b. analgesic for the pain management
    c. rapid transport to the nearest burn center
    d. preparation for possible seizure activity

38. The human body is a good conductor of electricity because:
    a. it can never be grounded.
    b. the body consists primarily of water.
    c. the body contains so many electrolytes.
    d. it has so many natural pathways for current travel.

39. Which electrical currents are the most dangerous?
    a. low-frequency AC
    b. high-frequency AC
    c. low-frequency DC
    d. all are equally dangerous

40. Which of the following is the most accurate about injuries from lightning strikes?
    a. Lightning rarely produces an exit wound.
    b. Lightning always produces an exit wound.
    c. Lightning always produces an entry wound.
    d. Electrical injuries from lightning are very common.

41. What is the most common entry point on the body for a current that produces an electrical burn?
    a. head
    b. feet
    c. chest
    d. hands

42. Select the skin condition that has the most resistance to electrical voltage.
    a. wet, intact skin
    b. dry, intact skin
    c. calloused palm
    d. mucous membrane

43. What is the significance of an electrical injury with two external burn injury locations?
    a. The patient received two separate shocks.
    b. Anything between the two locations may be injured.
    c. Two external burn injury locations indicate that the cause was direct current.
    d. Two external burn injury locations indicate that the cause was alternating current.

44. Each of the following is a common physiologic dysfunction associated with electrical burns, except:
    a. seizures.
    b. singed nasal hair.
    c. respiratory arrest.
    d. hearing impairment.

45. The very first action to take when responding to a call for an electrical burn is to:
    a. determine if the patient is unresponsive.
    b. stage the ambulance 50 meters from the location of the incident.
    c. wait for the fire department to determine if the scene is safe to enter.
    d. identify the source of the electricity before approaching the patient.

46. An exposure to ionizing radiation:
    a. cannot be seen, heard, or felt.
    b. can be felt, but not seen or heard.
    c. can be heard, but not seen or felt.
    d. can be seen, but not heard or felt.

47. A Geiger counter is a detection instrument that measures the RAD or:
    a. radiation absorbed dose.
    b. roentgen absorbed dose.
    c. rate of adverse discovery.
    d. rate admitted through the dermis.

48. Radiation sickness results when humans or animals are exposed:
    a. acutely in a single large exposure.
    b. to excessive doses of ionizing radiation.
    c. chronically, by exposure to dangerous radiation levels over a period of time.
    d. any of the above.

49. An incident involving exposure to ionizing radiation is referred as a "dirty accident" when the:
    a. patient was exposed to radioactive gas.
    b. patient's source of exposure was a fire.
    c. patient was exposed to radioactive smoke or dust.
    d. patient is contaminated and is an exposure hazard for rescuers.

50. Which of the following is most accurate about the signs and symptoms of overexposure to ionizing radiation?
    a. Many signs and symptoms are the same as those seen with radiation therapy for cancer.
    b. Signs and symptoms are only associated with overexposure to gamma rays.
    c. Signs and symptoms are very different from those seen with radiation therapy for cancer.
    d. The patient will not develop signs and symptoms until several days after an overexposure to ionizing radiation.

51. _____ is/are especially sensitive to radiation.
    a. Platelets
    b. Hemoglobin
    c. Red blood cells
    d. White blood cells

52. When you suspect that your patient has been overexposed to ionizing radiation, the primary focus of care is:
    a. finding and correcting life-threatening injuries.
    b. obtaining a RAD reading with a Geiger counter.
    c. transporting the patient to a level 1 trauma center.
    d. decontaminating the rescuers as soon as possible.

53. Which of the following does not affect a rescuer's potential for exposure to radiation?
    a. distance from the source of exposure
    b. length of time near the source of exposure
    c. the amount of radioactive material present
    d. the age and physical condition of the rescuer

54. Why should the EMT-I rapidly remove all of a burn victim's clothing?
   a. The patient is easier to flush with all clothing removed.
   b. He must ensure that no embers or smoldering portions can burn the patient further.
   c. It is easier to estimate the rule of nines when the clothing is removed.
   d. Completing a detailed physical exam is easier with the clothing removed.

55. When should the EMT-I suspect that a burn injury is possible child abuse?
   a. when the history is inconsistent with the injuries
   b. when the burns are located on the front of the body
   c. when the burns are located on the back of the body
   d. when the body surface area of the burn is more than 27 percent

Chapter 14 Answer Form

	A	B	C	D			A	B	C	D
1.	❏	❏	❏	❏		25.	❏	❏	❏	❏
2.	❏	❏	❏	❏		26.	❏	❏	❏	❏
3.	❏	❏	❏	❏		27.	❏	❏	❏	❏
4.	❏	❏	❏	❏		28.	❏	❏	❏	❏
5.	❏	❏	❏	❏		29.	❏	❏	❏	❏
6.	❏	❏	❏	❏		30.	❏	❏	❏	❏
7.	❏	❏	❏	❏		31.	❏	❏	❏	❏
8.	❏	❏	❏	❏		32.	❏	❏	❏	❏
9.	❏	❏	❏	❏		33.	❏	❏	❏	❏
10.	❏	❏	❏	❏		34.	❏	❏	❏	❏
11.	❏	❏	❏	❏		35.	❏	❏	❏	❏
12.	❏	❏	❏	❏		36.	❏	❏	❏	❏
13.	❏	❏	❏	❏		37.	❏	❏	❏	❏
14.	❏	❏	❏	❏		38.	❏	❏	❏	❏
15.	❏	❏	❏	❏		39.	❏	❏	❏	❏
16.	❏	❏	❏	❏		40.	❏	❏	❏	❏
17.	❏	❏	❏	❏		41.	❏	❏	❏	❏
18.	❏	❏	❏	❏		42.	❏	❏	❏	❏
19.	❏	❏	❏	❏		43.	❏	❏	❏	❏
20.	❏	❏	❏	❏		44.	❏	❏	❏	❏
21.	❏	❏	❏	❏		45.	❏	❏	❏	❏
22.	❏	❏	❏	❏		46.	❏	❏	❏	❏
23.	❏	❏	❏	❏		47.	❏	❏	❏	❏
24.	❏	❏	❏	❏		48.	❏	❏	❏	❏

	A	B	C	D			A	B	C	D
49.	❏	❏	❏	❏		53.	❏	❏	❏	❏
50.	❏	❏	❏	❏		54.	❏	❏	❏	❏
51.	❏	❏	❏	❏		55.	❏	❏	❏	❏
52.	❏	❏	❏	❏						

CHAPTER

Thoracic Trauma

1. Chest injuries are the _____ leading cause of trauma death in the United States.
   a. first
   b. second
   c. third
   d. fourth

2. The space in the chest between the pleural sacs of the lungs is the:
   a. peritoneum.
   b. pericardium.
   c. mediastinum.
   d. retroperitoneum.

3. Moments before a car collides, almost instinctively, the patient takes a deep breath and closes the glottic opening. If the impact results in chest compression, it can instantly cause a:
   a. glottic injury.
   b. pneumothorax.
   c. diaphragmatic injury.
   d. tension pneumothorax.

4. What type of chest trauma may impair cardiac output?
   a. vascular damage
   b. bleeding intercostal artery
   c. increased intrapleural pressure
   d. any of the above

5. When a traumatic injury causes CO_2 retention, the _____, which monitor CO_2 levels in the blood, will respond accordingly.
   a. pleurae
   b. alveoli
   c. baroreceptors
   d. chemoreceptors

6. When a chest injury results in internal hemorrhage, the blood loss can be significant, as the chest cavity can hold _____ ml of blood.
   a. 1,000–1,500
   b. 2,000–3,000
   c. 3,000–4,000
   d. 4,000–5,000

7. Chest pain that is sharp and clearly worsened by breathing is most likely to be caused by a/an:
   a. injury to the heart.
   b. esophageal injury.
   c. diaphragmatic injury.
   d. lung or chest wall problem.

8. Chest wall injuries include each of the following, except:
   a. atelectasis.
   b. rib fractures.
   c. flail segment.
   d. sternal contusion.

9. Rib fractures frequently occur with blunt trauma chest injuries and are most common in which ribs?
   a. 3 to 6.
   b. 4 to 9.
   c. 6 to 10.
   d. 10 to 12.

10. The paradoxical moment of a flail segment of the chest wall is:
    a. difficult to detect or stabilize in the prehospital setting.
    b. minimal when the flail segment is small, because of muscle spasm.
    c. minimal when the flair segment is large, because of muscle spasm.
    d. prominent in all instances, regardless of the number of ribs involved.

11. Sternal fractures are associated with high mortality because:
    a. the most common MOI is a motor vehicle crash.
    b. a patient with a sternal fracture is difficult to intubate.
    c. of the associated injuries that occur to the organs under the sternum.
    d. the significant force needed to fracture the sternum is transmitted to the spine.

12. While you are assessing a conscious victim of a drive-by shooting, you discover a hole in the upper right chest that appears to be the entrance gunshot wound (GSW). Your next action is to:

    a. assess the back for an exit wound.

    b. cover the wound with a trauma dressing.

    c. cover the wound with your gloved hand.

    d. roll the patient onto the right side to occlude the opening.

13. A lung collapses because of increased intrapulmonary pressure. This condition is called a:

    a. hemopneumothorax.

    b. open pneumothorax.

    c. simple pneumothorax.

    d. tension pneumothorax.

14. Your patient was thrown from a horse and landed on a rock. She tells you that she felt her ribs crack, and feels like she cannot breathe. She is pale and diaphoretic. She is working hard to breathe and her lung sounds are decreased on the left side. The chest has no open wounds and the lower chest is dull on percussion. What type of chest trauma do you suspect?

    a. hemothorax

    b. simple pneumothorax

    c. tension pneumothorax

    d. pericardial tamponade

15. (Continuing with the preceding question) Your crew administers high-flow oxygen and quickly immobilizes the patient on a long backboard. As you obtain vital signs and begin transport to the trauma center, she appears to be getting worse. She is cyanotic, struggling to breathe, and hypotensive. What action do you take next?

    a. Intubate and reassess.

    b. Obtain a pulse oximetry reading.

    c. Start an IV and administer a fluid challenge.

    d. Assist ventilations with a bag mask.

16. The patient with a pulmonary contusion is a high-priority patient requiring rapid transport, because this injury:

    a. is associated with 95 percent mortality.

    b. is associated with severe thoracic injuries.

    c. causes the chest wall to become unstable.

    d. always progresses to a tension pneumothorax.

17. When the myocardium experiences a contusion, there is hemorrhage with edema, which causes:

    a. cellular injury.

    b. congestive heart failure.

    c. decreased breath sounds.

    d. subcutaneous emphysema.

18. When blunt trauma to the heart causes blood to fill the pericardial sac, which of the following signs can be observed?

    a. dyspnea and hypertension

    b. tracheal deviation with normal SpO_2

    c. hypotension with distended neck veins

    d. decreased breath sounds and coughing up blood

19. You suspect that your patient has a pericardial tamponade from a closed chest injury. Your care for the patient includes airway and ventilation control with high-flow oxygen and:

    a. IV fluid challenge.

    b. pericardiocentesis.

    c. chest decompression.

    d. cardiac compressions.

20. Your transportation considerations for the patient with a suspected pericardial tamponade include:

    a. early notification to the ED.

    b. transport to the nearest ED.

    c. gentle handling and transport.

    d. rapid transport to a level one trauma center.

21. A vascular injury involving separation of the aortic intima and media is called a:

    a. dissection or rupture.

    b. vena cava disconnection.

    c. division of the pulmonary veins.

    d. parting of the pulmonary arteries.

22. What is the effect of an expanding hematoma in the chest?

    a. The patient develops pain in the left shoulder.

    b. The expansion compresses the great vessels.

    c. Bowel sounds become decreased or absent.

    d. A black-and-blue discoloration becomes apparent on the back.

23. The patient with a suspected rupture of the aorta is critical and can die very quickly. Treatment by the EMT-I includes:

    a. rapid but gentle transport to the nearest hospital.

    b. chest decompression and positive pressure ventilation.

    c. IV access and administration of a vasopressor (epinephrine).

    d. insertion of a nasogastric tube to relieve pressure from the hematoma.

24. The pathophysiology of a diaphragmatic injury involves organs of:

    a. the chest only.

    b. the abdomen only.

    c. the chest and abdomen.

    d. neither the chest nor the abdomen.

25. You are listening to the breath sounds of a patient who was stabbed in the upper abdomen. You hear bowel sounds in the base of the right lung, so you suspect that the patient has which of the following injuries?

    a. esophageal
    b. diaphragmatic
    c. aortic dissection
    d. tracheobronchial

26. In the management of a patient with a suspected diaphragmatic injury, which of the following actions should the EMT-I avoid?

    a. Trendelenburg position
    b. palpation of the abdomen
    c. positive pressure ventilation
    d. percussion of the abdomen or thorax

27. A 20-year-old male was stabbed in the upper chest, near the neck, during an attempted robbery. He is conscious, spitting up bright red blood, has obvious respiratory distress, and has significant subcutaneous emphysema in the neck and upper chest. Which of the following is most likely the patient's primary injury?

    a. esophageal tear
    b. traumatic asphyxia
    c. diaphragmatic rupture
    d. tracheobronchial laceration

28. (Continuing with the preceding question) In addition to the respiratory distress associated with this type of thoracic injury, which of the following life-threatening conditions can you expect the patient to develop rather quickly?

    a. petechial hemorrhage
    b. tension pneumothorax
    c. hemorrhage of the conjunctiva
    d. hoarseness and difficulty swallowing

29. (Continuing with the two preceding questions) You control external bleeding with direct pressure and your partner obtains the following vital signs: respiratory rate, 38/labored; decreased lung sounds on the right; pulse rate 130/weak and thready; BP, 80/48; skin CTC is cyanotic, moist, and cool. In addition to high-flow oxygen administration, emergency treatment includes:

    a. IV fluid challenge.
    b. the use of a tourniquet.
    c. chest decompression.
    d. bilateral chest decompression.

30. When a patient develops hypotension after being extricated from a crushing force on the chest, such as being pinned against a wall by a forklift, the primary injury is:

    a. esophageal.
    b. aortic rupture.
    c. tracheobronchial.
    d. traumatic asphyxia.

31. A primary concern for a patient with esophageal injury is the:

    a. development of pain and fever.
    b. need for thoracic needle decompression.
    c. associated injuries to the surrounding organs.
    d. development of hoarseness and difficulty swallowing.

32. The least common MOI of an esophageal injury is:

    a. blunt trauma.
    b. stabbing bullet.
    c. penetrating missile.
    d. penetrating knife wound.

33. Your patient is 14 years old and he is trapped under a load of particle board. The load shifted unexpectedly and has pinned his entire body; only his neck and head are exposed. He is complaining of severe difficulty breathing and states that his body feels numb. What type of chest injury is associated with this type of MOI?

    a. esophageal
    b. aortic rupture
    c. tracheobronchial
    d. traumatic asphyxia

34. (Continuing with the preceding question) After the load is lifted off the patient's torso, the first component of emergency care is:

    a. IV fluids.
    b. to intubate the patient.
    c. airway management.
    d. spinal immobilization.

35. When sudden compression forces squeeze the chest so that the chest is unable to expand, you would expect to see:

    a. tracheal deviation.
    b. signs of hypotension.
    c. the jugular veins engorge.
    d. subcutaneous emphysema.

36. You are performing a rapid trauma exam on a critical patient who was involved in a high-speed MVC. The patient appears to be in shock, and you suspect that the patient has a pulmonary contusion. How much blood loss from a pulmonary contusion can you estimate the patient will have?

    a. 250–500 ml
    b. 500–1,000 ml
    c. 1,000–1,500 ml
    d. 2,000–3,000 ml

37. The presence of rib fractures increases the risk of mortality in which age group?

    a. pediatric
    b. early adult
    c. middle-aged adult
    d. elderly

38. Your patient is a 20-year-old, petite female who was the driver of a vehicle involved in a moderate-speed collision in an intersection. She was not belted in, but had no loss of consciousness, though she is complaining of neck and left shoulder pain, difficulty breathing, and sternal pain. Her vital signs are: respiratory rate, 30/labored, with diminished breath sounds in the left apex; pulse rate, 110/regular; BP, 118/74; skin CTC is pink, warm, and dry. What do you suspect is the cause of her dyspnea?

    a. sternal contusion
    b. simple pneumothorax
    c. possible fractured rib(s)
    d. any of the above

39. (Continuing with the preceding question) The patient is administered high-concentration oxygen, extricated from the vehicle, and immobilized on a long backboard. As the patient is moved into the ambulance, she continues to complain of difficulty breathing. The next action you take is to:

    a. perform a detailed physical exam.
    b. perform a focused exam of the chest.
    c. start two large-bore IVs and administer a fluid bolus.
    d. assist ventilations with a bag mask and obtain an SpO$_2$ reading.

40. A driver loses control of his vehicle on ice and hits a tree head-on. Considering the MOI, which of the following describes the "third collision"?

    a. the impact of the car striking the tree
    b. the impact of the patient striking the steering wheel
    c. the impact of the mediastinum striking the chest wall
    d. the impact of objects in the vehicle striking the windshield

41. Blast injuries have multiple phases, with different energy patterns and potential for injury. Which phase is associated with a pressure wave that can cause major effects on the lungs?

    a. primary
    b. secondary
    c. tertiary
    d. quaternary or fourth

42. Which of the following findings at a trauma scene should give the EMT-I an "index of suspicion" that the patient may have a serious chest injury?

    a. cracked windshield
    b. dashboard intrusion
    c. bent rear-view mirror
    d. cracked steering wheel

43. The visiting nurse called EMS for an elderly patient who has chest pain. Ever since falling out of bed several hours ago, the patient has complained of chest pain under the right arm, especially with movement. The nurse is concerned because his oxygen saturation is only 86 percent and normally it is near 100 percent. What is the most likely cause of the decreased oxygen saturation?

    a. flail segment
    b. hypotension
    c. hypoventilation
    d. increased intrathoracic pressure

44. (Continuing with the preceding question) In addition to administering high-concentration oxygen, what is the quickest way to improve the patient's oxygenation?

    a. Stabilize the injury site.
    b. Administer an IV fluid bolus.
    c. Encourage the patient to breathe deeper.
    d. Perform a thoracic chest decompression.

45. When the throat or upper chest is perforated, tears to the _____ may occur.

    a. esophagus
    b. diaphragm
    c. pericardium
    d. pleural space

Chapter 15 Answer Form

	A	B	C	D			A	B	C	D
1.	❏	❏	❏	❏		24.	❏	❏	❏	❏
2.	❏	❏	❏	❏		25.	❏	❏	❏	❏
3.	❏	❏	❏	❏		26.	❏	❏	❏	❏
4.	❏	❏	❏	❏		27.	❏	❏	❏	❏
5.	❏	❏	❏	❏		28.	❏	❏	❏	❏
6.	❏	❏	❏	❏		29.	❏	❏	❏	❏
7.	❏	❏	❏	❏		30.	❏	❏	❏	❏
8.	❏	❏	❏	❏		31.	❏	❏	❏	❏
9.	❏	❏	❏	❏		32.	❏	❏	❏	❏
10.	❏	❏	❏	❏		33.	❏	❏	❏	❏
11.	❏	❏	❏	❏		34.	❏	❏	❏	❏
12.	❏	❏	❏	❏		35.	❏	❏	❏	❏
13.	❏	❏	❏	❏		36.	❏	❏	❏	❏
14.	❏	❏	❏	❏		37.	❏	❏	❏	❏
15.	❏	❏	❏	❏		38.	❏	❏	❏	❏
16.	❏	❏	❏	❏		39.	❏	❏	❏	❏
17.	❏	❏	❏	❏		40.	❏	❏	❏	❏
18.	❏	❏	❏	❏		41.	❏	❏	❏	❏
19.	❏	❏	❏	❏		42.	❏	❏	❏	❏
20.	❏	❏	❏	❏		43.	❏	❏	❏	❏
21.	❏	❏	❏	❏		44.	❏	❏	❏	❏
22.	❏	❏	❏	❏		45.	❏	❏	❏	❏
23.	❏	❏	❏	❏						

Medical/Behavioral Emergencies and Obstetrics/Gynecology

CHAPTER 16

Respiratory Emergencies

1. Each healthy alveolus is surrounded by a:
   a. chemoreceptor.
   b. pulmonary vein.
   c. pulmonary capillary.
   d. supply of lactic acid.

2. Which of the following statements about the pathology of ventilation is most correct?
   a. Ventilation and oxygenation are always interrelated.
   b. Ventilation is the movement of oxygen into the lungs.
   c. Ventilation is controlled by the cerebral cortex in the brain.
   d. Ventilation and oxygenation are not always interrelated.

3. Which of the following conditions can cause a disruption of the pulmonary circulation to alveolar gas flow that creates a ventilation-perfusion mismatch?
   a. epiglottitis
   b. laryngeal edema
   c. narcotic overdose
   d. pulmonary embolism

4. A 24-year-old female called EMS because she has no way of getting to the hospital. She has been sick for three days with muscle aches, fever, chills, sore throat, and an earache. She has a nonproductive cough and developed wheezing earlier today. She has no history of asthma and denies smoking. What do you suspect is causing her wheeze?
   a. She has developed COPD.
   b. She is an undiagnosed asthmatic.
   c. She has early signs of pulmonary edema.
   d. She has developed an upper respiratory infection.

5. Which of the following airway or ventilation techniques is appropriate for the patient presenting with anxiety and hyperventilation?
   a. Administer oxygen by non-rebreather mask (NRB).
   b. Administer an aerosolized bronchodilator by a nebulizer.
   c. Have the patient breathe into a paper bag for 2 minutes.
   d. Coach the patient to slow the breathing rate, but do not administer oxygen.

6. The non-rebreather mask can provide high-concentration oxygen with a high volume for the patient:
   a. who is apneic.
   b. without a gag reflex.
   c. with a poor tidal volume.
   d. who has a good respiratory effort.

7. With medical direction, which of the following medications can the EMT-I administer to the patient who is experiencing a severe asthma attack?
   a. oxygen only
   b. aerosolized albuterol and IV epinephrine
   c. aerosolized albuterol and subcutaneous epinephrine
   d. subcutaneous epinephrine and intramuscular (IM) or intravenous (IV) Benadryl

8. You are obtaining a focused history and performing a physical exam on a 63-year-old male. He has a chief complaint of difficulty breathing and a history of smoking and emphysema. He is anxious, cyanotic, and slightly confused about his past medical history. Of the following diagnostic information, which is helpful in making treatment decisions for this patient?
   a. PO_2 and SpO_2
   b. SpO_2 and ECG
   c. temperature and ECG
   d. blood sugar level and SpO_2

9. Patients in distress with restrictive airway disease may be observed doing pursed-lip breathing. This is a defense mechanism that helps improve oxygenation by:

   a. decreasing resistance to inspiratory airflow.
   b. stimulating cilia in the lungs to sweep out mucus.
   c. creating airway pressures that keep the alveoli open.
   d. creating airway pressures that decrease pulmonary hypertension.

10. Your patient describes recurrent productive coughing for several months of the year, over the past two or more consecutive years. You have learned that an overgrowth of airway mucous glands and excess secretion of mucus most likely result from:

    a. lung cancer.
    b. bronchial asthma.
    c. chronic bronchitis.
    d. chronic pneumonia.

11. When the lung tissue is damaged so that elastic recoil is lost, as seen with emphysema, the patient experiences:

    a. resistance to expiratory airflow.
    b. resistance to inspiratory airflow.
    c. partial upper airway obstruction.
    d. venous distention and pulmonary edema.

12. What is the first consideration for the EMT-I when managing a patient with pneumonia?

    a. The patient with pneumonia is contagious.
    b. The patient with pneumonia needs antibiotic therapy.
    c. The patient with pneumonia typically has a concurrent pulmonary disease.
    d. The patient with pneumonia will require continuous nebulizer treatments during transport.

13. The local nursing home is requesting transportation of a 89-year-old female with low SpO$_2$ readings (in the 80s). You perform a physical exam and find that the patient has distended neck veins (JVD), wet crackles in the bases of her lungs, peripheral edema, and ascites. Her vital signs are: respiratory rate, 32; pulse rate, 90/irregular; BP, 160/100; skin CTC is cyanotic, warm, and dry. Based on your findings, what is this patient's past medical history?

    a. pneumonia
    b. lung cancer
    c. right-sided heart failure
    d. obstructive airway disease

14. While at work, a 26-year-old male suddenly developed sharp chest pain and shortness of breath. A coworker tells you that the patient had been sick with a cold for a couple of days. He has been coughing more frequently since the pain began, and states that the pain is in the right chest. The patient has no significant past medical history except for 16 years of smoking. Vital signs are: respiratory rate, 30/diminished on the right side; pulse rate, 106/regular; BP, 134/78; skin CTC is warm, moist, and good color. What do you suspect is the patient's problem?

    a. pulmonary embolism
    b. acute myocardial infarction
    c. spontaneous pneumothorax
    d. new onset of bronchial asthma

15. Blood clots are a common cause of pulmonary thromboembolism. There are other causes of pulmonary emboli, which include all of the following except:

    a. tumor tissue.
    b. amniotic fluid.
    c. IV medications.
    d. fat and air bubbles.

16. Dispatch has sent you on a call for difficulty breathing. When you arrive, you find an elderly female in severe respiratory distress. Her head is nodding and she does not respond to you. While you are listening to her lung sounds, she stops breathing, though she still has a pulse. Your partner ventilates her using a bag mask device as you prepare to intubate the patient. Your first attempt is unsuccessful. When you look in the airway a second time, you see that the vocal cords and surrounding muscles appear to be in spasm. What is the most likely cause of the laryngeal spasm?

    a. epiglottitis
    b. loss of gag reflex
    c. excess mucus production
    d. an overly aggressive intubation attempt

17. You have responded to a call for a cardiac arrest and upon arrival quickly confirm that the patient is apneic and pulseless. Citizen CPR is resumed as you obtain an ECG and find asystole, a nonshockable rhythm. As you prepare to intubate the patient, you ask your partner to place the patient in the "sniffing" position, to:

    a. prevent gastric distention.
    b. prevent right mainstem intubation.
    c. prevent vomiting and aspiration.
    d. help you visualize the vocal cords.

18. You have a young, asthmatic patient who is in severe respiratory distress, and are considering intubating her. Because she is still conscious, you have decided to intubate her nasally, but her condition is deteriorating rapidly. At what point of this patient's deterioration is nasal intubation contraindicated in airway management?

   a. respiratory arrest
   b. unresponsiveness
   c. respiratory rate between 6 and 12
   d. SpO_2 reading of less than 80 percent

19. You have successfully intubated a patient who was in respiratory arrest following an anaphylactic reaction. Which diagnostic device can you use now that will provide an $EtCO_2$ reading in two forms, one that is a number and one that is a wave form or graph?

   a. capnometer
   b. capnograph
   c. pulse oximeter
   d. colorimetric device

20. Your crew was dispatched for a seizure call. When you arrive, the patient is postictal. You begin your assessment and obtain vital signs. During the focused physical exam, the patient begins seizing again and has clenched teeth. You decide to insert a nasal pharyngeal airway (NPA). Before you insert the NPA, you lubricate the tube with a _____ gel because _____.

   a. petroleum; it is biodegradable
   b. water-soluble; it is less irritating to airway tissues
   c. water-soluble; it will numb and shrink the airway tissues
   d. hydrocarbon-based; it will not cause chemical aspiration pneumonia.

Chapter 16 Answer Form

	A	B	C	D			A	B	C	D
1.	❏	❏	❏	❏		11.	❏	❏	❏	❏
2.	❏	❏	❏	❏		12.	❏	❏	❏	❏
3.	❏	❏	❏	❏		13.	❏	❏	❏	❏
4.	❏	❏	❏	❏		14.	❏	❏	❏	❏
5.	❏	❏	❏	❏		15.	❏	❏	❏	❏
6.	❏	❏	❏	❏		16.	❏	❏	❏	❏
7.	❏	❏	❏	❏		17.	❏	❏	❏	❏
8.	❏	❏	❏	❏		18.	❏	❏	❏	❏
9.	❏	❏	❏	❏		19.	❏	❏	❏	❏
10.	❏	❏	❏	❏		20.	❏	❏	❏	❏

CHAPTER

17

Cardiovascular Emergencies

1. The morbidity and mortality associated with cardio-vascular disease:
   a. are the same as for hepatitis.
   b. are the same as for HIV/AIDS.
   c. have been unchanged for the past decade.
   d. have improved because of improvements in treatments.

2. The pacemaker cells of the heart, which determine the heart's normal rate and rhythm, are located in the:
   a. sinoatrial node.
   b. atrioventricular node.
   c. bundle of His.
   d. Purkinje fibers.

3. EMT-Is can significantly reduce their own risk of developing cardiovascular disease by:
   a. reducing sodium intake.
   b. drinking 8 or more glasses of water every day.
   c. consuming diet sodas, without caffeine, instead of regular soda.
   d. avoiding any carbonated beverages.

4. Of the many risk factors for developing cardiac dis-ease, which one is known to double the risk of having a heart attack?
   a. stress
   b. male gender
   c. cigarette smoking
   d. sedentary lifestyle

5. The components of assessment for the patient with possible cardiovascular compromise include:
   a. obtaining a focused history, vital signs, ECG, and blood samples.
   b. listening to lung sounds and heart tones, and administering oxygen and nitroglycerin.
   c. obtaining serial vital signs, instituting pain management, and transporting to the appropriate facility.
   d. giving early notification to the ED, completing a thrombolytic checklist, and starting two IVs.

6. The P-R interval of the normal ECG complex corre-lates to the:
   a. repolarization of the ventricles.
   b. impulse through the atria into the AV node.
   c. depolarization of the atria before contraction.
   d. depolarization of the ventricles before contraction.

7. When the ECG records a tachycardic rhythm above 180 in an elderly adult, the EMT-I should suspect that the:
   a. heart is not adequately filling the ventricles.
   b. patient is at high risk for sudden cardiac arrest.
   c. patient is noncompliant with a heart medication.
   d. ECG shows premature ventricular complexes (PVCs).

8. For the EMT-I to accurately calculate the heart rate from an ECG recording, the:
   a. rhythm should be regular.
   b. rhythm must be normal sinus.
   c. rate cannot be more than 100 nor less than 60.
   d. rhythm cannot be generated by an artificial pacemaker.

9. One limitation on calculation of the heart rate from an ECG is the presence of a:
   a. pulse deficit.
   b. pulsus paradoxus.
   c. serious symptom such as chest pain.
   d. presence of an implanted pacemaker.

10. When reading an ECG strip, the regularity of the rhythm can quickly be determined by:
    a. assessing the R-R interval.
    b. discounting the presence of premature complexes.
    c. counting the number of P waves in a 6-second strip.
    d. counting the number of R waves in a 6-second strip.

11. Electrical impulses are measured for duration. On ECG paper, one large box represents _____ seconds.
    a. 0.2
    b. 2.0
    c. 0.04
    d. 0.05

12. A patient who is apneic and pulseless should be defibrillated when the ECG recording shows:
    a. asystole.
    b. ventricular tachycardia.
    c. pulseless electrical activity (PEA).
    d. implanted ventricular pacemaker spike.

13. EMS was dispatched for a 68-year-old female who fainted. When you arrive, she is supine on the floor. She is conscious, pale, diaphoretic, and has chest pain. After administering oxygen, you determine that she is hypotensive, with a BP of 80/40, and has a sinus bradycardia of 48. Before contacting medical control, which of the following interventions can the EMT-I use to help improve the patient's condition?
    a. Start an IV and administer a fluid bolus.
    b. Sedate the patient and apply external pacing.
    c. Start an IV and administer a dose of atropine.
    d. Administer aspirin and nitroglycerin for the chest pain.

14. Why would a person who has never had a heart attack need an implanted defibrillation device?
    a. The person has unstable angina.
    b. The patient has had two coronary artery bypasses.
    c. The person has heart disease that causes irregular pacemaker activity.
    d. The person is over 50 years of age and has a significant family history of heart disease.

15. A person who frequently develops chest pain upon exertion and takes nitroglycerin for relief is most likely experiencing:
    a. stable angina.
    b. unstable angina.
    c. acute ischemia.
    d. acute myocardial infarction.

16. Which of the following conditions can produce signs and symptoms similar to angina or an MI?
    a. hiatal hernia and gastric reflux
    b. pulmonary embolism and pneumothorax
    c. aortic dissection and esophageal rupture
    d. any of the above

17. Which of the following is the most common mechanism by which the heart muscle suffers tissue death from a lack of oxygen?
    a. hemorrhagic shock
    b. spasms in the coronary arteries
    c. narrowing of the coronary arteries
    d. occlusion of a coronary artery from a thrombus

18. When the EMT-I is treating a patient whom she suspects is having a heart attack, she must be alert for and prepared to manage possible complications that may arise. Which of the following conditions rarely develops within the first hour of the onset of symptoms of a heart attack?
    a. cardiac arrest
    b. cardiogenic shock
    c. pulmonary embolism
    d. congestive heart failure

19. Why is the OPQRST history of chest pain so important?
    a. It can be used to differentiate an old MI from a new AMI.
    b. It is one of three primary components used to make a cardiac diagnosis.
    c. It can help predict if a patient will go into cardiac arrest before arriving at the ED.
    d. It helps a patient in denial come to terms with the possibility that he or she is having an MI.

20. Some patients will have an MI without the classic symptoms of chest, neck, or arm pain. These patients often have symptoms that are considered atypical. Which of the following is an atypical symptom associated with an MI?
    a. syncope
    b. weakness
    c. shortness of breath
    d. all of the above

21. A patient with a history of angina developed chest pain today while watching television. Usually his chest pain is relieved by rest and one dose of nitroglycerin. Today he took three doses and got no relief. What is your first consideration for this patient?
    a. The nitroglycerin is old or expired.
    b. The patient is experiencing cardiac ischemia.
    c. The patient's stable angina became unstable today.
    d. The patient has a new onset of congestive heart failure.

22. (Continuing with the preceding question) The patient appears sick, pale, and sweaty. He is short of breath when you ask him questions about his pain and history. His pain is substernal and radiates to his jaw with a severity of 9/10. His vital signs are: respiratory rate 28/labored; pulse rate 64/irregular; BP 184/78. His SpO_2 is 96 percent and his ECG is sinus with PVCs. With permission from medical control, what pharmacological agents can the EMT-I use to treat this patient?
    a. nitrates and aspirin
    b. nitrates and narcotics
    c. nitrates and antiarrhythmics
    d. nitrates and antihypertensives

23. (Continuing with the two preceding questions) With permission of medical control, you have administered one dose of the pharmacological agents. The patient's pain has not decreased, and he continues to look very sick. You reassure the patient as you move him to the ambulance. Once in the ambulance, you ensure that the oxygen is on, the IV is running well, and:

a. discreetly prepare for the possibility that the patient may go into cardiac arrest.

b. explain to the patient that it may become necessary to intubate him, and obtain permission to do so.

c. ask the patient if he has any advance directives and have him explain them to you.

d. reestablish communications with medical control and discuss the use of additional pharmacologicals should the patient go into cardiac arrest.

24. The two major problems associated with heart failure are that cardiac output decreases and:

a. blood backs up in the arterial system.

b. blood backs up in the venous system.

c. fluids accumulate in the pericardial sac.

d. myocardial ischemia and tissue death occur.

25. Which of the following is a cardiac cause of acute pulmonary edema?

a. narcotic overdose

b. exacerbation of COPD

c. inhalation of a toxic substance

d. exacerbation of paroxysmal nocturnal dyspnea

26. The signs and symptoms of acute pulmonary edema (APE) may include shortness of breath, jugular vein distention (JVD), cardiac dysrhythmias, crackles in the bases of the lungs, and chest discomfort. These signs and symptoms often make it difficult to differentiate APE from:

a. unstable angina.

b. cardiogenic shock.

c. an exacerbation of COPD.

d. abdominal aortic aneurysm.

27. A person with advanced heart failure may awaken during the night with a sudden episode of severe shortness of breath. This condition is called paroxysmal nocturnal dyspnea (PND) and occurs because:

a. the patient forgot to take her diuretic.

b. the patient has to sleep in a sitting position.

c. the patient became hypertensive during the night.

d. blood pools in the lungs and causes pulmonary congestion.

28. A hypertensive emergency is a life-threatening condition that can cause serious organ damage. The organs most likely to be at risk from a hypertensive emergency are the:

a. eyes, heart, and brain.

b. brain, heart, and lungs.

c. eyes, ears, and kidneys.

d. brain, heart, and kidneys.

29. A hypertensive emergency is defined as a sudden and severe increase in blood pressure that:

a. rises above 220 systolic or 120 diastolic.

b. rises above both 240 systolic and 120 diastolic.

c. is associated with other life-threatening emergencies.

d. can lead to serious, irreversible, end-organ damage.

30. A woman who is in her third trimester of pregnancy has her sister call EMS when the pregnant woman suddenly develops double vision and begins vomiting. The pregnancy has been normal so far, and the patient has no significant past medical history. The patient looks sick, is confused, and complains of epigastric pain. Her vital signs are: respiratory rate 22/regular; pulse rate 110/regular; BP 190/100; blood sugar level 164 mg/dL; SpO_2 98 percent. What do you suspect is the problem with this patient?

a. stroke

b. eclampsia

c. preeclampsia

d. pulmonary embolism

31. (Continuing with the preceding question) The EMT-I's management plan for this patient includes administering high-flow oxygen and:

a. performing a stroke score and starting an IV.

b. being prepared for the patient to go into cardiac arrest.

c. starting an IV, and administering one dose of nitroglycerin.

d. starting an IV, and reassessing the patient every 5 minutes.

32. The husband of a 65-year-old female saw his wife collapse suddenly. He states that before she passed out, she complained of chest pain. Now she is responsive to pain, cyanotic, and cool to the touch. Her vital signs are: respiratory rate 34/shallow; pulse rate 98/weak and regular; BP 60/30. Her blood sugar level is 140 mg/dL, SpO_2 is 88 percent, and ECG is abnormal with wide QRS complexes. What do you suspect is the patient's problem?

a. She is having a massive MI.

b. She has a ruptured aortic aneurysm.

c. She has a ruptured thoracic aneurysm.

d. She is experiencing a pulmonary embolism.

33. (Continuing with the preceding question) The patient's lung sounds are slightly diminished in the bases. You administer high-flow oxygen and elevate the patient's legs. Your partner starts an IV while you contact medical control to advise them of your critical patient. Which of the following orders do you expect to receive?

    a. No medication orders, just rapid transport.
    b. Administer a fluid bolus and treat for shock.
    c. Attempt a nasal intubation to secure the airway.
    d. Administer one dose of epinephrine 0.5 mg IV push.

34. The most severe form of heart failure due to left ventricular malfunction is called:

    a. massive MI.
    b. cardiogenic shock.
    c. cardiac tamponade.
    d. acute pulmonary edema.

35. A term for the sudden stopping of the pumping action of the heart is:

    a. asystole.
    b. resuscitation.
    c. cardiac arrest.
    d. ventricular fibrillation.

36. It is 9:30 a.m. when a call for a cardiac arrest comes in. A male in his 40s waves you to the side door of the residence. When you get closer, he tells you that he found his father unresponsive on the bedroom floor. The son talked to his father on the phone yesterday. When you enter the bedroom, you see the father lying on his side. He is blue-gray in the face and neck. The room is very warm and so is the patient. What action do you take next?

    a. Attach an AED and push "Analyze."
    b. Ask the son if his father has any advance directives.
    c. Rapidly assess the patient for signs of irreversible death.
    d. Start CPR while your partner attaches an AED and prepares to analyze the patient.

37. You have been dispatched with the local fire department for a cardiac arrest. When you arrive, first responders are performing CPR and attaching an AED to an elderly male. You quickly verify pulselessness and observe as the AED analyzes the patient's rhythm. No shock is advised and CPR is resumed. A family member is present and obviously very upset. You determine that the patient was seen alive two hours ago and that she has an advance directive stating that the patient does not want to be kept alive with life support equipment. How should you proceed now?

    a. Direct the first responders to stop CPR and ask dispatch to send the coroner.
    b. Continue resuscitation efforts, begin transport to the nearest ED, and contact medical control for orders.
    c. Continue resuscitation efforts while you contact medical control and request an order to terminate the code.
    d. Direct the first responders to stop CPR, cover the patient with a sheet, and turn the patient over to the police.

38. Until defibrillation is available at the patient's side, the single most effective treatment for the victim of sudden cardiac arrest is:

    a. perfect CPR.
    b. IV epinephrine.
    c. fluid administration.
    d. endotracheal intubation.

39. The patient you are treating for a suspected MI has had significant relief of his chest pain after receiving high-flow oxygen and two nitroglycerin pills. His vital signs after treatment are: respiratory rate 18/regular; pulse rate 74/regular; BP 140/90; skin CTC is warm and moist with good color. As you prepare him for transport, he asks for a drink of water, because the oxygen has made his mouth dry. How should you handle his request?

    a. Contact medical control and discuss the request.
    b. Give nothing by mouth, because people with myocardial ischemia often have nausea.
    c. Let him have a sip of water; it will not cause any harm and will make the patient feel better.
    d. Only if medical control grants permission to administer aspirin, let the patient have a sip of water with the aspirin.

40. Your first call of the shift is a cardiac arrest; your partner is a paramedic. Once the patient is intubated or an IV is started, the patient will be given emergency cardiac medications. With permission from medical control, which of the following drugs would you be able to assist the paramedic in administering to the patient?

    a. epinephrine by IV only
    b. only epinephrine, either IV or ET
    c. epinephrine, atropine, and an antidysrhythmic by IV
    d. epinephrine, atropine, and an antidysrhythmic by IV or ET

41. Your patient is a 48-year-old female with a complaint of palpitations and shortness of breath. She has had palpitations for two hours and now is feeling very anxious. This feeling has occurred before, but has never lasted this long. She takes an antihypertensive and has no allergies to medications. Her vital signs are: respiratory rate 26/regular; pulse rate too fast to count; BP 100/56; skin CTC is pale, warm, and dry. Which of the following ECG rhythms could not produce the patient's symptoms?

    a. atrial fibrillation
    b. ventricular fibrillation
    c. ventricular tachycardia
    d. supraventricular tachycardia

42. Thrombolytic drugs provide the greatest benefit to a patient experiencing an MI when the:

    a. patient is under the age of 60.
    b. patient is having a first heart attack.
    c. infarct is located in the left coronary artery.
    d. patient is able to receive therapy within 4 hours.

43. You and your crew are standing by at a local high school baseball game. A commotion over at home plate catches your attention, and you see a young player lying on the ground. Another player says the patient was hit in the chest with a ball and then collapsed. The patient is not breathing and has no pulse. CPR is started and the AED is attached. With this MOI, what rhythm do you suspect the AED will analyze?

    a. asystole
    b. ventricular fibrillation
    c. pulseless electrical activity
    d. supraventricular tachycardia

44. Which of the following statements about an ECG is most correct?

    a. For the patient experiencing chest pain, an ECG can rule out an MI.
    b. A normal ECG means that the patient with chest pain is experiencing angina.
    c. The patient with heart disease will always have an abnormal ECG.
    d. Obtaining an ECG does not take priority over care for life-threatening injuries.

45. The patient you are treating for a complaint of chest pain has experienced complete relief with oxygen and three doses of nitroglycerin. As you reassess her vital signs, you see her wince as if she is in pain. You ask her if she has had a return of chest pain and she says no, but now she has an intense headache. You tell her that headaches are a normal side effect of nitroglycerin and occur because nitro:

    a. constricts the cerebral blood vessels.
    b. causes spasms in cerebral vascular smooth muscle.
    c. dilates blood vessels that increase blood flow to the head.
    d. causes the blood pressure to drop and drains blood from the head.

Chapter 17 Answer Form

	A	B	C	D		A	B	C	D
1.	❏	❏	❏	❏	24.	❏	❏	❏	❏
2.	❏	❏	❏	❏	25.	❏	❏	❏	❏
3.	❏	❏	❏	❏	26.	❏	❏	❏	❏
4.	❏	❏	❏	❏	27.	❏	❏	❏	❏
5.	❏	❏	❏	❏	28.	❏	❏	❏	❏
6.	❏	❏	❏	❏	29.	❏	❏	❏	❏
7.	❏	❏	❏	❏	30.	❏	❏	❏	❏
8.	❏	❏	❏	❏	31.	❏	❏	❏	❏
9.	❏	❏	❏	❏	32.	❏	❏	❏	❏
10.	❏	❏	❏	❏	33.	❏	❏	❏	❏
11.	❏	❏	❏	❏	34.	❏	❏	❏	❏
12.	❏	❏	❏	❏	35.	❏	❏	❏	❏
13.	❏	❏	❏	❏	36.	❏	❏	❏	❏
14.	❏	❏	❏	❏	37.	❏	❏	❏	❏
15.	❏	❏	❏	❏	38.	❏	❏	❏	❏
16.	❏	❏	❏	❏	39.	❏	❏	❏	❏
17.	❏	❏	❏	❏	40.	❏	❏	❏	❏
18.	❏	❏	❏	❏	41.	❏	❏	❏	❏
19.	❏	❏	❏	❏	42.	❏	❏	❏	❏
20.	❏	❏	❏	❏	43.	❏	❏	❏	❏
21.	❏	❏	❏	❏	44.	❏	❏	❏	❏
22.	❏	❏	❏	❏	45.	❏	❏	❏	❏
23.	❏	❏	❏	❏					

CHAPTER

18

Diabetic Emergencies

1. Diabetes mellitus is a chronic disease of the endocrine system which is caused by a:
   a. loss of counterregulatory hormones.
   b. changes in the production of epinephrine.
   c. decrease in the secretion of insulin.
   d. decrease in the secretion of glucagon.

2. The hormone insulin lowers blood sugar by:
   a. breaking down protein into amino acids.
   b. stimulating new production of sugar by the liver.
   c. moving sugar molecules from the blood into the cells.
   d. moving sugar molecules from the cells into the blood.

3. When a person's insulin supply becomes inadequate, the result is:
   a. liver failure.
   b. neuropathy.
   c. dehydration.
   d. cell starvation.

4. Because glucose is the sole source of nutrition for the central nervous system (CNS), a significant fall in blood sugar levels will cause:
   a. increased lipid levels.
   b. altered mental status.
   c. coronary artery disease.
   d. silent myocardial infarction.

5. When a diabetic emergency is suspected, and there is no way to obtain a quick blood sugar level reading, the EMT-I should:
   a. support the airway, breathing, circulation, and begin rapid transport.
   b. treat the patient for hypoglycemia until a blood sugar level reading is obtained.
   c. treat the patient for hyperglycemia until a blood sugar level reading is obtained.
   d. support the airway, breathing, and circulation until a blood sugar level reading is obtained.

6. When the body is malnourished, it begins to metabolize fat. This process produces ketones. Excess ketone production is a problem because:
   a. it raises insulin levels in the body.
   b. it disrupts the acid-base balance in the body.
   c. the body can become overhydrated, which can lead to hyponatremia.
   d. the amount of glucagon and epinephrine present in the body may become decreased.

7. When the insulin level becomes too high, the effects on the body include:
   a. ketoacidosis.
   b. frequent urination.
   c. decreased blood sugar level.
   d. hyperosmolar hyperglycemic nonketotic coma.

8. The pathophysiology of hyperglycemia involves:
   a. the production of ketones.
   b. the development of acidosis.
   c. abnormally high blood sugar.
   d. excessive insulin production.

9. Which of the following statements about hyperglycemia is most accurate?
   a. The onset of hyperglycemia is usually rapid.
   b. Hyperglycemia always produces diabetic ketoacidosis (DKA).
   c. A patient with hyperglycemia may have no immediate symptoms.
   d. Hyperglycemia stimulates the release of glucagon and epinephrine.

10. The primary goal in the treatment of the patient with hyperglycemia is to:
    a. correct dehydration.
    b. stop ketone production.
    c. treat cardiac dysrhythmias.
    d. correct glucose intolerance.

11. Your unit is dispatched for an unresponsive patient with a history of known insulin-dependent diabetes. When you arrive at the residence, the patient is lying on a couch, conscious but confused. His airway is open and he is breathing adequately. You see vomitus on his face and chest. His wife tells you that he was acting like his sugar was low, so she administered a shot of glucagon. How should you proceed next?

    a. Obtain a blood sugar level reading before doing anything else.
    b. Conduct the initial assessment and determine the patient's priority.
    c. Confirm that the patient is insulin-dependent and administer oral glucose.
    d. Administer high-flow oxygen and ask the wife to bring you the empty glucagon syringe.

12. (Continuing with the preceding question) When you talk to the patient, you find that he knows his name and where he is, but is confused about the day of the week and what is happening right now. His blood sugar level is 54 mg/dL, and his vital signs are: respiratory rate 16/regular; pulse rate 90/regular; BP 136/80; skin CTC is cool and moist with good color. Management of this patient includes:

    a. administering high-flow oxygen and waiting for the glucagon to take effect.
    b. starting an IV, drawing blood samples, and (if your protocol permits) administering D50.
    c. administering oral glucose only until the blood sugar reading is 80 mg/dL or higher.
    d. encourage the patient to consume a drink with lots of sugar and eat carbohydrates.

13. You have been dispatched on a call for a 70-year-old male patient with stroke symptoms. Your general impression is that of a confused elderly male with slurred speech. His friend called EMS when the patient failed to meet him for breakfast; he went to the patient's house and could not get the patient to get up. There is no indication that the patient is a diabetic, and the friend is unaware of his medical history. You find no life threats during your initial assessment. How should you proceed next?

    a. Perform a prehospital stroke score.
    b. Administer oral glucose and start an IV.
    c. Administer high-flow oxygen and obtain a blood sugar level reading.
    d. Administer high-flow oxygen, start an IV, and perform a stroke exam.

14. (Continuing with the preceding question) The patient is unable to answer any questions or follow your instructions. His vital signs are: respiratory rate 26, with wheezing; pulse rate 106/regular; BP 114/60; skin CTC is hot, moist, and flushed. The blood sugar level is 48 mg/dL. Management of this patient includes oxygen and:

    a. oral glucose only.
    b. IV, fluid bolus, and oral glucose.
    c. IV, D50 (per local protocol), or oral glucose.
    d. oral glucose, and assistance with a metered dose inhaler.

15. The local nursing home has requested transport of a 78-year-old female patient to the ED. She has a history of hypertension, a pacemaker, and diabetes. Today she is confused, weak, and has vomited twice. Her labs came back with a glucose level of 390 mg/dL, so she is going to be admitted. The patient opens her eyes when you touch her, but does not speak. Her respirations are deep and rapid, her distal pulse is weak and rapid, her BP is 180/100, and her skin is hot, dry, and flushed. What do you suspect is causing the abnormal vital signs?

    a. shock
    b. hyperglycemia
    c. hyperglycemia with diabetic ketoacidosis
    d. hyperglycemic hyperosmolar nonketotic coma

16. (Continuing with the preceding question) How do you plan to manage this patient?

    a. Administer oxygen and do a routine transport.
    b. Administer oxygen, IV, and fluid bolus (per local protocol).
    c. Administer oxygen, IV, and D50 (per local protocol) or oral glucose.
    d. Administer oxygen and assist ventilations with a bag mask.

17. Which of the following symptoms is frequently associated with hyperglycemia with DKA?

    a. anxiety
    b. chest pain
    c. abdominal pain
    d. vision disturbance

18. Your unit is dispatched to an unknown problem at a private residence. When you arrive, a family member leads you to an unconscious 56-year-old male lying on the kitchen floor. The patient is pale, cold, and lying in urine. He has slow, shallow, snoring respirations and no distal pulse. The carotid pulse is slow and regular. The family tells you that he was fine last night at bedtime and that he is an insulin-dependent diabetic with a cardiac history. What action do you take next?

    a. Obtain a blood sugar level reading right away.
    b. Obtain an ECG or attach the AED to the patient.
    c. Insert an airway adjunct and assist the patient's ventilations.
    d. Remove the patient's wet clothing before taking any other steps.

19. (Continuing with the preceding question) Additional help arrives and several things happen quickly. The patient is moved from the cold floor to your stretcher. His initial SpO_2 is 86 percent, his ECG is sinus bradycardia at 56, and his blood sugar level is 24 mg/dL. Two crew members are having difficulty obtaining IV access. What action do you take next?

    a. Begin to rewarm the patient.
    b. Contact medical control for instructions.
    c. Intubate the patient and begin rapid transport.
    d. Determine if the patient keeps glucagon in the residence.

20. One ampule of D50 is the standard IV dose of high-concentration dextrose for a patient with a hypoglycemic emergency. What is the concentration of this dose?

    a. 25 grams of dextrose in 25 cc
    b. 50 grams of dextrose in 50 cc
    c. 100 grams of dextrose in 50 cc
    d. 25 grams of dextrose diluted in 50 cc

Chapter 18 Answer Form

	A	B	C	D			A	B	C	D
1.	❏	❏	❏	❏		11.	❏	❏	❏	❏
2.	❏	❏	❏	❏		12.	❏	❏	❏	❏
3.	❏	❏	❏	❏		13.	❏	❏	❏	❏
4.	❏	❏	❏	❏		14.	❏	❏	❏	❏
5.	❏	❏	❏	❏		15.	❏	❏	❏	❏
6.	❏	❏	❏	❏		16.	❏	❏	❏	❏
7.	❏	❏	❏	❏		17.	❏	❏	❏	❏
8.	❏	❏	❏	❏		18.	❏	❏	❏	❏
9.	❏	❏	❏	❏		19.	❏	❏	❏	❏
10.	❏	❏	❏	❏		20.	❏	❏	❏	❏

CHAPTER 19

Allergic Reactions

1. A foreign substance that causes the production of antibodies when introduced to the body is an:
   a. insect.
   b. antigen.
   c. immunity.
   d. anaphylactic reaction.

2. An overreaction of the immune system to an antigen, which causes a variety of symptoms ranging from mild to severe and life-threatening, is called:
   a. an allergen.
   b. anaphylaxis.
   c. autoimmunity.
   d. an allergic reaction.

3. When an antigen reacts with the antibodies on mast cells, there is a release of histamines and other mediators resulting in:
   a. immunity.
   b. an allergic reaction.
   c. an immune response.
   d. adrenalin insufficiency.

4. When chemicals are released from mast cells as a result of an antibody trigger, and the body experiences progressive shock from severe vasodilation, this condition is called:
   a. immunity.
   b. anaphylaxis.
   c. a protein response.
   d. histamine transmission.

5. A trigger for an allergic reaction that enters the body by ingestion is an:
   a. allergen.
   b. antibody.
   c. immunity.
   d. anaphylactic reaction.

6. A hypersensitivity reaction involving antibodies that trigger bronchoconstriction and cardiovascular collapse is:
   a. urticaria.
   b. anaphylaxis.
   c. isoimmunity.
   d. an immune response.

7. A bee sting is an example of an antigen that enters the body through which route?
   a. topical
   b. injection
   c. ingestion
   d. absorption

8. During your interview with a patient, as part of the SAMPLE history, the patient tells you he is allergic to sulfa. Through what route of exposure did the patient most likely identify sulfa as an allergen?
   a. topical
   b. injection
   c. ingestion
   d. inhalation

9. You are reassessing a 28-year-old male who had a syncopal event. In the initial assessment he was alert and denied dyspnea or chest pain. His vital signs are: respiratory rate 18/non-labored; heart rate 70/regular and strong; BP 110/60. His ECG is NSR, and glucose is 82 mg/dL. He describes a history of fainting when emotionally upset. The patient now complains of shortness of breath and has a red skin rash and inflammation around the area of the electrodes. What is most likely happening to the patient?
   a. He is having an allergic reaction to latex.
   b. He is exhibiting an acquired immunity.
   c. He is about to experience another syncopal event.
   d. He is exhibiting urticaria, which is associated with emotional stress.

10. When a patient experiences hives as a result of exposure to an antigen, the route of exposure was most likely:

    a. absorbed through the skin.
    b. due to a sting or injection.
    c. caused by inhalation.
    d. the method of entry into the body bears no relation to the presence of hives.

11. Common antigens associated with anaphylaxis include:

    a. poison ivy, perfume, and animal dander.
    b. pollen, chocolate, cosmetics, and shellfish.
    c. peanuts, insect stings, snake bites, and poison ivy.
    d. antibiotics, insect stings, blood products, and foods.

12. The mediators that are released from mast cells in response to an antigen-antibody reaction are located in the skin, respiratory tract, and _____. Therefore, the most common findings in anaphylaxis are hives, wheezing, and _____.

    a. brain; confusion
    b. GI tract; abdominal pain
    c. myocardium; weak pulse
    d. capillary beds; pulmonary edema

13. Anaphylactic shock occurs following an abnormal immune system response or overresponse causing:

    a. hives and swelling with normal vital signs.
    b. vascular dilation and plasma loss into tissues.
    c. itching and rash with no respiratory symptoms.
    d. tingling sensation on the skin and vascular constriction.

14. A 34-year-old male came to your EMS station stating that he was stung multiple times while mowing the lawn. He thinks he stepped on a wasp nest in the ground. He has red welts on his legs, arm, face, and neck. He denies swelling of the mouth, tongue, or throat, but is having difficulty breathing and is experiencing chest tightness. He is not allergic to bees. His skin CTC is pale, warm, and moist. His vital signs are: respiratory rate 24, with clear lung sounds; heart rate 110/regular and weak; BP 110/60. The ECG shows sinus tachycardia, and SpO_2 is 100 percent. What is this patient's condition?

    a. The patient is in anaphylactic shock and is critical.
    b. The patient is progressing to anaphylaxis and is potentially unstable.
    c. The patient has signs and symptoms of an allergic reaction and is potentially unstable.
    d. The patient has signs and symptoms of an allergic reaction, but, because he is not allergic to bees, he is stable.

15. EMS was called for an allergic reaction. The patient is alert and complaining of itchy, watery eyes, runny nose, and headache. The symptoms began shortly after she arrived at work. The patient denies having any allergies. A coworker gave her over-the-counter (OTC) Benadryl 10 minutes ago. Her skin CTC is warm, moist, and flushed. Her vital signs are: respiratory rate 22/nonlabored, with clear lung sounds; heart rate 86/regular; BP 144/90. The ECG is NSR, and SpO_2 is 96 percent. What is the patient's condition?

    a. Because the patient has no known allergies, she is stable.
    b. She has signs and symptoms of anaphylactic reaction.
    c. She has signs and symptoms of an allergic reaction and appears stable.
    d. She has signs and symptoms of an allergic reaction and appears unstable.

16. (Continuing with the preceding question) What emergency care is appropriate for this patient?

    a. high-flow oxygen, IV access, and 25 mg Benadryl
    b. high-flow oxygen, position of comfort, reassurance, and supportive care
    c. subcutaneous epinephrine, IV access with fluid bolus, and 25 mg Benadryl
    d. observe the patient for 30 minutes for signs of progressive allergic reaction; if none develops, refer her to her own physician

17. You are treating a patient who is experiencing an anaphylactic reaction. Medical control has authorized you to administer an antihistamine as part of your pharmacological interventions. Which medication will you administer?

    a. albuterol
    b. dopamine
    c. epinephrine
    d. diphenhydramine

18. Which medication is the primary bronchodilator used to manage a patient who is experiencing anaphylaxis?

    a. albuterol
    b. Benadryl
    c. Solu-Medrol
    d. epinephrine

19. When an anaphylactic reaction is prolonged, the patient may experience:

    a. an acquired immunity.
    b. peripheral vascular constriction.
    c. dysrhythmias and cardiogenic shock.
    d. abdominal cramping, vomiting, and diarrhea.

20. How does the administration of antihistamines alone affect the patient who is having ongoing anaphylactic reactions?

    a. The administration of antihistamines is never recommended for ongoing anaphylactic reactions.

    b. Antihistamines will block the histamines released from mast cells and reverse the progression of anaphylactic shock.

    c. Multiple doses of antihistamines given at appropriate intervals will decrease the vascular permeability and prevent shock.

    d. Antihistamines do not block all of the mediators released in an immune response, so this treatment could potentially be fatal.

21. When a patient experiences cardiovascular collapse from anaphylaxis, is the administration of epinephrine appropriate?

    a. Yes; however, the dose must be doubled.

    b. No; the patient needs fluids and dopamine.

    c. Yes; use IV epinephrine because subcutaneous epinephrine may be ineffective.

    d. No; because the peripheral circulation will be so poor that the epinephrine will not reach the target organs in time.

22. When the body's immune response overreacts and releases chemical substances, what findings associated with the upper airway may the EMT-I make?

    a. obstruction due to swelling

    b. wheezing due to bronchoconstriction

    c. pulmonary edema due to leaking alveoli

    d. urticaria due to plasma leaking into the tissues

23. You are dispatched to a dental office for an unresponsive 24-year-old male. Within minutes after receiving a local anesthetic for a dental procedure, the patient complained of severe difficulty breathing, turned cyanotic, and became unresponsive. The patient's airway is open, but his tongue appears swollen, there is no air movement, and his carotid pulse is weak and very slow. The first action in the care of this patient is to:

    a. manage the airway.

    b. obtain venous access.

    c. administer epinephrine.

    d. attach an AED or therapy cables.

24. You are called for an allergic reaction in a 14-year-old patient with a known allergy to peanuts who has had an exposure. The patient has an epinephrine auto-injector, which she used when she felt her throat swelling. Now the swelling is reduced, but she is having palpitations. The patient tells you that she had an anaphylactic reaction two years ago and now she always carries the auto-injector with her. Skin CTC is warm, dry, and flushed. Vital signs are: respiratory rate 24, with clear lung sounds; heart rate 120/regular; BP 128/78. The ECG shows sinus tachycardia, and SpO$_2$ is 98 percent. What is the patient's condition, and how should she be managed?

    a. Palpitations are normal in allergy patients, so her condition is stable.

    b. The patient is critical, because of the palpitations and her past history of anaphylaxis.

    c. The patient is potentially unstable, and you should assume that she may progress to anaphylaxis as she has in the past.

    d. The swelling is less, so the epinephrine is working; palpitations are normal with epinephrine use, so the patient is stable.

25. You are dispatched to an 18-year-old who is sick. Your general impression is of a young woman with obvious facial swelling. She is very upset and thinks she is having a reaction to something from the hair salon. She denies difficulty breathing or swelling of the throat, tongue, or lips. Skin CTC is red, with swelling on the forehead and face. Vital signs are: respiratory rate 18/nonlabored; heart rate of 90/regular; BP of 118/84; ECG is NSR, and SpO$_2$ is 100 percent. What emergency treatment is most appropriate for this patient?

    a. oxygen, IV fluids, and supportive care

    b. oxygen, supportive care, and antihistamines

    c. subcutaneous epinephrine, oxygen, and IV fluids

    d. oxygen, SQ epinephrine, IV fluids, and antihistamines

Chapter 19 Answer Form

	A	B	C	D
1.	❏	❏	❏	❏
2.	❏	❏	❏	❏
3.	❏	❏	❏	❏
4.	❏	❏	❏	❏
5.	❏	❏	❏	❏
6.	❏	❏	❏	❏
7.	❏	❏	❏	❏
8.	❏	❏	❏	❏
9.	❏	❏	❏	❏
10.	❏	❏	❏	❏
11.	❏	❏	❏	❏
12.	❏	❏	❏	❏
13.	❏	❏	❏	❏

	A	B	C	D
14.	❏	❏	❏	❏
15.	❏	❏	❏	❏
16.	❏	❏	❏	❏
17.	❏	❏	❏	❏
18.	❏	❏	❏	❏
19.	❏	❏	❏	❏
20.	❏	❏	❏	❏
21.	❏	❏	❏	❏
22.	❏	❏	❏	❏
23.	❏	❏	❏	❏
24.	❏	❏	❏	❏
25.	❏	❏	❏	❏

CHAPTER

20

Poisoning/Overdose Emergencies

1. You are assessing a patient with a complaint of severe abdominal pain. His symptoms of diarrhea and vomiting began during the night and have persisted until late morning. The patient believes he may have food poisoning. What personal protective equipment (PPE) and safety concerns do you have regarding this patient?

   a. gloves for assessing and moving the patient, and an emesis basin for the patient

   b. gloves for the EMT-I and an oxygen mask for the patient, to prevent the spread of airborne particles

   c. gloves and eye protection for the EMT-I, to prevent exposure to the patient's body substances

   d. gloves for the EMT-I, handwashing and removal of any soiled clothing for the patient before he is moved

2. In which of the following situations should the EMT-I call the poison control center directly?

   a. only when the suspected poisoning involves a child patient

   b. only after following the first-aid instructions on the container

   c. when the substance has been identified, even if the patient has no symptoms

   d. only when the suspected poisoning is intentional (suicide) and symptoms have developed

3. Shortness of breath and coughing are common signs and symptoms of poisoning associated with which route of entry into the body?

   a. injection

   b. ingestion

   c. inhalation

   d. absorption

4. A poison control center is an emergency telephone service available 24 hours a day, 7 days a week, for the purpose of:

   a. providing information about treating poisonings.

   b. providing services to reduce child injury and illness.

   c. protecting consumers by identifying hazards in packaging and recalled items.

   d. providing emergency treatment advice for all kinds of poison exposures at a nominal cost to the patient.

5. The American Association of Poison Control Centers (AAPCC) has 61 poison centers in the United States. When you call the number 1-800-222-1222, the AAPCC operator will redirect you to the closest or most appropriate poison control center based on:

   a. age and gender of your patient.

   b. the number of patients with the same exposure.

   c. which toxic substances are specific to your region.

   d. the prior number of accidental poisonings in your region.

6. It is 2:00 a.m. and your unit is dispatched to a call for a 30-year-old sick person. You arrive at a single-family residence, where a woman meets you at the door. She is confused, complaining of headache, and states that she cannot awaken her family. There is no sign of smoke or unusual odors in the doorway or on the woman. What action(s) should you take next?

   a. Begin a search of the residence for the family members.

   b. Advise dispatch to send the fire department and the police.

   c. Enter the residence and complete an initial assessment of the woman.

   d. Bring the woman to your ambulance to obtain a focused history and physical exam.

7. You are assessing a 4-year-old female who sustained a snakebite on her leg. Her mother says she came into the kitchen because she heard her daughter scream, then cry; the mother then saw a snake crawl behind the refrigerator. The child is crying, her skin color is good, and the wound appears swollen and discolored. Animal control is on the way to secure the snake. You begin emergency care for the bite, which includes:

   a. cleaning the site with soap and water.

   b. elevating the extremity and applying cold packs to the bite.

   c. applying constricting bands above and below the bite marks.

   d. with gloves on, scraping the site to remove any venom.

8. A patient with a known sensitivity to poison oak has called EMS because he had an accidental repeat exposure and has no transportation. The affected area involves both lower legs, which look red and swollen. The patient is complaining of severe itching, and a closer look reveals the formation of small blisters. The emergency care for this exposure begins with:

    a. applying activated charcoal to the area with blisters.
    b. removing any contaminated clothing and flushing all exposed areas with water.
    c. applying calamine lotion over the affected areas and 2 inches into the unaffected area.
    d. washing the affected area with soap and water, wrapping the area with dry dressings, and applying cold packs for the itching.

9. Deep and rapid breathing, abdominal pain, fever, dehydration, and ringing in the ears are associated with an overdose of:

    a. aspirin.
    b. cocaine.
    c. mushrooms.
    d. acetaminophen.

10. (Continuing with the preceding question) The emergency care for a possible overdose patient with the symptoms previously described includes management of the ABCs and:

    a. active cooling.
    b. pain management.
    c. avoiding induced vomiting.
    d. administration of activated charcoal.

11. The most common poisonings by overdose, which cause nausea, vomiting, and abdominal pain, occur from nonprescription pain medications such as:

    a. alcohol (e.g., ethanol).
    b. marijuana.
    c. mushrooms.
    d. acetaminophen.

12. An unresponsive male is lying in bed in his basement bedroom. His mother called when she could not waken him. The last time she saw him awake was the previous day. The patient is cool and dry to the touch, pale, and has the following vital signs: respiratory rate 6/shallow; pulse rate 58/weak; and BP 80/40. When you listen to lung sounds, you discover that the patient is wearing multiple analgesic transdermal patches. What is the major priority for this patient?

    a. preventing seizures and aspiration
    b. ensuring that he has an open airway and assisting ventilations
    c. starting an IV and administering naloxone as soon as possible
    d. moving the patient out of the basement into a warm, ventilated area

13. (Continuing with the preceding question) While you begin care for the patient, your partner performs a rapid physical exam and discovers that the patient has more analgesic patches on his back and all his extremities. What is the major priority for you and your partner in the care of this patient?

    a. opening as many windows as possible to increase ventilation of the area
    b. notifying dispatch that you have a suicide attempt, and requesting that police be sent to the scene
    c. wearing the appropriate PPE during removal of the transdermal patches and continuing care of the patient
    d. trying to determine if the patient was depressed or has a history of attempted suicide

14. A psychological craving for a chemical agent, resulting from abuse or addiction, is called:

    a. tolerance.
    b. craving.
    c. drug dependence.
    d. drug or substance abuse.

15. You suspect a possible carbon monoxide poisoning, because more than one family member presents with similar signs and symptoms (headache, nausea, and body aches). The first step in the care of these patients is to:

    a. get everyone out of the residence.
    b. administer oxygen to family members with symptoms.
    c. call for the fire department to get a CO reading in the residence.
    d. administer oxygen to everyone in the residence, whether or not they have symptoms.

Chapter 20 Answer Form

	A	B	C	D
1.	❏	❏	❏	❏
2.	❏	❏	❏	❏
3.	❏	❏	❏	❏
4.	❏	❏	❏	❏
5.	❏	❏	❏	❏
6.	❏	❏	❏	❏
7.	❏	❏	❏	❏
8.	❏	❏	❏	❏

	A	B	C	D
9.	❏	❏	❏	❏
10.	❏	❏	❏	❏
11.	❏	❏	❏	❏
12.	❏	❏	❏	❏
13.	❏	❏	❏	❏
14.	❏	❏	❏	❏
15.	❏	❏	❏	❏

CHAPTER

21

Neurological Emergencies

1. When part of the blood and oxygen supply to brain cells is cut off, a "brain attack" or stroke occurs. One way this condition develops is when an artery becomes blocked. Another way this occurs is when a/an:

   a. epileptic seizure persists.
   b. artery in the brain ruptures.
   c. patient with diabetes experiences a prolonged hypoglycemic event.
   d. acute myocardial infarction occurs in the inferior wall of the left ventricle.

2. The major difference between a stroke and a mini-stroke (TIA) is:

   a. time and speed of onset.
   b. that a TIA has no lasting effect.
   c. that the causes of each are different.
   d. size and location of the affected area of the brain.

3. A neurological emergency that is caused by an infectious disease may result in complications such as blindness, deafness, and cognitive deficits. _____ could cause such an emergency.

   a. A tumor
   b. Meningitis
   c. Spina bifida
   d. Cerebral palsy

4. Which of the following signs and symptoms are not typically associated with a neurological emergency?

   a. abnormal respirations
   b. substernal chest pain
   c. headache or weakness
   d. vision, speech, or motor disturbances

5. When a patient is experiencing a stroke, time becomes a significant factor in patient recovery. Which of the following treatment considerations is the least important in the prehospital phase of care of a patient who is having a stroke?

   a. starting two IVs
   b. giving early notification to the ED
   c. ruling out hypoglycemia with blood glucose testing
   d. transporting to a facility with thrombolytic therapy ability

6. Which of the following suggests that a stroke is the result of a thrombus?

   a. The onset of symptoms is rapid.
   b. The onset of symptoms is gradual.
   c. The onset of symptoms began with a loss of consciousness.
   d. A change in speech is the patient's primary symptom.

7. The treatment of a patient with a suspected transient ischemic attack is:

   a. guided by severity and the time of onset of signs and symptoms.
   b. the same as for a patient with a suspected cerebrovascular attack (CVA).
   c. more aggressive than that for a patient with a suspected CVA.
   d. more conservative than that for a patient with a suspected CVA.

8. The family of a patient with special needs has called EMS for transportation. The patient, who has a history of a terminal brain tumor, has had a sudden change in condition. The nurse on the scene reports that the patient's blood pressure is rising, his breathing pattern is suddenly changing, and his heart rate is decreasing. What do these findings suggest?

   a. neurological posturing
   b. intracerebral hemorrhage
   c. rising intracranial pressure
   d. falling intracranial pressure

9. Many prescription medications can cause a patient to experience a syncopal event. Which of the following drugs is not typically a cause of syncope?

   a. nitrates
   b. beta blockers
   c. antihypertensives
   d. epinephrine auto-injector

10. The patient you are assessing has a sudden onset of confusion and weakness. His wife called EMS shortly after the symptoms began. You suspect that the patient may be experiencing a stroke, so you perform a stroke assessment. Which three factors do you assess?

    a. speech, pronator drift, and grimace

    b. ability to walk, grip strength, and vision disturbances

    c. headache, loss of consciousness, and abnormal speech

    d. SpO_2 reading, blood glucose reading, and pronator drift

11. Dispatch has sent you to a call for a 16-year-old who is having seizures. When you arrive, the patient is having a generalized seizure and the caretaker reports that this is the third seizure today. The patient has a history of seizures and takes medication for the condition. You confirm that there has been no traumatic injury as a result of the seizures today and begin to assess and manage the airway. Which of the following actions do you begin with?

    a. suction and insert an OPA

    b. use your stethoscope listen to lung sounds

    c. administer oxygen with a NRB mask at 10 lpm

    d. open the airway; if that is not possible, insert an NPA

12. You are assessing a patient who appears to be awaking after a syncopal event. The patient is confused and is not answering questions appropriately. The patient is wearing a Medic Alert bracelet which indicates that he is diabetic and epileptic. Your partner obtains vital signs while you consider the cause of the unconsciousness. What two things must you rule out first to help you figure out what is happening with the patient?

    a. hypoxia and hypoglycemia

    b. traumatic injury and incontinence

    c. abnormal ECG and hypoglycemia

    d. witnesses' accounts of seizure activity and how long seizure activity lasted

13. Chronic repetitive seizures (idiopathic epilepsy) are one of the most frequent causes of seizures in which two age groups?

    a. infants and toddlers

    b. children and adolescents

    c. adolescents and young adults

    d. young adults and older adults

14. Your crew was dispatched for a syncopal event. When you arrive, the patient is beginning to regain consciousness. Her eyes are closed, but she pulls her arm away as you assess her pulse. You speak to her and she opens her eyes. What is the typical response from a patient who awakens among strangers?

    a. fright

    b. anger

    c. confusion

    d. embarrassment

15. Stroke patients often understand what is happening to them, but are unable to communicate because of a neurological deficit. An example of this is aphasia, which means the patient has:

    a. a pronator drift in one or both arms.

    b. a loss of muscle coordination and balance.

    c. impaired vision, with weakness and spasticity.

    d. lost the ability to speak, because of a defect in or loss of language function.

Chapter 21 Answer Form

	A	B	C	D			A	B	C	D
1.	❑	❑	❑	❑		9.	❑	❑	❑	❑
2.	❑	❑	❑	❑		10.	❑	❑	❑	❑
3.	❑	❑	❑	❑		11.	❑	❑	❑	❑
4.	❑	❑	❑	❑		12.	❑	❑	❑	❑
5.	❑	❑	❑	❑		13.	❑	❑	❑	❑
6.	❑	❑	❑	❑		14.	❑	❑	❑	❑
7.	❑	❑	❑	❑		15.	❑	❑	❑	❑
8.	❑	❑	❑	❑						

CHAPTER 22

Nontraumatic Abdominal Emergencies

1. A patient who vomits blood that has the appearance of coffee grounds is most likely:
   a. bleeding in the lower GI tract.
   b. digesting blood in the stomach.
   c. in a state of hypovolemic shock.
   d. in need of an IV fluid bolus of more than 1,000 cc.

2. A patient tells you that he experiences abdominal pain after eating fatty foods. Which of the following conditions is provoked by this practice?
   a. gastritis
   b. peptic ulcer
   c. lactose intolerance
   d. gallbladder disease

3. Which of the following causes of acute abdominal pain is not typically considered a life-threatening condition?
   a. acute myocardial infarction (AMI)
   b. gastroenteritis
   c. ruptured viscus
   d. ruptured abdominal aortic aneurysm

4. Many causes of abdominal pain do not originate in the abdomen. Which of the following causes of abdominal pain does originate inside the abdomen?
   a. AMI
   b. hepatitis
   c. pneumonia
   d. kidney failure

5. A 24-year-old male has a chief complaint of acute lower right abdominal pain that began 2 hours ago. He is lying very still and denies shortness of breath or chest pain. He states that he has not felt well for a couple of days. He hasn't had much of an appetite, but denies nausea or vomiting. Which of the following conditions should be suspected, given these symptoms?
   a. obstruction
   b. appendicitis
   c. kidney stone
   d. urinary tract infection

6. You are dispatched on an EMS call for a sick person. Upon arrival, you find a 70-year-old female sitting at the kitchen table. She is alert, although she has her head down on the table. She is very pale, diaphoretic, and says that suddenly she felt very weak. She denies difficulty breathing, chest pain, or abdominal pain. She has no significant past medical history and takes no medications. Her husband confirms the information and adds that she has had a head cold for two days. The patient has no distal pulse. What action should you take next?
   a. Administer high-flow oxygen.
   b. Obtain a blood glucose reading and attach the AED.
   c. Ask about vomiting and last bowel movement.
   d. Lay her supine on the floor and elevate her legs.

7. Why must ectopic pregnancy be ruled out in a female presenting with acute abdominal pain?
   a. An ectopic pregnancy can rupture, creating life-threatening bleeding.
   b. An AMI can present with the same symptoms as a ruptured ectopic pregnancy.
   c. Acute abdominal pain in the female is associated with projectile vomiting and high risk of aspiration.
   d. A ruptured abdominal aortic aneurysm can present with the same symptoms as a ruptured ectopic pregnancy.

8. A local physician's office has requested transport of a 68-year-old female with tearing abdominal pain radiating through to the back. Her symptoms began two weeks ago and today they are becoming severely intense. She denies shortness of breath, chest pain, nausea, or vomiting, but has pain in both thighs. This patient should be transported to rule out:
   a. kidney stones.
   b. bowel obstruction.
   c. ectopic pregnancy.
   d. abdominal aortic aneurysm.

9. The patient you are transporting for evaluation of acute abdominal pain is in severe distress. He did not allow you to palpate his abdomen because of the intense pain he is experiencing. During the transport, you see that his pain becomes worse with each bump in the road. This type of pain response is similar to:
   a. referred pain.
   b. rebound tenderness.
   c. orthostatic sensitivity.
   d. musculoskeletal pain.

10. Your patient has an abdominal obstruction and is awaiting surgery. He tells you he is currently experiencing severe abdominal pain. He is lying very still with his legs flexed and he is guarding his abdomen. This type of pain is:
    a. referred.
    b. somatic.
    c. visceral.
    d. psychosomatic.

11. A 16-year-old female has been diagnosed with acute appendicitis. She is complaining of intermittent abdominal pain with cramps. She is pale, diaphoretic, and nauseated. This type of pain is:
    a. referred.
    b. somatic.
    c. visceral.
    d. psychosomatic.

12. You are assessing a 64-year-old male who is lying in bed with a complaint of weakness and rectal bleeding. The patient appears extremely pale, is short of breath, and has no distal pulse. A focused physical exam of this patient will include each of the following, except:
    a. an orthostatic exam.
    b. a pulmonary exam.
    c. a cardiovascular exam.
    d. palpation of the abdomen.

13. (Continuing with the preceding question) Your physical examination reveals a rapid carotid pulse, clear lung sounds, diffuse pain in both lower abdominal quadrants, and no peripheral edema. Vital signs are: respiratory rate 26; pulse rate 118/regular; and BP 80/40. Management of this patient begins with high-flow oxygen and:
    a. treating for shock.
    b. listening for bowel sounds.
    c. placing the patient in the supine position with legs elevated.
    d. obtaining a stool sample for the hospital.

14. A patient with pain in the upper right quadrant has tenderness on palpation. His chief complaint is malaise and weakness for several days, with nausea and vomiting. He tells you that he has lost weight recently because he has lost his appetite. Which of the following conditions do you suspect the patient may have?
    a. kidney failure
    b. acid reflux disease
    c. a bowel obstruction
    d. an infectious disease

15. (Continuing with the preceding question) The patient also tells you that he has had night sweats and fever. His urine has been dark-colored and his stool is loose and clay-colored. You suspect he may have hepatitis. What physical finding, if present, can help confirm your suspicions?
    a. stiff neck
    b. needle marks
    c. yellow eyes or skin
    d. bruising on the torso

Chapter 22 Answer Form

	A	B	C	D			A	B	C	D
1.	❑	❑	❑	❑		9.	❑	❑	❑	❑
2.	❑	❑	❑	❑		10.	❑	❑	❑	❑
3.	❑	❑	❑	❑		11.	❑	❑	❑	❑
4.	❑	❑	❑	❑		12.	❑	❑	❑	❑
5.	❑	❑	❑	❑		13.	❑	❑	❑	❑
6.	❑	❑	❑	❑		14.	❑	❑	❑	❑
7.	❑	❑	❑	❑		15.	❑	❑	❑	❑
8.	❑	❑	❑	❑						

CHAPTER 23

Environmental Emergencies

1. An example of an environmental emergency is a:
   a. trauma condition exacerbated by chronic alcoholism.
   b. medical condition caused by poor health in the elderly.
   c. trauma condition caused by certain prescription medications.
   d. medical condition exacerbated by below-average temperatures.

2. Which of the following is likely to predispose an individual to an environmental emergency?
   a. fatigue
   b. diabetes
   c. infancy or young age
   d. all of the above

3. Late at night, an elderly woman fell in her kitchen and was unable to get up. Her daughter came by the next day when her mother did not answer phone calls. The patient is confused and incontinent of urine, neither of which is normal for her. After ruling out hypoxia and hypoglycemia, which of the following should you consider as a possible cause of the abnormal findings?
   a. mild hypothermia
   b. mild hyperthermia
   c. severe hypothermia
   d. severe hyperthermia

4. Environmental factors that may complicate treatment or transport decisions include:
   a. terrain.
   b. climate.
   c. season.
   d. all of the above.

5. The four primary types of environmental illnesses are heat illness, cold illness,
   a. frostbite, and burns.
   b. metabolic illness, and thermoregulation.
   c. pressurization illnesses, and localized injuries.
   d. decompression sickness, and high-altitude illness.

6. *Severe hypothermia* is defined as the presence of signs and symptoms with a core body temperature (CBT) below:
   a. 30°C/86°F.
   b. 32°C/88°F.
   c. 34°C/90°F.
   d. 36°C/92°F.

7. Which method of monitoring a patient's core body temperature is considered the most reliable?
   a. oral
   b. rectal
   c. axillary
   d. tympanic

8. The body has the ability to dissipate heat by _____ mechanism(s).
   a. one
   b. two
   c. three
   d. four

9. When the body senses heat loss, it begins to generate heat through metabolic reactions and through:
   a. radiation.
   b. muscular activity.
   c. dilating peripheral blood vessels.
   d. increasing the respiratory and heart rates.

10. The most common cold disorder is:
    a. frostnip.
    b. frostbite.
    c. shivering.
    d. hypothermia.

11. Which of the following is a common predisposing factor associated with heat and cold disorders?
    a. arthritis
    b. pregnancy
    c. hypertension
    d. thyroid disease

12. Certain over-the-counter medications can predispose individuals to heat illness because these drugs affect the ability to sweat and dissipate heat. One such medication type is:
    a. antihistamines.
    b. antihypertensives.
    c. caffeinated products.
    d. products containing aspirin.

13. *Heat illness* is defined as an increased core body temperature because of:
    a. an excessive loss of sodium and potassium.
    b. a normal fluid loss with an electrolyte imbalance.
    c. excessive sodium loss and increased potassium.
    d. the body's inability to adequately dissipate heat.

14. A young couple is moving from one apartment to another on a warm spring day. They have been going nonstop since early morning. In the afternoon, the male begins to experience heat cramps, nausea, and heavy sweating. He finally stops to rest when he feels the muscles in his arms and legs twitching, and soon thereafter the twitching is followed by painful spasms. The cause of his heat cramps is:
    a. inadequate acclimatization.
    b. an excessive loss of potassium.
    c. a malfunction in the thermoregulatory center.
    d. an excessive loss of salt and water in the sweat.

15. Heat illness can develop quickly or over one to two days; it manifests various signs and symptoms. The sign or symptom indicating that a heat illness has become an extreme medical emergency is the development of:
    a. extreme thirst.
    b. weakness and fatigue.
    c. an altered level of consciousness.
    d. decreased or absent sweating.

16. To help prevent heat illness when in a warm environment, one should maintain an adequate fluid intake by:
    a. drinking only when thirsty.
    b. drinking regardless of thirst.
    c. avoiding any type of diuretic.
    d. avoiding nonprescription diuretics.

17. Which of the following is most accurate about heat exhaustion?
    a. There is a low incidence of heat exhaustion in young children.
    b. Heat cramps are a warning sign and always precede heat exhaustion.
    c. The patient with heat exhaustion will have signs and symptoms of shock.
    d. The patient with heat exhaustion will have a normal or slightly elevated temperature.

18. Which of the following is most accurate about the difference between fever and heat stroke?
    a. Both fever and heat stroke may cause an altered mental status.
    b. Fever is an abnormal response of an intact thermoregulatory system.
    c. Heat stroke is a normal response of an intact thermoregulatory system.
    d. Fever is an abnormal response to the release of chemicals called pyrogens.

19. In the patient with heat illness, an IV fluid bolus of 500 ml normal saline helps to correct dehydration and:
    a. may cause nausea and vomiting.
    b. may cause mild pulmonary edema.
    c. often decreases the pain from heat cramps.
    d. rapidly cools the patient from the inside out.

20. You are dispatched to the local indoor ice skating rink for a sick person. When you arrive, you are taken to a 14-year-old male dressed in hockey gear. The patient is conscious and alert but looks ill. He is pale, warm, and diaphoretic, and complains of abdominal pain and weakness. He has been sick with a cold for the past week, but felt better this morning and so decided to go to hockey practice. Your partner obtains vital signs and you begin treating the patient by:
    a. starting an IV of normal saline.
    b. giving the patient sips of cool water.
    c. removing some of the patient's clothing.
    d. laying the patient on the ice to begin rapid cooling.

21. (Continuing with the preceding question) The patient's vital signs are: respiratory rate 22/nonlabored; pulse rate 112/regular; and BP 96/50. He feels light-headed when you move him to the stretcher. Except for the recent cold, he has no significant past medical history, and has only taken over-the-counter cold medications. What is this patient's primary problem?
    a. He has a fever.
    b. He is dehydrated.
    c. He has signs and symptoms of heat stroke.
    d. He has signs and symptoms of heat cramps.

22. Hypothermia is a condition in which the core body temperature falls to less than 95°F, due to increased heat loss from the body or:
    a. inadequate nutrition.
    b. hyperthyroid disease.
    c. decreased production of heat.
    d. intolerance to cold temperatures.

23. Which of the following factors predisposes a patient to hypothermia?
    a. children aged 4 to 6
    b. overexertion in cold temperatures
    c. any patient with a history of chronic back pain
    d. any elderly person living alone with a chronic disease

24. To help prevent hypothermia when participating in outdoor activities, which of the following should be avoided?
    a. adequate nutrition
    b. limited exposure time
    c. alcohol and tobacco use
    d. wearing the proper clothing

25. The differences between mild and severe hypothermia are the presence of signs and symptoms and:
    a. type of cooling process.
    b. the core body temperature.
    c. the patient's past medical history.
    d. speed of onset of signs and symptoms.

26. An elderly patient has fallen on a tile floor at home and is unable to get up. If left alone overnight, what type of hypothermia is this person prone to develop?
    a. acute
    b. chronic
    c. relative
    d. immersion

27. Which of the following initial signs or symptoms are typically associated with mild hypothermia?
    a. cardiac irritability
    b. speech disturbances
    c. altered mental status
    d. loss of fine motor control

28. Your patient, who has a history of dementia, was found lying in a wet bed in the morning by a home health aide. The aide states that the patient is more confused than normal and does not know where he is. The patient appears uninjured, but smells of urine. His vital signs, blood glucose reading, and ECG are normal. What finding most reliably rules out hypothermia in this patient?
    a. core body temperature
    b. the increased alteration in mental status
    c. the ambient temperature of the house
    d. the amount of time the patient was in the wet bed

29. While performing CPR on a patient with severe hypothermia, the rescuers should:
    a. use normal chest compressions and ventilation.
    b. use modified chest compression and normal ventilation.
    c. avoid the use of an AED until the core body temperature is above 86°F.
    d. avoid the use of an AED until the core body temperature is above 92°F.

30. A hiker came out of the woods in cold winter conditions. He is mildly hypothermic and has frostbite on toes of both feet. The nearest hospital is 40 minutes away. In the ambulance, his wet clothing is removed, high-flow oxygen is administered, and a blanket wrap is used to cover the patient. Specific care for the feet includes:
    a. splinting only.
    b. slow rewarming with hot packs.
    c. gently rubbing the toes with alcohol.
    d. packing the feet in snow to prevent rapid warming.

31. A *near-drowning episode* is defined as:
    a. a submersion lasting more than 10 minutes.
    b. a submersion episode in cold water at less than 80°F.
    c. a submersion episode with at least transient recovery.
    d. death due to asphyxiation during an immersion episode.

32. Which of the following statements about near-drowning is most correct?
    a. Victims of near-drowning in salt water recover better.
    b. The near-drowning victim will always be hypothermic.
    c. Upon initial assessment, the patient may appear normal.
    d. Alcohol is a factor in more than 50 percent of near-drowning episodes.

33. In what way can hypothermia play a protective role in a near-drowning?
    a. Cold may decrease cerebral metabolism.
    b. The colder the water, the less hypoxic the patient will become.
    c. The colder the water, the less brain damage the victim will have.
    d. Cold may cause a laryngeal spasm, leading to a dry drowning.

34. The best predictor of severity of damage to the victim of near-drowning is the:
    a. depth of submersion.
    b. length the submersion lasted.
    c. age and gender of the victim.
    d. time to the first spontaneous breath.

35. A victim of near-drowning is pulled out of salt water by lifeguards. The patient is coughing up water, appears pale, and is confused. One of the lifeguards provides rescue breaths with a pocket mask, which stimulates the patient to cough and breathe. An initial assessment of the patient includes:
    a. obtaining a core body temperature.
    b. obtaining respiratory and pulse rates.
    c. assessing lung sounds and pupillary reaction.
    d. assessing lung sounds and quality of the pulse.

36. (Continuing with the preceding question) You administer high-flow oxygen and the patient becomes more alert. His vital signs are: respiratory rate 26/labored with audible wheezing; pulse rate 124/regular; BP 110/66; skin CTC reveals a cyanotic face and neck, cool extremities with goose bumps, and shivering. In addition to warming the patient, you will start an IV of:

    a. normal saline at a rate to keep the vein open.
    b. one-half normal saline at a rate to keep the vein open.
    c. normal saline with large bore and administer a fluid bolus.
    d. one-half normal saline with a large bore and administer a fluid bolus.

37. A scuba diver is exposed to atmospheric pressure changes during a dive. As a diver descends, the gases contained in her lungs will:

    a. expand.
    b. contract.
    c. dissolve.
    d. dissipate.

38. Altitude sickness occurs as a result of decreased atmospheric pressure. The clinical findings associated with all forms of altitude sickness:

    a. include altered mental status and hypotension.
    b. may include rash, joint pain, and congestive heart failure.
    c. occur because of the body's abnormal response to hypoxia at altitude.
    d. occur because of the presence of air bubbles in the central circulation.

39. You are interviewing a patient who developed stroke symptoms with loss of sensation in the right extremities. He also complains of shoulder and neck pain ever since returning from a diving trip 10 days ago. He denies shortness of breath or chest pain. How should you proceed with the focused physical exam?

    a. Complete a pulmonary and cardiac exam.
    b. Complete a neuro exam, including the prehospital stroke score.
    c. Assess range of motion in the neck, shoulders, and all extremities.
    d. Assess all affected areas of the body for subcutaneous emphysema.

40. (Continuing with the preceding question) The patient states that his wife was with him on all the dives and has not had any pain or symptoms, so he was waiting for the pain to resolve, but today he developed the loss of sensation in the right extremities. His vital signs are: respiratory rate 18/regular; pulse rate 68/regular; and BP 146/90. Skin CTC is warm, dry, and pink. What are the treatment considerations for this patient?

    a. Transport the patient to the nearest stroke center.
    b. Consult medical control about hyperbaric therapy.
    c. Transport to any facility the patient chooses will be appropriate.
    d. Obtain a glucose reading before making any transportation decisions.

Chapter 23 Answer Form

	A	B	C	D
1.	❏	❏	❏	❏
2.	❏	❏	❏	❏
3.	❏	❏	❏	❏
4.	❏	❏	❏	❏
5.	❏	❏	❏	❏
6.	❏	❏	❏	❏
7.	❏	❏	❏	❏
8.	❏	❏	❏	❏
9.	❏	❏	❏	❏
10.	❏	❏	❏	❏
11.	❏	❏	❏	❏
12.	❏	❏	❏	❏
13.	❏	❏	❏	❏
14.	❏	❏	❏	❏
15.	❏	❏	❏	❏
16.	❏	❏	❏	❏
17.	❏	❏	❏	❏
18.	❏	❏	❏	❏
19.	❏	❏	❏	❏
20.	❏	❏	❏	❏

	A	B	C	D
21.	❏	❏	❏	❏
22.	❏	❏	❏	❏
23.	❏	❏	❏	❏
24.	❏	❏	❏	❏
25.	❏	❏	❏	❏
26.	❏	❏	❏	❏
27.	❏	❏	❏	❏
28.	❏	❏	❏	❏
29.	❏	❏	❏	❏
30.	❏	❏	❏	❏
31.	❏	❏	❏	❏
32.	❏	❏	❏	❏
33.	❏	❏	❏	❏
34.	❏	❏	❏	❏
35.	❏	❏	❏	❏
36.	❏	❏	❏	❏
37.	❏	❏	❏	❏
38.	❏	❏	❏	❏
39.	❏	❏	❏	❏
40.	❏	❏	❏	❏

CHAPTER 24

Behavioral Emergencies

1. Many factors can alter the behavior of any ill or injured person, whether or not the person has a history of a behavioral disorder. The factor that makes an experience a behavioral emergency for the person is:
   a. the use of alcohol.
   b. the excessive use of drugs.
   c. that person's reaction to a crisis.
   d. the presence of a chemical imbalance.

2. Which of the following is most accurate about the pathophysiology of behavioral and psychiatric disorders?
   a. A person's surroundings cause behavioral disorders.
   b. Behavioral disorders are caused by a genetic problem.
   c. Multiple factors cause both behavioral and psychiatric disorders.
   d. Psychiatric disorders are caused by chemical alterations in the brain.

3. Therapeutic interviewing techniques are used with emotionally disturbed patients to establish rapport, maintain calm, and encourage the patient to cooperate. An example of a therapeutic interviewing technique is:
   a. limiting interruptions when listening to the patient.
   b. avoiding any specific questions about the immediate problem.
   c. keeping your questions very specific to the patient's past medical history.
   d. getting the patient to actively listen to your supportive and empathetic dialogue.

4. Which of the following should be avoided during the physical assessment of the patient with a behavioral emergency?
   a. Surround the patient with plenty of people.
   b. Approach the patient slowly and purposefully.
   c. Limit physical assessment to obtaining vital signs.
   d. Provide rapid intervention for life-threatening conditions.

5. A simple and effective technique used to obtain information from a disturbed patient is:
   a. always agreeing with the patient.
   b. being honest with the patient.
   c. telling the patient what he or she wants to hear.
   d. having physical assistance ready and using it as needed.

6. Age and sex factors that increase the risk of a person becoming suicidal include being a:
   a. male less than 19 years of age.
   b. male between 19 and 45 years of age.
   c. female less than 19 years of age.
   d. female between 19 and 45 years of age.

7. You are managing a patient with a behavioral emergency. The family is present and wants to stay with the patient during the transport. A general guideline is to:
   a. allow the relatives to stay only if the patient consents.
   b. not allow the relatives to stay under any circumstances.
   c. contact medical control for advice, as each case is unique.
   d. allow the relatives to stay only when the patient will not cooperate otherwise.

8. The EMT-I is responsible for knowing each of the following medicolegal aspects of management of the emotionally disturbed patient, except:
   a. crisis intervention.
   b. psychiatric diagnosis.
   c. transport without consent.
   d. alcohol and drug detoxification.

9. There are times when patients must be transported for evaluation even if they do not consent. Which of the following persons should the EMT-I transport against the patient's will?
   a. a person with dementia
   b. a person with altered mental status
   c. a person in police custody for abuse
   d. a person with a history of paranoia of hospitals

10. If it should become necessary to physically restrain a patient, humane restraints should be used. Which of the following is a humane restraining device?
    a. metal handcuffs
    b. plastic handcuffs
    c. leather restraints
    d. cord or rope wrap

11. Before attempting to physically restrain a patient, you must make certain that it is legal for you to do so. Then you must:
    a. have enough personnel to complete the task.
    b. be sure that the patient wants to harm himself or herself.
    c. obtain consent from the patient's family or caretaker.
    d. confirm that the patient does not have a history of seizures.

12. The police are with a patient who says that he "hears voices." The officer reports that for the last 2 hours, the patient has been ranting a story that cannot possible be real and that currently he does not appear to have a concept of reality. Initially the patient was hyperactive. During the last 30 minutes he has become calm and cooperative. What behavioral emergency is the patient exhibiting?
    a. paranoia
    b. neurosis
    c. psychosis
    d. acute depression

13. (Continuing with the preceding question) You obtain more information from the officer and observe the patient. Which of the following clues suggests that the patient may develop violent behavior?
    a. crying and sobbing
    b. pacing back and forth
    c. disheveled appearance
    d. persistent mumbling in monotone phrases

14. A patient has fears out of proportion to reality that compel the patient to avoid the feared object or situation and may interfere with normal daily activities. This disorder is called:
    a. a phobia.
    b. a neurosis.
    c. paranoia.
    d. psychosis.

15. You are assessing a 16-year-old female who took 10 aspirins in an effort to harm herself. She changed her mind and called 9-1-1 shortly after ingesting the aspirin. She is alert and oriented, with no specific complaint. She does describe recent activities associated with depression, such as difficulty sleeping, loss of appetite, and weight loss. Which term would you use to describe what has occurred with this patient?
    a. suicide failure
    b. suicidal gesture
    c. suicide attempt
    d. successful suicide

Chapter 24 Answer Form

	A	B	C	D		A	B	C	D
1.	❏	❏	❏	❏	9.	❏	❏	❏	❏
2.	❏	❏	❏	❏	10.	❏	❏	❏	❏
3.	❏	❏	❏	❏	11.	❏	❏	❏	❏
4.	❏	❏	❏	❏	12.	❏	❏	❏	❏
5.	❏	❏	❏	❏	13.	❏	❏	❏	❏
6.	❏	❏	❏	❏	14.	❏	❏	❏	❏
7.	❏	❏	❏	❏	15.	❏	❏	❏	❏
8.	❏	❏	❏	❏					

CHAPTER 25

Gynecological Emergencies

1. Which of the following hormones induces the development of female sexual characteristics and stimulates bone and muscle growth?

   a. estrogen
   b. vasopressin
   c. testosterone
   d. progesterone

2. The assessment of a female patient with a complaint of abnormal vaginal bleeding and cramping includes a focused physical examination of the:

   a. pelvis.
   b. rectum.
   c. abdomen.
   d. symphysis pubis.

3. The most common chief complaint of a patient with a gynecological emergency is:

   a. fever.
   b. nausea.
   c. abdominal pain.
   d. abnormal vaginal bleeding.

4. After managing the ABCs, the general approach to care of the female patient with acute abdominal pain or vaginal bleeding is:

   a. to suspect and treat for shock.
   b. IV access and pain management.
   c. high-flow oxygen and rapid transport.
   d. early notification to the ED for a possible surgical patient.

5. When the cervix is infected with a sexually transmitted disease, the infection can spread to internal organs. This condition is called:

   a. cystitis.
   b. implantation.
   c. endometriosis.
   d. pelvic inflammatory disease (PID).

6. When an ovarian cyst ruptures, typically the patient will experience sudden, sharp pelvic pain. The pain is caused by:

   a. stretching of the ovarian membrane.
   b. fluids from the rupture irritating the peritoneum.
   c. sagging of the tissues extending from the rupture.
   d. pressure on the uterus by the fluids from the rupture.

7. EMS was called for a 32-year-old female who collapsed at work. The patient is lying on the floor, alert now and complaining of feeling dizzy before and after the fainting episode. She denies difficulty breathing or chest pain, but has had pressure in the pelvic area all day. She is currently having an irregular period, but last month it was normal. She denies having any vaginal bleeding or discharge. What condition must be ruled out first with this patient?

   a. ovarian torsion
   b. ectopic pregnancy
   c. ruptured ovarian cyst
   d. pelvic inflammatory disease

8. (Continuing with the preceding question) The patient denies being pregnant, but has endometriosis. She takes no medications and is allergic to sulfa drugs. Her vital signs are: respiratory rate 20/nonlabored; pulse rate 106/regular; and BP 116/66. Skin CTC is pale, warm, and moist. Management of this patient includes administration of high-flow oxygen and:

   a. position of comfort, then transport to the nearest facility.
   b. supine position, IV access, and transport to the appropriate facility.
   c. left lateral recumbent position, and preparation for projectile vomiting.
   d. psychological support, IV access, and transport to the patient's gynecologist.

9. Physical signs that may be noted on the victim of an assault include:
   a. swelling of the labia.
   b. new lacerations of the perineum.
   c. defensive wounds on the extremities.
   d. any of the above.

10. Management of the victim of sexual assault begins with managing any life-threatening injuries. Thereafter, the focus of care is:
    a. to clean, dress, and cover all external wounds.
    b. aimed at preserving any potential evidence.
    c. directed toward providing emotional support.
    d. to rule out the possibility of disease transmission.

11. The victim of a sexual assault is unwilling to allow assessment. She is alert and extremely anxious, her breathing appears unlabored, and her skin color is good. What can you do to persuade her to allow you to help?
    a. Protect her privacy and modesty.
    b. Do nothing until the patient is ready.
    c. Maintain direct eye contact when talking with the patient.
    d. Encourage the patient to call a trusted friend to stay with her.

12. Which of the following methods can the EMT-I use to help preserve evidence from the victim of a sexual assault, without minimizing appropriate care?
    a. Do not remove any clothing from the victim.
    b. Handle the victim's clothing as little as possible.
    c. Do not ask the patient any questions about the attacker.
    d. Place the victim's clothing in a red bag and take it to the hospital.

13. Which of the following findings may indicate sexual abuse?
    a. pain during urination
    b. acute abdominal pain during the menstrual period
    c. irregular periods and vaginal discharge with an odor
    d. an elderly patient with signs and symptoms of an STD

14. The most common bacterial STD, in both men and women, is frequently present with no symptoms and can be treated with antibiotics. This condition is:
    a. AIDS.
    b. syphilis.
    c. hepatitis.
    d. chlamydia.

15. The 28-day cycle of changes in the endometrium in response to sexual hormone levels is the:
    a. ovarian cycle.
    b. gestation cycle.
    c. menstrual cycle.
    d. implantation phase.

Chapter 25 Answer Form

	A	B	C	D		A	B	C	D
1.	❑	❑	❑	❑	9.	❑	❑	❑	❑
2.	❑	❑	❑	❑	10.	❑	❑	❑	❑
3.	❑	❑	❑	❑	11.	❑	❑	❑	❑
4.	❑	❑	❑	❑	12.	❑	❑	❑	❑
5.	❑	❑	❑	❑	13.	❑	❑	❑	❑
6.	❑	❑	❑	❑	14.	❑	❑	❑	❑
7.	❑	❑	❑	❑	15.	❑	❑	❑	❑
8.	❑	❑	❑	❑					

CHAPTER

26

Obstetrical Emergencies

1. The development of the placenta begins with the:
   a. release of estrogen following menses.
   b. secretory phase of the menstrual cycle.
   c. release of progesterone during the ovarian cycle.
   d. implantation of the fertilized egg in the endometrium.

2. Which of the following is considered an abnormal event during pregnancy?
   a. The heart rate increases by 10–20 beats per minute.
   b. The blood pressure increases during the second trimester.
   c. The blood pressure decreases during the second trimester.
   d. The circulating blood volume increases by nearly 50 percent.

3. When assessing the vital signs of a pregnant patient, the EMT-I should:
   a. count the pulse rate for a full minute.
   b. position the patient with both her legs elevated.
   c. consider the normal changes in vital signs that occur during pregnancy.
   d. always obtain a blood pressure reading on both arms.

4. During which stage of labor does the cervix dilate in preparation for delivery?
   a. 1
   b. 2
   c. 3
   d. 4

5. Which of the following presentations is an example of an abnormal delivery?
   a. the vaginal delivery of twins
   b. the baby's head passes through the cervix first
   c. the baby's buttocks pass through the cervix first
   d. the baby's head presents face-up at the vaginal opening

6. Which of the following conditions is a serious complication when present during pregnancy or delivery?
   a. hypertension
   b. urinary frequency
   c. swelling of the hands
   d. new varicose veins in the legs

7. A female at 22 weeks' gestation is experiencing sudden pelvic pain, which she describes as severe with constant pain and intermittent contractions. She states that the baby is moving and denies any vaginal bleeding or discharge. Which life-threatening condition must be considered early with this patient?
   a. placenta previa
   b. abruptio placenta
   c. spontaneous abortion
   d. the onset of gestational diabetes

8. You are assessing a female in the late third trimester who is having contractions. Which of the following signs indicates that the patient is close to delivery?
   a. regular contractions
   b. irregular contractions
   c. bowel movement during a contraction
   d. slow leak of fluid from the vaginal opening

9. Your patient was the driver of a motor vehicle that was involved in a collision in an intersection. Her complaint is neck and low back pain. She is in the third trimester of her first pregnancy. Immobilization and transportation concerns for this patient include:
   a. no additional concerns related to the pregnancy.
   b. the possibility of inducing supine hypotension syndrome.
   c. worsening the patient's back pain with the use of a long backboard.
   d. the possibility of inducing pregnancy-associated hypertension during immobilization.

10. Your patient is in very active labor. Her membranes have ruptured and crowning is visible. While you prepare the mother for delivery, you have your partner coach the mother through the contractions. She will coach the mother by:

    a. instructing the mother not to push during contractions.
    b. having the mother arch her back during each contraction.
    c. telling the mother to breathe rapidly during the contraction to avoid pushing too hard.
    d. telling the mother to push with the contractions and then breathe deeply in between.

11. Tearing of the perineum is common in childbirth. One method the EMT-I can use to minimize the risk of tearing is to:

    a. coach the mother to push only during contractions.
    b. place both hands on the baby's head to keep it from exploding out of the vaginal opening.
    c. press a 5 × 9 inch gauze pad over the perineum with a gloved hand during delivery of the baby's head.
    d. place a pillow under the mother's buttocks and a gloved hand over the perineum during delivery of the baby's head.

12. During childbirth, after delivery of the baby's head, the next step for the EMT-I is to:

    a. assess an APGAR score.
    b. assist the baby to turn on its side.
    c. look for a cord wrapped around the baby's neck.
    d. place a gloved hand over the perineum to prevent tearing.

13. Once the baby has been delivered and the umbilical cord has been cut, it is easier to manage and assess the baby. Until the cord is cut, the EMT-I should keep the baby at or below the level of the vaginal opening to prevent:

    a. hypoxia in the baby.
    b. hypotension in the baby.
    c. hypothermia in the baby.
    d. hypotension in the mother.

14. Which of the following is most accurate about delivery of the placenta?

    a. The clamp attached to the cord near the placenta should be removed.
    b. The clamp attached to the cord near the placenta should not be removed.
    c. The placenta should be kept warm and dry if delivered before you arrive at the ED.
    d. Contractions for delivery of the placenta are more severe than contractions for delivery of the baby.

15. Minor vaginal bleeding is normal after delivery of the placenta. When bleeding is heavy, the EMT-I should massage the fundus of the uterus to slow bleeding. Another way to slow bleeding is to:

    a. place ice packs on the mother's abdomen.
    b. allow the baby to suckle the mother's breast.
    c. place direct pressure on the fundus of the uterus.
    d. pack the vaginal opening with a trauma dressing.

16. EMS is dispatched to a residence where a home delivery is in progress with a midwife present. The midwife tells you that the mother is in active labor and that the crowning is abnormal, with the baby's arm presenting at the vaginal opening. This type of delivery:

    a. typically requires a cesarean section.
    b. can be completed at the residence with your help.
    c. is often associated with preeclampsia and eclampsia.
    d. has a high risk of mortality for both the baby and the mother.

17. You are obtaining a focused history from a patient who is 10 weeks pregnant and complains of abdominal pain and vaginal bleeding. Her pregnancy history is gravida −3 and para −2. How many children has she given birth to?

    a. 2
    b. 3
    c. 4
    d. 5

18. A first-time mother has been in labor for 2 hours. The pregnancy is at 39 weeks and has been normal. She has no significant past medical history. She has suddenly developed shortness of breath and right-sided chest pain that increases with a deep breath. She is very anxious and has the following vital signs: respiratory rate 30; pulse rate 100/regular; and BP 124/76. Which of the following life-threatening conditions must the EMT-I consider immediately?

    a. fractured ribs
    b. asthma attack
    c. placenta previa
    d. pulmonary embolism

19. Meconium, which is the first bowel movement of the baby, may be present in the fluids during birth. The presence of meconium usually indicates that the baby:

    a. is premature.
    b. will need resuscitation.
    c. will develop neonatal jaundice.
    d. has experienced or is experiencing fetal distress.

20. Which of the following factors associated with premature birth and low birth weight is avoidable?

    a. premature labor
    b. gestational diabetes
    c. maternal use of tobacco
    d. hypertension syndromes

21. You are preparing to assist in the delivery of a full-term baby. The mother has had three full-term babies with no complications. She called EMS because this labor has progressed faster than she anticipated and she is still waiting for a relative to come and watch her other children. How many patients will require your attention for this call?

    a. 1
    b. 2
    c. 4
    d. 5

22. (Continuing with the preceding question) In addition to gloves, what is the minimum personal protective equipment you will need to assist in the delivery of this baby?

    a. eye protection and a gown
    b. two umbilical clamps and two plastic bags
    c. eye protection and clean towels or sheets
    d. face mask, eye protection, and two plastic bags

23. The EMT-I's approach to physical examination of the pregnant patient should be calm, comforting, and reassuring. One way of demonstrating compassion and consideration for the pregnant patient during the physical exam is to:

    a. protect the patient's modesty and privacy.
    b. avoid asking questions that may embarrass her.
    c. avoid asking questions that may embarrass you or your crew.
    d. obtain a thorough and complete history before performing the physical exam.

24. You and your partner are assisting in the delivery of a full-term baby. Your partner is an EMT-B who has never assisted with childbirth and is uncertain about how to help. How should you approach the delivery with your inexperienced partner?

    a. Allow your partner to care for the mother, but not the baby.
    b. Have your partner observe but not participate in the delivery.
    c. Coach your partner and explain the management steps in the delivery.
    d. Do not tell the patient that your partner has no prior experience with childbirth.

25. You are transporting a 28-year-old female who is in labor. Through your assessment, you have determined that the delivery is not imminent. As you prepare the patient for transport, you have her lie on the stretcher in the left lateral recumbent position (on her left side), because:

    a. this is the best position to listen for fetal heart tones.
    b. this is the best position to obtain vital signs on a pregnant patient.
    c. if she becomes nauseated and vomits, your uniform will not be soiled.
    d. the weight of the fetus will be off the mother's vena cava, allowing adequate blood return to her heart.

Chapter 26 Answer Form

	A	B	C	D		A	B	C	D
1.	❑	❑	❑	❑	14.	❑	❑	❑	❑
2.	❑	❑	❑	❑	15.	❑	❑	❑	❑
3.	❑	❑	❑	❑	16.	❑	❑	❑	❑
4.	❑	❑	❑	❑	17.	❑	❑	❑	❑
5.	❑	❑	❑	❑	18.	❑	❑	❑	❑
6.	❑	❑	❑	❑	19.	❑	❑	❑	❑
7.	❑	❑	❑	❑	20.	❑	❑	❑	❑
8.	❑	❑	❑	❑	21.	❑	❑	❑	❑
9.	❑	❑	❑	❑	22.	❑	❑	❑	❑
10.	❑	❑	❑	❑	23.	❑	❑	❑	❑
11.	❑	❑	❑	❑	24.	❑	❑	❑	❑
12.	❑	❑	❑	❑	25.	❑	❑	❑	❑
13.	❑	❑	❑	❑					

Infants, Children, and Geriatrics

CHAPTER

27

Neonatal Resuscitation

1. Until 6 weeks of age, a baby is considered a:
   a. neonate.
   b. newborn.
   c. premature.
   d. embryonic.

2. The term used in reference to the mother during labor is:
   a. antepartum.
   b. intrapartum.
   c. extrauterine.
   d. pre-embryonic.

3. Which of the following is most accurate about antepartum factors that can affect childbirth?
   a. The antepartum factors that affect childbirth can be avoided or prevented.
   b. Not all antepartum factors that affect childbirth can be avoided or prevented.
   c. Diabetes and hypertension syndromes are two antepartum factors that can affect childbirth.
   d. Having given birth to three or more children is an antepartum factor that can affect childbirth.

4. New onset of third-trimester vaginal bleeding is dangerous for the mother and the baby. The EMT-I should recognize this as a high-risk factor for both patients, suspect it, and treat the mother for:
   a. placenta previa.
   b. prolapsed cord.
   c. premature labor.
   d. abnormal limb presentation.

5. The newborn assessment that is performed immediately after birth evaluates respiratory effort, heart rate, and:
   a. length.
   b. weight.
   c. skin color.
   d. blood pressure.

6. The EMT-I who is assisting with childbirth must be prepared to assist a newborn that may be in distress after birth. The primary equipment needed to assist a distressed newborn includes:
   a. length-based tape (Broselow).
   b. airway and ventilation equipment.
   c. heart rate monitor and pulse oximeter.
   d. vascular access equipment and resuscitation medications.

7. The Apgar score is a well-accepted method for evaluating newborns:
   a. immediately after birth.
   b. at 1 minute and 1 hour after birth.
   c. immediately and 30 minutes after birth.
   d. at 1 minute and 5 minutes after birth.

8. Your unit has been dispatched to a pregnancy call. When you arrive, you quickly determine that the baby has been delivered, but the cord is still attached. As your partner opens the obstetric (OB) kit and prepares to cut the cord, you calculate the Apgar score. The baby is moving and crying, and coughs occasionally. Her skin is pink on the body, but her extremities are blue, and the pulse is 130. What is her Apgar score?
   a. 7
   b. 8
   c. 9
   d. 10

9. Which of the following signs is an indication for the EMT-I to provide ventilatory assistance to a neonate?
   a. tachypnea
   b. sternal retractions
   c. grunting and cyanosis
   d. all of the above

10. Which of the following airway and ventilation equipment is more appropriate for an older child than for the premature neonate?
    a. bulb syringe
    b. bag mask
    c. oropharyngeal airway
    d. cuffed endotracheal tube

11. A newborn with signs of respiratory distress is not improving even with high-concentration oxygenation and assisted ventilations. You are anticipating the possibility of having to perform chest compressions. When would chest compression be appropriate for a newborn?

a. when the heart rate falls below or remains below 100 beats per minute

b. when the respiratory rate falls below or remains below 20 breaths per minutes

c. when ventilations by endotracheal intubation fail to improve signs of respiratory distress

d. when the heart rate falls below 60 bpm despite adequate assisted ventilations for 30 seconds

12. The compression/ventilation ratio for a newborn during resuscitation is:

a. the same for BLS and ALS providers.

b. different when two rescuers are involved.

c. different when only one rescuer is involved.

d. different for BLS than for ALS providers.

13. Which of the following is an indication that a newborn's condition is improving with chest compressions and ventilations?

a. warm and dry skin

b. increased heart rate

c. absence of meconium in the airway

d. visible chest rise and fall with ventilations

14. You have just assisted in the delivery of a premature baby. Using a bulb syringe, you cleared the airway, and you are positive there was no meconium. As you warm and dry the baby, you see that she is slow to respond. What action do you take next?

a. Provide blow-by oxygen.

b. Assist ventilation using a bag mask.

c. Stimulate the baby by continuing to warm and dry her.

d. Intubate the baby, then suction the lower airway for possible meconium.

15. (Continuing with the preceding question) Which technique is appropriate for the action you selected?

a. Let oxygen blow by the face, rather than placing a mask on the face.

b. Use a newborn bag mask without a pop-off valve to assist ventilations.

c. Flick the bottom of the feet, using your fingers, or rub the back.

d. Using a #3 endotracheal tube, intubate the baby and use a meconium aspirator attached to a suction unit.

16. While assisting a newborn's ventilations with a bag mask, you watch for improvement by assessing for signs of adequate perfusion and respiratory effort. When the baby shows improvement, the next action you should take is to:

a. obtain a blood pressure.

b. stop ventilations and continue to keep the baby warm.

c. slowly decrease the rate and pressure of the ventilations.

d. provide humidified oxygenation using a simple face mask.

17. The initial steps of neonatal resuscitation include each of the following, except:

a. intubation.

b. suctioning the airway.

c. providing oxygenation.

d. assisting with ventilations.

18. The EMT-I will know that a distressed neonate has improved with the use of blow-by oxygenation when the baby:

a. is flaccid.

b. has sternal retractions.

c. is grunting and cyanotic.

d. has a heart rate above 160 bpm.

19. In which of the following circumstances should the newly born patient be rapidly transported to the hospital?

a. when the first Apgar score is 7

b. when the second Apgar score is 10

c. when the baby's heart rate is 80 bpm after drying and warming

d. when the baby's respiratory rate is 40/minute after drying and warming

20. The risk factors for aspiration of meconium include inappropriately managing the newborn's airway and:

a. a postterm baby.

b. a premature baby.

c. not recognizing the presence of meconium in a distressed baby.

d. the mother's use of medications during delivery.

21. If meconium is present at birth and the newly born takes its first breath through the mouth, the meconium can be aspirated into the lungs, causing:

a. them to collapse.

b. pulmonary emboli.

c. bronchospasm and atelectasis.

d. small airway obstruction and aspiration pneumonia.

22. While assisting with a delivery, you observe meconium staining in the fluids as the mother pushes during contractions. This is a clear indication of:

a. fetal distress.

b. preterm gestation.

c. postterm gestation.

d. aspirated meconium.

23. The ALS management of particulate meconium includes effectively clearing the baby's airway:
    a. by using a bulb syringe.
    b. by using a French catheter.
    c. with an ET tube and meconium aspirator.
    d. by using your smallest finger to sweep the mouth clear.

24. The condition in which hypoxia and persistent fetal circulation continue after birth, causing the newborn to become apneic and bradycardic, is called:
    a. primary apnea.
    b. secondary apnea.
    c. apnea of infancy.
    d. apnea of prematurity.

25. Which of the following signs indicates actual fetal distress?
    a. bradycardia
    b. fetal movement
    c. leaking amniotic fluid
    d. increased movement felt by the mother

26. Chest compressions should be provided when life-threatening bradycardia in the newborn falls below the rate of:
    a. 40 bpm.
    b. 60 bpm.
    c. 80 bpm.
    d. 100 bpm.

27. Immediately after the first Apgar score is evaluated on the newborn, a heart rate of 90 would be scored as _____ points.
    a. 0
    b. 1
    c. 2
    d. 3

28. _____ prevent(s) the alveoli (air sacs) from collapsing when a newborn inhales.
    a. Surfactant
    b. Drying and warmth
    c. Suctioning and stimulation
    d. Warm ambient temperatures

29. The premature newborn is at risk for developing hypoxia because of poorly developed lungs and:
    a. low birth weight.
    b. immature respiratory muscles.
    c. excessive amounts of surfactant.
    d. the increased frequency of meconium aspiration.

30. Neonates are prone to gastric and fluid distention due to immature digestive systems. The abdominal distention causes:
    a. belly breathing.
    b. hyperventilation.
    c. electrolyte imbalances.
    d. decreased lung capacity.

31. The most common complication of intubation associated with the neonate is:
    a. barotrauma.
    b. pneumothorax.
    c. a misplaced tube.
    d. abdominal distention.

32. Neonates can lose body heat rapidly because they:
    a. cannot easily stop shivering once they are warm.
    b. have a large amount of fat in relation to their muscle mass.
    c. have a large body surface area in relation to their weight.
    d. have a small body surface area in relation to their weight.

33. The EMT-I can help prevent heat loss in the newly born by:
    a. having the mother hold the baby.
    b. letting the mother breast-feed the baby.
    c. quickly drying the baby and removing wet linens.
    d. placing a heat pack on top of the head and under the arms.

34. The EMT-I should suspect possible hypothermia in the neonate when the mental status is not alert and the:
    a. baby is shivering.
    b. baby is postterm.
    c. ambient temperature is cool.
    d. baby's skin appears yellowish.

35. When the EMT-I suspects that a newborn is hypothermic, in addition to warming the baby she must be prepared to:
    a. manage vomiting and diarrhea.
    b. set up a temporary incubator for the transport.
    c. assess for and manage hypoxia and hypoglycemia.
    d. assess and compare oral and rectal temperatures.

36. The leading cause of cardiac arrest in the neonate is:
    a. respiratory arrest.
    b. fetal alcohol syndrome.
    c. prolonged suction postdelivery.
    d. trauma from the birthing process.

37. In the newborn, resuscitation chest compressions are provided:
    a. before the umbilical cord is cut.
    b. only after the baby fails a second Apgar score.
    c. at a rate of 15 compressions to 2 ventilations.
    d. after aggressive assisted ventilations are begun.

38. The first level of care for neonatal resuscitation include which steps of care?
    a. Administer epinephrine.
    b. Begin chest compressions.
    c. Dry, warm, suction, and stimulate.
    d. Provide positive pressure ventilations.

39. The essential elements of postarrest stabilization in the neonate are:
   a. warmth and oxygenation.
   b. oxygenation and fluid administration.
   c. suction and continued stimulation.
   d. prevention of hypoglycemia and seizures.

40. Which of the following actions is inappropriate for the EMT-I when caring for a neonate in critical condition who will not survive?
   a. expressing empathy
   b. avoiding any attempt to minimize the loss
   c. offering the family the opportunity to ask questions
   d. answering your cell phone while attending to the needs of the family

41. What is the emotional effect on the parents of a critically ill neonate when the EMT-I fails to learn the child's name?
   a. The EMT-I may appear rude.
   b. The parents could be offended.
   c. The EMT-I may appear impersonal.
   d. Any of the above.

42. You are about to begin transport of a neonate who is in cardiac arrest. You suspect that SIDS is the cause of the arrest. What action is appropriate to take with the parents before transporting the baby?
   a. Tell the parents to concentrate on their surviving children.
   b. Wait for the police to arrive to interview the parents at the residence.
   c. Tell them that their child is in asystole and that you need to leave immediately.
   d. Designate a provider to stay with the family to explain and answer questions.

43. Which of the following can help the parents or caregivers of an ill baby accept the role of the EMT-I and facilitate the giving and receiving of information?
   a. The EMT-I has a neat and professional appearance.
   b. The EMT-I introduces himself or herself to the parents right away.
   c. The dispatcher obtains key data and provides prearrival instructions.
   d. The EMT-I addresses the parents using appropriate titles and last names.

44. Your patient is 3 weeks old and appears to be very ill. The history from the mother indicates that the baby became sick suddenly. The father is extremely concerned and upset. In addition to managing the baby, what can you do to help the parents?
   a. Show sympathy for the parents.
   b. Let the mother attend to the father's distress.
   c. Be supportive and reassuring while caring for the baby.
   d. Include the parents in all aspects of assessment and treatment.

45. The most common causes of neonatal seizures are fever, infections, and:
   a. hypoxia.
   b. hypoglycemia.
   c. hyperthermia.
   d. low birth weight.

Chapter 27 Answer Form

	A	B	C	D		A	B	C	D
1.	❏	❏	❏	❏	24.	❏	❏	❏	❏
2.	❏	❏	❏	❏	25.	❏	❏	❏	❏
3.	❏	❏	❏	❏	26.	❏	❏	❏	❏
4.	❏	❏	❏	❏	27.	❏	❏	❏	❏
5.	❏	❏	❏	❏	28.	❏	❏	❏	❏
6.	❏	❏	❏	❏	29.	❏	❏	❏	❏
7.	❏	❏	❏	❏	30.	❏	❏	❏	❏
8.	❏	❏	❏	❏	31.	❏	❏	❏	❏
9.	❏	❏	❏	❏	32.	❏	❏	❏	❏
10.	❏	❏	❏	❏	33.	❏	❏	❏	❏
11.	❏	❏	❏	❏	34.	❏	❏	❏	❏
12.	❏	❏	❏	❏	35.	❏	❏	❏	❏
13.	❏	❏	❏	❏	36.	❏	❏	❏	❏
14.	❏	❏	❏	❏	37.	❏	❏	❏	❏
15.	❏	❏	❏	❏	38.	❏	❏	❏	❏
16.	❏	❏	❏	❏	39.	❏	❏	❏	❏
17.	❏	❏	❏	❏	40.	❏	❏	❏	❏
18.	❏	❏	❏	❏	41.	❏	❏	❏	❏
19.	❏	❏	❏	❏	42.	❏	❏	❏	❏
20.	❏	❏	❏	❏	43.	❏	❏	❏	❏
21.	❏	❏	❏	❏	44.	❏	❏	❏	❏
22.	❏	❏	❏	❏	45.	❏	❏	❏	❏
23.	❏	❏	❏	❏					

CHAPTER

28

Pediatrics

1. Which preventive measure can make the most difference in bicycle-related pediatric deaths?
   a. removing training wheels
   b. riding only on the sidewalk
   c. wearing a helmet when riding
   d. riding only with adult supervision

2. Unlike adults or older children, young children typically have a belly that protrudes because of:
   a. excess adipose tissue.
   b. an oversized large intestine.
   c. an oversized small intestine.
   d. immature abdominal muscles.

3. You need to perform a fingerstick for a blood sugar reading on a 5-year-old patient. What should you tell the child?
   a. Tell her it will hurt.
   b. Tell her not to cry.
   c. Tell her it won't hurt.
   d. Tell her she did not do anything wrong.

4. For the complex pediatric call, the EMT-I should have a plan that includes:
   a. managing the parent or caregiver first.
   b. managing emotionally distressed parents.
   c. the use of special pediatric transport child seats.
   d. the use of pediatric basic trauma life support (PBTLS).

5. What approach should the EMT-I use to keep both the child and the family calm when a critically injured child is causing a very emotional emergency scene?
   a. Maintain a calm approach.
   b. Use a command-and-directive approach.
   c. Maintain an aggressive, direct approach.
   d. Use a team approach to overwhelm and distract the family.

6. As a child grows older, his blood pressure will:
   a. increase.
   b. decrease.
   c. stay the same.
   d. be inconsistent.

7. One of the most important parameters used when assessing a pediatric patient's severity of illness or injury is:
   a. past medical history.
   b. the patient's general appearance.
   c. the first set of vital signs.
   d. body size and weight.

8. A sick or injured 5-year-old child requires positive pressure ventilation if her respiratory rate persists at a minimum rate above how many breaths per minute?
   a. 20
   b. 30
   c. 40
   d. 50

9. Using a blood pressure cuff that is too large for a child will:
   a. cause pain for the patient.
   b. cause a falsely low reading.
   c. cause a falsely high reading.
   d. embarrass the rescuer.

10. Children grow in four primary ways: physically, mentally, emotionally, and:
    a. socially.
    b. efficiently.
    c. economically.
    d. professionally.

11. Which airway adjunct is appropriate for an actively seizing 10-year-old male?
    a. oropharyngeal airway
    b. nasopharyngeal airway
    c. cuffed endotracheal tube
    d. uncuffed endotracheal tube

12. Which of the following is the most serious complication associated with improper use of an airway adjunct in an infant?
    a. hypoxia
    b. excessive drooling
    c. opening of the oropharynx
    d. bleeding from the soft palate

13. The appropriate ventilation device to use with a 4-year-old female who is intubated with a 4.0 uncuffed endotracheal tube is:

    a. a bag mask.
    b. a demand-valve resuscitator.
    c. an automatic transport ventilator (ATV).
    d. a flow-restricted, oxygen-powered ventilation device (FROPVD).

14. What effect does the onset of hypoxia have on children?

    a. They develop fever.
    b. They become dehydrated.
    c. Their breathing rate increases.
    d. Their breathing rate decreases.

15. When selecting the ET tube size for a small child, it is appropriate to:

    a. also have one size smaller and one size larger available.
    b. have two of each size available to choose from.
    c. consult medical control to confirm the appropriate size.
    d. document the size selected before inserting the device.

16. A common problem associated with ET tube placement in a small child is:

    a. gastric distention.
    b. gastric decompression.
    c. verifying tube placement.
    d. inability to visualize chest rise and fall.

17. Which of the following is the most accurate about pediatric respiratory distress?

    a. Cyanosis and mottling are early signs of respiratory distress.
    b. The respiratory rate itself is the best indicator of the severity of distress.
    c. Slow and gasping respirations are early signs of respiratory distress.
    d. A poor general appearance is a good indication of respiratory distress.

18. Respiratory failure occurs when the child is unable to:

    a. maintain a heart rate of 100 bpm or more.
    b. physically take a breath because of extreme fatigue.
    c. stop using accessory muscles of the neck and abdomen to breathe.
    d. maintain adequate O_2 and CO_2 levels in the blood to meet the body's needs.

19. The most common cause of cardiac arrest in children is:

    a. head injury.
    b. heart attack.
    c. respiratory arrest.
    d. fever and infection.

20. What is the leading medical complaint in children?

    a. fever
    b. vomiting
    c. diarrhea
    d. respiratory distress

21. The pediatric airway is proportionately smaller than the adult airway, which means that:

    a. children are easier to ventilate.
    b. the smaller airways are easier to suction.
    c. the tongue is never a possible cause of obstruction.
    d. even minor swelling in the airway can cause a complete obstruction.

22. When a 3-year-old suddenly develops respiratory distress or stridor, the EMT-I should suspect _____ first.

    a. croup
    b. epiglottitis
    c. an asthma attack
    d. an aspirated foreign body

23. For the small child with signs of respiratory distress, which of the following maneuvers should the EMT-I avoid, because it could cause a complete obstruction?

    a. startling the child
    b. manipulating the airway
    c. attempting to visualize the airway
    d. any of the above

24. Which of the following is an indication for gastric decompression in a child?

    a. hypoxia
    b. vomiting
    c. umbilical herniation
    d. endotracheal intubation

25. Which of the following respiratory conditions causes upper airway obstruction?

    a. croup
    b. asthma
    c. pneumonia
    d. bronchiolitis

26. What type of infection is most commonly associated with fever in children?

    a. viral
    b. fungal
    c. bacterial
    d. systemic

27. Croup may cause swelling of the _____, which can result in a partial airway obstruction.

    a. nares
    b. uvula
    c. tongue
    d. tissue under the epiglottis

28. A 2-year-old male has been sick with an ear infection for 2 days. He is taking antibiotics. At 10:00 p.m., he awoke with persistent coughing, a fever, and difficulty breathing. There is no drooling or wheezing, but he has nasal flaring. Which of the following conditions is most likely the cause of his problems?

    a. croup
    b. asthma
    c. bronchiolitis
    d. foreign body obstruction

29. (Continuing with the preceding question.) The initial management of this sick patient begins with high-flow oxygen (humidified if possible) and:

    a. examining the mouth and throat.
    b. getting him into the cool night air.
    c. calming him so he will be more comfortable.
    d. keeping him warm by wrapping him in blankets.

30. Which of the following is considered a cause of foreign body airway obstruction in the pediatric patient?

    a. asthma
    b. mucus
    c. epiglottitis
    d. meningitis

31. Once a foreign body has been removed from the airway and the patient is breathing adequately, there is still a risk of subsequent obstruction because of:

    a. tissue swelling.
    b. temporary hypoxia.
    c. transient asphyxia.
    d. all of the above.

32. Which of the following is an indication of a complete obstruction in a child with a suspected foreign body airway obstruction?

    a. stridor
    b. drooling
    c. wheezing
    d. unresponsiveness

33. At what age would the Heimlich maneuver (abdominal thrusts) be appropriate for a child who is choking and cannot expel the foreign object?

    a. 6 months and older
    b. 12 months and older
    c. the Heimlich maneuver is appropriate for any age
    d. the Heimlich maneuver is not appropriate for children less than 8 years of age

34. Which of the following is the most correct about children and epiglottitis?

    a. Epiglottitis is associated with a seal-like, barking cough.
    b. Epiglottitis occurs only in children less than 10 years of age.
    c. Epiglottitis is relatively rare, but is potentially life-threatening.
    d. Epiglottitis causes the tissue under the glottic opening to swell.

35. Epiglottitis is caused by:

    a. viral infection.
    b. fungal infection.
    c. traumatic injury.
    d. bacterial infection.

36. Which respiratory emergency is most common associated with drooling?

    a. croup
    b. epiglottitis
    c. bronchiolitis
    d. foreign body obstruction

37. When a child with severe respiratory distress has symptoms that could be associated with croup or epiglottitis, the EMT-I should:

    a. obtain a rectal temperature.
    b. provide rapid transport using lights and sirens.
    c. provide humidified oxygenation and keep the child calm.
    d. call medical control for help in making a specific diagnosis.

38. An 18-month-old infant has coughing, fever, tachypnea, rales, and consolidation in the left lower lobe. Which condition do you suspect?

    a. asthma
    b. epiglottitis
    c. pneumonia
    d. bronchiolitis

39. Allergies are most commonly associated with which respiratory emergency?

    a. asthma
    b. epiglottitis
    c. pneumonia
    d. bronchiolitis

40. Bronchiolitis typically occurs in children less than _____ years of age during the _____ seasons.

    a. 2; winter and spring
    b. 5; autumn and winter
    c. 8; spring and autumn
    d. 12; summer and winter

41. Which of the following conditions is produced by a viral infection and has symptoms that are often indistinguishable from those of asthma?
    a. epiglottitis
    b. pneumonia
    c. bronchiolitis
    d. foreign body obstruction

42. A patient with suspected pneumonia may have shallow respirations and decreased chest wall movement because:
    a. of carbon dioxide retention.
    b. this prevents fatigue and hypoxia.
    c. there is air trapping in the lungs.
    d. of sharp localized pain associated with movement.

43. A pediatrician's office has called for your ambulance to transport a child with pneumonia to the hospital. When you consider which PPE to use you take into account the incubation period for pneumonia, which is:
    a. 1 to 3 days.
    b. 5 to 7 days.
    c. 7 to 10 days.
    d. 2 weeks.

44. The treatment for a child with suspected pneumonia includes:
    a. keeping the child calm and providing high-concentration oxygen.
    b. being alert for air trapping and providing positive pressure ventilations.
    c. providing high-concentration oxygenation and warm packs on the chest.
    d. allowing the child to sit in tripod position and suctioning excessive drooling.

45. A child with early signs of asthma will attempt to compensate for air trapping by:
    a. coughing and drooling.
    b. decreasing the heart rate.
    c. increasing the rate and effort of breathing.
    d. decreasing expiratory wheezing and increasing inspiratory wheezing.

46. The third leading cause of preventable pediatric deaths in the United States is:
    a. burns.
    b. drowning.
    c. poisoning.
    d. bicycle accidents.

47. Aspiration pneumonia causes a foreign body lower airway obstruction in children as a result of:
    a. inhaling vomitus.
    b. uncontrolled seizures.
    c. severe local infection.
    d. severe system infection.

48. Which of the following signs or symptoms is an indication of a foreign body lower airway obstruction in a 2-year-old?
    a. drooling and coughing
    b. stridor and hoarseness
    c. sudden onset of unilateral wheezing
    d. sudden onset of a seal-like, barking cough

49. Which of the following is a major contributing factor to foreign body lower airway obstruction in children?
    a. asthma
    b. meningitis
    c. submersion
    d. abuse or neglect

50. Each of the following is a common cause of shock in infants and children, except:
    a. SIDS.
    b. burns.
    c. dehydration.
    d. poison ingestion.

51. One of the best indicators of the severity of shock in an infant or child is:
    a. mental status.
    b. the SpO_2 reading.
    c. the blood pressure.
    d. the past medical history.

52. Blood loss, even from a minor injury, is more significant in a child because:
    a. children have less blood volume.
    b. children get faint at the sight of blood.
    c. their blood loss is difficult to measure.
    d. children have immature coping mechanisms.

53. Infants compensate for shock by:
    a. decreasing insulin production.
    b. increasing thermoregulatory effort.
    c. increasing peripheral vascular resistance.
    d. increasing their heart and respiratory rates.

54. An infant has cold hands and feet in a warm ambient temperature. This finding may indicate:
    a. shock.
    b. poisoning.
    c. hypoglycemia.
    d. hyperglycemia.

55. A 4-year-old was struck by a vehicle and now has an altered mental status and signs of shock. On the scene, she was immobilized and given high-concentration oxygen by non-rebreather mask. Her vital signs are: respiratory rate 28/clear breath sounds; pulse rate 120 bpm/weak; and BP 90/60. Skin CTC is pale, cool extremities, and capillary refill of 5 seconds. What action is appropriate next?

    a. intubate
    b. begin CPR
    c. begin rapid transport
    d. establish IV access prior to transport

56. Your pediatric patient is in cardiac arrest with a rhythm of asystole or pulseless electrical activity (PEA). He fails to respond to initial airway, breathing, and circulation interventions. The first appropriate medication to administer is:

    a. insulin.
    b. atropine.
    c. glucagon.
    d. epinephrine.

57. The key factor for the management of a child in pulseless ventricular tachycardia or ventricular fibrillation is rapid:

    a. warming.
    b. transport.
    c. intubation.
    d. defibrillation.

58. When the EMT-I recognizes that a child has a dysrhythmia, the appropriate treatment will depend on the EMT-I's ability to:

    a. obtain vascular access.
    b. intubate and administer medications.
    c. recognize when the patient is stable or unstable.
    d. include the parents in deciding the treatment options.

59. The correct amount of joules, on the first shock, to defibrillate a child who is in ventricular fibrillation is:

    a. 200 J.
    b. 0.5 J per kilogram.
    c. 1 J per kilogram.
    d. 2 J per kilogram.

60. Which of the following conditions will *not* typically produce sinus tachycardia in infants?

    a. fever
    b. anxiety
    c. hypovolemia
    d. inadequate tissue oxygenation

61. Which of the following is of concern in a 2-month-old with tachycardia?

    a. strong crying
    b. rate of 200 bpm
    c. narrow QRS complex
    d. capillary refill of more than 2 seconds

62. A 6-month-old infant was born with a congenital heart defect. EMS was called because the child had been sick with a respiratory infection for the past few days, but today there was a significant change in the child's behavior. She is very restless and is sweaty. What finding is of immediate concern?

    a. wide QRS complex
    b. narrow QRS complex
    c. capillary refill of more than 2 seconds
    d. temperature of 102.5°F

63. Tachycardia, together with signs of poor perfusion, in the infant or child is associated with:

    a. sepsis.
    b. crying.
    c. seizures.
    d. cardiac arrest.

64. The primary cause of bradycardia in a child is:

    a. hypoxia.
    b. infection.
    c. hypovolemia.
    d. hypothermia.

65. The most common hypoxia induced pediatric dysrhythmia is:

    a. asystole.
    b. bradycardia.
    c. ventricular fibrillation.
    d. supraventricular tachycardia (SVT).

66. You are dispatched for a possible overdose to the home of a 14-month-old boy. The grandmother tells you that she found the baby chewing pills from her prescription heart medication about 30 minutes ago. The patient is unresponsive, breathing is shallow, skin color is cyanotic and mottled, capillary refill time is 4 seconds. Vital signs are: respiratory rate 16/irregular; pulse rate 56/regular; and BP is 60 systolic. What do you suspect is the problem?

    a. beta blocker ingestion
    b. full airway obstruction
    c. partial airway obstruction
    d. head injury from physical abuse

67. (Continuing with the preceding question) What are your first actions in the care of this patient?

    a. Ventilate with high-concentration oxygen.
    b. Obtain vascular access and administer epinephrine.
    c. Obtain an ECG, glucose reading, and temperature.
    d. Suction the airway and attempt to clear the foreign body obstruction.

68. (Continuing with the preceding two questions) After your initial actions, what should you reassess first to determine if your interventions are working?
    a. heart rate
    b. respiratory rate
    c. pulse oximetry
    d. capillary refill

69. When a bradycardia in a pediatric patient is not recognized quickly and treated appropriately, the effect will be:
    a. deterioration to asystole.
    b. onset of hypoxic seizures.
    c. a loss of peripheral vascular resistance.
    d. increased peripheral vascular resistance.

70. Which of the following is the most accurate about the compression/ventilation ratio of CPR for an infant?
    a. A ratio of 3:1 is most effective for infants.
    b. A ratio of 5:1 provides more ventilations per minute than a ratio of 15:2.
    c. A ratio of 15:2 provides more ventilations per minute than a ratio of 5:1.
    d. More compressions than ventilations are appropriate for infants.

71. Appropriate parameters for performing adequate CPR on an infant or child include:
    a. rate.
    b. depth.
    c. full chest recoil.
    d. all of the above.

72. How does ALS treatment for a pediatric cardiac arrest differ from treatment of an adult?
    a. Treatment is based on weight or size.
    b. Defibrillation is not used on children less than 8 years old.
    c. Epinephrine is the only medication used in pediatric cardiac arrest.
    d. Airway management for vomiting during a cardiac arrest is necessary only in adults.

73. In which age group are children most susceptible to seizures?
    a. newly born to neonate
    b. 3 months to 3 years
    c. 6 years to 12 years
    d. adolescence

74. Febrile seizures are caused by:
    a. electrolyte disturbances.
    b. a sudden, rapid rise in body temperature.
    c. a sudden rise in intracranial pressure.
    d. a rise in temperature to more than 101°F.

75. You have responded to a call for a possible seizure. The mother says that she was driving when she looked in the rear-view mirror at her son in his car seat. She states that his eyes were rolled back in his head and he appeared to have stopped breathing. By the time she pulled over to the side of the road, he was breathing again, but was very tired. She called 9-1-1. There is no history of seizures, but the child has been sick with an ear infection. He is hot to the touch and is drooling. What do you suspect is the cause of the apnea?
    a. hypoxia
    b. ear infection
    c. febrile seizure
    d. secretions in the airway

76. (Continuing with the preceding question) What is your management plan for this child?
    a. Administer high-concentration oxygen with assisted ventilations.
    b. Administer acetaminophen for the fever and infection.
    c. Suction the airway and remove excess clothing.
    d. Suction the airway and intubate.

77. The most dangerous diabetic problem in a pediatric patient is:
    a. a hypoglycemic event.
    b. a hyperglycemic event.
    c. new-onset diabetes mellitus type I.
    d. new-onset diabetes mellitus type II.

78. Hypoglycemia may be induced in a child by:
    a. overeating.
    b. giving the child aspirin.
    c. giving too much insulin.
    d. not giving enough insulin.

79. The normal range of blood glucose for a 5-year-old is _____ mg/dL.
    a. 50–100
    b. 80–120
    c. 80–140
    d. 100–120

80. The appropriate medication and dose for a 6-year-old who is experiencing a hypoglycemic event is:
    a. dextrose 5.5 percent/10 grams.
    b. dextrose 10 percent/10 grams.
    c. dextrose 25 percent/25 grams.
    d. dextrose 50 percent/25 grams.

81. Treatment of the pediatric patient who is experiencing hyperglycemia is directed at reducing the blood glucose level and:
    a. rehydration.
    b. hyperventilation.
    c. correcting hypoxia.
    d. alleviating muscle cramps.

82. Hyperglycemia in a child is often associated with:
    a. shortness of breath.
    b. increased physical stress.
    c. undiagnosed new onset of diabetes mellitus.
    d. giving too much insulin without adequate food intake.

83. The first clue that should make the EMT-I suspect that an illness is related to diabetes in a pediatric patient is:
    a. seizure activity.
    b. altered mental status.
    c. vomiting lasting more than 12 hours.
    d. a blood glucose reading of 200 mg/dL.

84. Signs and symptoms of diabetic ketoacidosis include:
    a. bradycardia and nausea.
    b. pale, moist, and cool skin.
    c. increased thirst and hunger.
    d. decreased thirst and hunger.

85. You must establish vascular access in a 4-year-old patient who needs a fluid bolus. At which site should you attempt access first?
    a. scalp vein
    b. saphenous vein
    c. antecubital fossa
    d. lateral aspect of the tibial tuberosity

86. Intraosseous infusion is inappropriate in which of the following instances?
    a. a 2-year-old in severe shock
    b. a 6-month-old's suspected SIDS death
    c. a 3-year-old with epiglottitis who is crying
    d. a 4-year-old who was found in water and is in cardiac arrest

87. One of the major complications of vascular access in the pediatric patient in the prehospital setting is _____, which can actually worsen the patient's condition.
    a. pain
    b. sepsis
    c. phlebitis
    d. pulmonary embolism

88. The most lethal mechanism of injury in children is _____, which cause(s) head injury.
    a. falls
    b. drownings
    c. sports-related
    d. gunshot wounds

89. One major anatomical difference between children and adults is softer bones. This significant difference must be considered when caring for child victims of traumatic injury, because:
    a. broken bones will heal much faster in a child.
    b. broken bones are easier to assess in a child.
    c. a child's bones are better able to protect the underlying organs.
    d. a child's bones cannot protect the underlying organs as effectively as in an adult.

90. The most important intervention the EMT-I can provide for a pediatric patient with a head injury is:
    a. to keep the child from having a seizure.
    b. management of the airway and ventilation.
    c. to determine if the child was wearing a helmet.
    d. cervical stabilization and immobilization of the spine.

91. Which of the following statements about immobilizing a child with suspected spinal injury in a child safety seat is most accurate?
    a. Safety seats can be used as an immobilization device only when the child is stable and less than 2 years of age.
    b. Safety seats should never be used to immobilize a child with a suspected spinal injury.
    c. When the patient is stable, the safety seat can be used as an immobilization device even when there is damage to the safety seat.
    d. The patient must be in stable condition, and the safety seat must be adequately secured in the ambulance when used as an immobilization device.

92. Which two IV fluids are preferred for field resuscitation of the hypovolemic child?
    a. D5W and normal saline
    b. plasmanate and dextran
    c. normal saline and Ringer's lactate
    d. Ringer's lactate and hypertonic saline

93. What two fracture sites are most often associated with significant blood loss?
    a. hip and skull
    b. skull and femur
    c. skull and pelvis
    d. femur and pelvis

94. You are assessing a 4-year-old female who had been choking when EMS was called. Currently she has no distress. When you listen to lung sounds, you observe that the child has a large, yellowish-green bruise on her back. How old is the bruise?
    a. new today
    b. two days
    c. about a week
    d. one month

95. You are immobilizing an 18-month-old infant who fell down a flight of stairs. What technique can you use to keep the proportionately large head of the child in proper alignment?

    a. Flex the head forward slightly.

    b. Extend the head backward slightly.

    c. Place a towel under the infant's shoulders.

    d. Lay the child on a blanket first, then pad the voids.

96. A 3-year-old fell from a second-story window and appears to have a serious head injury. Blood and cerebrospinal fluid (CSF) are draining from the right ear. What type of skull fracture do you suspect the patient has?

    a. basilar

    b. frontal

    c. occipital

    d. temporal

97. An uncle who exposes himself to or fondles a 6-year-old niece is guilty of:

    a. child neglect.

    b. sexual abuse.

    c. physical abuse.

    d. failure to provide a safe environment.

98. Which of the following is an example of child neglect?

    a. denying a child proper nourishment

    b. exposing a child to pornography on the Internet

    c. multiple bruises of various ages on a child

    d. an injured child who is not comforted by a parent

99. The number of reported incidents of child abuse in the United States is:

    a. greatly overreported.

    b. more than 3 million reports a year.

    c. more than 6 million reports a year.

    d. more than 10 million reports a year.

100. What is the most common type of injury associated with child abuse?

    a. fractures

    b. brain injury

    c. soft tissue injury

    d. internal hemorrhage

101. The initial assessment and focused physical exam of a suspected child abuse victim is:

    a. performed in a more guarded manner.

    b. the same as for any other ill or injured child.

    c. directed at the most common site of injury, the head.

    d. best completed in the ambulance, apart from the suspected abuser.

102. The unexpected death of an infant from an unexplained cause is:

    a. Reyes syndrome.

    b. a potential homicide.

    c. apnea of infancy (AOI).

    d. defined as sudden infant death syndrome (SIDS).

103. Emotional reactions by the parents to the death of their child may include:

    a. guilt and blame.

    b. anger and frustration.

    c. shock and disbelief.

    d. all of the above.

104. The greatest incidence of SIDS occurs during which months?

    a. spring

    b. summer

    c. winter

    d. autumn

105. The cause of SIDS is unknown and:

    a. there are no symptoms.

    b. a family history of SIDS is not a risk factor.

    c. it only occurs in infants less than 6 months of age.

    d. it only occurs in infants greater than 6 months of age.

106. You are dispatched for an infant cardiac arrest. Upon arrival, it is apparent that the child has been dead for a while. The parents are insisting that you do anything possible for the child. What should you do?

    a. Provide hope and reassurance.

    b. Avoid approaching the parents.

    c. Consider that the parents are to blame.

    d. Provide psychological support to the parents or caregivers.

107. In addition to providing psychological and emotional support for the parents of a baby who has died of SIDS, the EMT-I must:

    a. consider the effect on the responders.

    b. evaluate any other children in the residence.

    c. complete a special incident report for the police.

    d. provide specific information about the call for research.

108. During which developmental age might a child believe that his or her illness or injury is a punishment for being bad?

    a. infant

    b. toddler

    c. school age

    d. adolescent

109. A child does not like to be touched by strangers or separated from his parents or caregivers. In what developmental age group is this child most likely to be?

    a. newborn
    b. infant
    c. toddler
    d. school age

110. Why should a teenage patient sometimes be interviewed without a parent or caregiver present?

    a. The patient will have more autonomy.
    b. The patient may be more open with you.
    c. You may be able to alleviate separation anxiety without the parents present.
    d. The patient will respect you more because you are treating her like an adult.

Chapter 28 Answer Form

	A	B	C	D			A	B	C	D
1.	❏	❏	❏	❏		26.	❏	❏	❏	❏
2.	❏	❏	❏	❏		27.	❏	❏	❏	❏
3.	❏	❏	❏	❏		28.	❏	❏	❏	❏
4.	❏	❏	❏	❏		29.	❏	❏	❏	❏
5.	❏	❏	❏	❏		30.	❏	❏	❏	❏
6.	❏	❏	❏	❏		31.	❏	❏	❏	❏
7.	❏	❏	❏	❏		32.	❏	❏	❏	❏
8.	❏	❏	❏	❏		33.	❏	❏	❏	❏
9.	❏	❏	❏	❏		34.	❏	❏	❏	❏
10.	❏	❏	❏	❏		35.	❏	❏	❏	❏
11.	❏	❏	❏	❏		36.	❏	❏	❏	❏
12.	❏	❏	❏	❏		37.	❏	❏	❏	❏
13.	❏	❏	❏	❏		38.	❏	❏	❏	❏
14.	❏	❏	❏	❏		39.	❏	❏	❏	❏
15.	❏	❏	❏	❏		40.	❏	❏	❏	❏
16.	❏	❏	❏	❏		41.	❏	❏	❏	❏
17.	❏	❏	❏	❏		42.	❏	❏	❏	❏
18.	❏	❏	❏	❏		43.	❏	❏	❏	❏
19.	❏	❏	❏	❏		44.	❏	❏	❏	❏
20.	❏	❏	❏	❏		45.	❏	❏	❏	❏
21.	❏	❏	❏	❏		46.	❏	❏	❏	❏
22.	❏	❏	❏	❏		47.	❏	❏	❏	❏
23.	❏	❏	❏	❏		48.	❏	❏	❏	❏
24.	❏	❏	❏	❏		49.	❏	❏	❏	❏
25.	❏	❏	❏	❏		50.	❏	❏	❏	❏

	A	B	C	D			A	B	C	D
51.	❏	❏	❏	❏		81.	❏	❏	❏	❏
52.	❏	❏	❏	❏		82.	❏	❏	❏	❏
53.	❏	❏	❏	❏		83.	❏	❏	❏	❏
54.	❏	❏	❏	❏		84.	❏	❏	❏	❏
55.	❏	❏	❏	❏		85.	❏	❏	❏	❏
56.	❏	❏	❏	❏		86.	❏	❏	❏	❏
57.	❏	❏	❏	❏		87.	❏	❏	❏	❏
58.	❏	❏	❏	❏		88.	❏	❏	❏	❏
59.	❏	❏	❏	❏		89.	❏	❏	❏	❏
60.	❏	❏	❏	❏		90.	❏	❏	❏	❏
61.	❏	❏	❏	❏		91.	❏	❏	❏	❏
62.	❏	❏	❏	❏		92.	❏	❏	❏	❏
63.	❏	❏	❏	❏		93.	❏	❏	❏	❏
64.	❏	❏	❏	❏		94.	❏	❏	❏	❏
65.	❏	❏	❏	❏		95.	❏	❏	❏	❏
66.	❏	❏	❏	❏		96.	❏	❏	❏	❏
67.	❏	❏	❏	❏		97.	❏	❏	❏	❏
68.	❏	❏	❏	❏		98.	❏	❏	❏	❏
69.	❏	❏	❏	❏		99.	❏	❏	❏	❏
70.	❏	❏	❏	❏		100.	❏	❏	❏	❏
71.	❏	❏	❏	❏		101.	❏	❏	❏	❏
72.	❏	❏	❏	❏		102.	❏	❏	❏	❏
73.	❏	❏	❏	❏		103.	❏	❏	❏	❏
74.	❏	❏	❏	❏		104.	❏	❏	❏	❏
75.	❏	❏	❏	❏		105.	❏	❏	❏	❏
76.	❏	❏	❏	❏		106.	❏	❏	❏	❏
77.	❏	❏	❏	❏		107.	❏	❏	❏	❏
78.	❏	❏	❏	❏		108.	❏	❏	❏	❏
79.	❏	❏	❏	❏		109.	❏	❏	❏	❏
80.	❏	❏	❏	❏		110.	❏	❏	❏	❏

CHAPTER

Geriatrics

1. Where elderly patients live is often a function of how well they can perform activities of daily living. Select the task that is *not* considered an activity of daily living.
   a. baking
   b. bathing
   c. grooming
   d. ambulating

2. Which of the following resources available to the elderly patient living at home is run under medical supervision?
   a. adult day care
   b. social day care
   c. nutrition services
   d. hospice programs

3. Which of the following physiologic changes is abnormal or inconsistent with the aging process?
   a. development of dementia
   b. decreased brain mass
   c. altered temperature regulation
   d. conduction system abnormalities

4. As a person ages, a decreased catecholamine response affects the ability of the heart to:
   a. resist the effects of coronary artery disease.
   b. keep the normal pacemaker functioning properly.
   c. regulate the strength of contractions during exertion.
   d. increase the rate in response to stress and exercise.

5. The risk of falls and motor vehicle collisions is higher in the elderly population primarily because of:
   a. declining immune function.
   b. declining cognitive functioning.
   c. reduced sight and sluggish reflexes.
   d. reduced hearing and color blindness.

6. As a result of age-related changes to the genitourinary system, the patient may have:
   a. incontinence.
   b. decreased blood flow.
   c. increased elimination of waste.
   d. decreased urinary tract infections.

7. Your patient has a hearing impairment and appears to be confused. What can you do to give psychological support when such factors make assessment difficult?
   a. Respect the patient's modesty.
   b. Explain to the patient what you are doing.
   c. Plan on taking extra time to complete your tasks.
   d. All of the above.

8. While performing a physical examination on an elderly patient, the EMT-I must use a gentle technique so as not to:
   a. cause the patient any additional injury.
   b. force the patient to receive unwanted care.
   c. overwhelm the patient with specialized exam equipment.
   d. cause concern for any family member or caretaker who may be observing.

9. The most common complications of osteoporosis include spinal fractures and:
   a. stroke.
   b. hip fractures.
   c. deep vein thrombosis.
   d. pulmonary embolism.

10. Why do elderly patients sometimes develop drug toxicity from a prescribed medication even when they take the exact amount prescribed at the right time?
    a. Diseases can slow the absorption of the medication, leaving too much in the system.
    b. Many medications cause constipation, which prevents proper elimination of medications.
    c. Gastrointestinal problems, which are chronic in the elderly, can cause malabsorption of medications.
    d. Many elderly patients have undiagnosed thyroid disease, which causes problems with metabolism.

11. Compliance with a medication regimen is a common problem in the elderly because:
    a. they skip doses to save money.
    b. they forget to take their medications.
    c. they have few resources to obtain more medications.
    d. all of the above.

12. As a rule, body systems become less effective with aging. The musculoskeletal system is directly affected by:
    a. increased bone density.
    b. increased muscle tone.
    c. increased sense of balance.
    d. decreased muscle and bone mass.

13. You are assessing a 69-year-old female with a chief complaint of difficulty breathing that has been getting worse over the past 2 days. She is overweight, has a history of congestive heart failure, and does not move much from her recliner except to use the bathroom. She also has new pleuritic chest pain and describes chronic pain in the lower left leg. Which of the following conditions should you suspect first?
    a. pneumonia
    b. emphysema
    c. chronic bronchitis
    d. pulmonary embolism

14. Common emergencies in Parkinson's patients result from all of the following, except:
    a. falls.
    b. dementia.
    c. difficulty swallowing.
    d. unilateral facial paralysis.

15. You are obtaining a focused history from a 68-year-old male with a new GI bleed. Which of his medications could be the cause of the GI bleed?
    a. Colace
    b. codeine
    c. ibuprofen
    d. oxycodone

16. You are dispatched to a nursing home for a traumatic injury. The patient is an 81-year-old male, who is sitting on the floor with a laceration on his forehead from a fall. His chief complaint is pain at the site of the injury. He is alert and says "I just tipped back and fell down." He denies shortness of breath, chest pain, dizziness, and loss of consciousness. The nurse leaves to get his paperwork. While you consider the possible causes of the fall, you begin to treat the patient by:
    a. controlling the bleeding.
    b. laying the patient supine on the floor.
    c. providing manual cervical immobilization.
    d. administering high-concentration oxygen.

17. (Continuing with the preceding question) Your partner obtains the following vital signs: respiratory rate 22/nonlabored; pulse rate 54/regular; and BP 130/50. Skin signs are pale, warm, and dry. During the rapid trauma exam, your partner finds that the patient also injured his left knee. The nurse returns with the paperwork, which includes a list of his medications, and states that the patient had knee surgery 4 days ago. He is taking a beta blocker for hypertension, analgesia for arthritis, and a stool softener. With the information you have so far, what is the most likely cause of the fall?
    a. The analgesia could have made the patient uncoordinated.
    b. The beta blocker could be slowing the heart rate, causing weakness.
    c. The patient cannot ambulate effectively because of the recent surgery.
    d. There is not enough information to narrow down the cause of the fall.

18. Because the elderly often have problems metabolizing medications, the EMT-I should assume that a patient's medication could be contributing to just about any health problem. Which of the following types of medication requires frequent monitoring by testing the levels in the blood?
    a. the antibiotic amoxicillin
    b. the antidiuretic furosemide
    c. the antidysrhythmic digitalis
    d. the antihypertensive ramipril

19. Your patient's daughter called EMS because she found her mother confused when she stopped in for today's visit. She describes finding her mother sitting in a warm bedroom, in bed, with several layers of clothing on but still shivering and cold to the touch. When there is no obvious environmental explanation, the EMT-I should assume that hypothermia in the elderly is caused by:
    a. hypoglycemia.
    b. hypothyroidism.
    c. severe infection.
    d. adverse medication reaction.

20. Physiological changes in the respiratory system that occur with aging include a decrease in airway cilia and diminished cough and gag reflexes. These changes increase the risk of:
    a. sustaining rib fractures with coughing.
    b. obtaining infectious pulmonary diseases.
    c. diminishing the inflammatory response.
    d. lung shrinkage (atrophy) and compliance.

21. When caring for an elderly patient who was injured in a fall, your critical actions must include:
    a. searching for an underlying medical cause of the fall.
    b. determining if the patient has been hospitalized recently.
    c. transporting the patient to a hospital that specializes in geriatrics.
    d. determining if the patient has had any similar falls in the last 6 months.

22. Semi-independent living, with meals and some medical monitoring provided for the resident, is an example of what type of nursing home?
    a. skilled nursing facility
    b. residential care facility
    c. senior retirement facility
    d. intermediate care facility

23. How do affective disorders such as forgetfulness or difficulty following directions increase the risk of injury in the elderly?
    a. They obscure normal physiological changes.
    b. They interfere with the tasks of daily living.
    c. They limit the caretaker's ability to access the patient.
    d. They increase the risk of developing concurrent illnesses.

24. Your patient has a terminal condition and has been placed on palliative care. This means that the patient:
    a. is living in a hospice community.
    b. does not wish to be resuscitated.
    c. is receiving care to relieve suffering.
    d. does not wish to receive emergency care.

25. When assessing an elderly patient who has fallen, do not forget the possibility of neglect or abuse. The most common abusers of the elderly are:
    a. friends.
    b. family.
    c. landlords.
    d. neighbors.

Chapter 29 Answer Form

	A	B	C	D
1.	❑	❑	❑	❑
2.	❑	❑	❑	❑
3.	❑	❑	❑	❑
4.	❑	❑	❑	❑
5.	❑	❑	❑	❑
6.	❑	❑	❑	❑
7.	❑	❑	❑	❑
8.	❑	❑	❑	❑
9.	❑	❑	❑	❑
10.	❑	❑	❑	❑
11.	❑	❑	❑	❑
12.	❑	❑	❑	❑
13.	❑	❑	❑	❑

	A	B	C	D
14.	❑	❑	❑	❑
15.	❑	❑	❑	❑
16.	❑	❑	❑	❑
17.	❑	❑	❑	❑
18.	❑	❑	❑	❑
19.	❑	❑	❑	❑
20.	❑	❑	❑	❑
21.	❑	❑	❑	❑
22.	❑	❑	❑	❑
23.	❑	❑	❑	❑
24.	❑	❑	❑	❑
25.	❑	❑	❑	❑

CHAPTER

30

Assessment-Based Management

1. Assessment is the cornerstone of patient care and is critical to:
   a. the EMT-I's attitude.
   b. arranging protocols.
   c. manpower considerations.
   d. the decision-making process.

2. Which of the following can lead to the EMT-I obstructing the assessment process?
   a. being nonjudgmental and objective
   b. classifying patients by their social status
   c. having an unbiased attitude about a patient
   d. approaching a patient with an impartial mindset

3. The prehospital assessment of a patient may be hindered when a patient is uncooperative. One of the most common reasons for an ill or injured patient to be uncooperative is:
   a. hypoxia.
   b. modesty.
   c. arrogance.
   d. tunnel vision.

4. Labeling a patient is a serious problem because it is unfair to the patient and:
   a. can lead to protocol violations.
   b. the patient can be improperly exposed.
   c. the patient may not get the full medical attention deserved.
   d. may influence the next caregiver to think about the patient in the same way.

5. Environmental distractions can make it difficult for the EMT-I to complete a thorough assessment. What can the EMT-I do to better focus on the assessment when such distractions are present?
   a. Have the EMS supervisor respond to the scene to help.
   b. Ask the patient what has worked best for her in the past.
   c. Follow a regular sequence when performing an assessment.
   d. Wait until the patient is in the ambulance to perform the assessment.

6. When an EMS crew consists of two or more members, the EMT-I can ensure that the assessment process is efficient by:
   a. assessing by committee.
   b. interviewing the patient herself.
   c. performing the entire assessment herself.
   d. delegating management tasks to crew members.

7. During the call, the EMT-I will gather information, and then evaluate and process that information to:
   a. diagnose a patient's illness or injury.
   b. provide the definitive care the patient requires.
   c. make the appropriate patient management decisions.
   d. improve the quality of life for a patient with a chronic disease.

8. The team leader is usually the EMT-I who will:
   a. give the patient presentation at the ED.
   b. act as the triage group leader at an MCI.
   c. drive the crew and patient to the hospital.
   d. decontaminate the ambulance after a call.

9. What equipment should the EMT-I bring to the side of every patient?
   a. no more than two pieces of equipment per crew member
   b. the minimal amount of equipment needed to run a cardiac arrest
   c. the type of call will help determine what equipment to bring to the patient
   d. any equipment needed to conduct the initial assessment and manage the ABCs.

10. Your unit is dispatched for a 20-year-old female with injuries from a dog bite. While en route to the call, you discuss with your partner what you will do once you arrive at the residence. What minimal equipment will you initially need for this call?

   a. hemorrhage control items, ice pack, and a splint
   b. Mace, leather gloves, and equipment to manage the ABCs
   c. dog treats, eye protection, and equipment to manage the ABCs
   d. equipment to conduct the initial assessment and manage the ABCs

11. The EMT-I's general approach for the patient who is experiencing a medical emergency includes:

   a. diagnosing the patient's illness.
   b. maintaining a calm, orderly demeanor.
   c. providing definitive care to the patient.
   d. carrying the least amount of equipment possible to the patient.

12. When speaking on a portable radio, the EMT-I must:

   a. request permission to transmit.
   b. encode the message prior to speaking.
   c. depress the microphone button for a moment before speaking.
   d. decode the message prior to depressing the microphone button.

13. The general approach to use with a patient who is complaining of chest pain is to:

   a. administer nitroglycerin as soon as possible, to help relieve the pain.
   b. manage the patient as if the pain is cardiac pain, until proven otherwise.
   c. aggressively manage the patient as if he may deteriorate into cardiac arrest.
   d. attempt to find another cause of the chest pain before treating the patient for a cardiac problem.

14. Which of the following is the most correct about the general approach to the patient in cardiac arrest (with either a medical or a traumatic cause)?

   a. Only a pediatric cardiac arrest is transported by helicopter.
   b. Only a medical cardiac arrest is transported by helicopter.
   c. Only a traumatic cardiac arrest is transported by helicopter.
   d. Cardiac arrest patients are generally not transported by helicopter.

15. The patient who presents with acute abdominal pain should get nothing by mouth (NPO), because the emergent condition may require surgery and:

   a. pain medication works best on an empty stomach.
   b. stomach contents impede diagnostic testing.
   c. the release of digestive enzymes often worsens the condition.
   d. the use of pain medication is contraindicated on a full stomach.

16. The initial treatment of a patient presenting with gastrointestinal bleeding begins with the administration of high-concentration oxygen and:

   a. pain management.
   b. treatment for shock.
   c. nasogastric tube placement.
   d. rapid transport to the nearest ED.

17. The general approach to management of the patient presenting with an altered mental status is to:

   a. look for evidence of recent trauma.
   b. determine if the patient is intoxicated.
   c. determine if the patient is having a stroke.
   d. rule out hypoxia and hypoglycemia as soon as possible.

18. What should the EMT-I's first priority be in any respiratory emergency?

   a. doing a scene size-up
   b. administering high-concentration oxygen
   c. recognizing signs of imminent respiratory arrest
   d. distinguishing an airway obstruction as upper or lower

19. When managing a trauma patient or patients, the EMT-I should ensure that the assessment progresses quickly and effectively by:

   a. completing a detailed physical exam for non-life- or limb-threatening injuries.
   b. making the appropriate decision regarding the application of a cervical collar.
   c. fully understanding the mechanism of injury (MOI) before treating the patient.
   d. ensuring that the scene is safe, completing a scene size-up, and evaluating the MOI.

20. The general approach to management of the patient who presents with an allergic reaction is to:

   a. rapidly administer subcutaneous epinephrine.
   b. determine the need for albuterol and corticosteroids.
   c. rapidly determine if the patient's symptoms are life-threatening.
   d. determine if the patient has ever had a severe allergic reaction in the past.

21. The key to obtaining an accurate patient assessment and providing the most appropriate medical care to a pediatric patient is to:

a. approach the patient as you would an adult.

b. modify your approach according to the age of the patient.

c. include the parent or caregiver in every aspect of assessment.

d. include a thorough survey of the child's home environment in your assessment.

22. The high-level clinical decision-making skills that the EMT-I uses in patient management draw on a combination of sources, including the patient's history, the physical examination findings, recognition of patterns, the EMT-I's field impression, and:

a. interpretation of ECG rhythm strips.

b. unbiased documentation of all patient care.

c. comprehension of existing BLS or ALS treatment protocols.

d. all of the above.

23. The key to performing an effective and complete patient assessment on all patients is to:

a. complete a detailed physical examination.

b. be organized and systematic in your approach.

c. demonstrate empathy and therapeutic communication.

d. get a complete health history before leaving the scene.

24. The general approach to management of the elderly patient who is experiencing a medical or traumatic emergency is to:

a. consider that serious problems are often taken too lightly.

b. remember that normal physiological changes can obscure findings during the assessment.

c. assess functional or physical limitations as part of prehospital management.

d. be concerned about all of the above.

25. How can the EMT-I use protocols in critical decision making regarding patient care?

a. Protocols are used as guidelines for care.

b. Protocols are the standard of care and should never be deviated from.

c. Protocols are a cookbook list of what the EMT-I must do on every call.

d. Protocols help the EMT-I arrive at the appropriate field impression of a patient.

26. Your unit was dispatched, with fire department first responders, for a call of difficulty breathing. When you arrive at the residence, the first responders are placing a non-rebreather mask on an elderly male who is in bed, unresponsive and gasping for breath. You come closer and assess that his airway is open and clear. With auscultation, you find that there is no air movement, the distal pulse is weak and fast, and his skin CTC is pale, warm, and dry. The patient's home is five minutes from a hospital. What steps do you take next?

a. Quickly move the patient to the ambulance for rapid transport.

b. Insert an NPA and replace the non-rebreather mask on the patient.

c. Attempt to insert an OPA and be prepared to suction if the patient vomits.

d. Begin ventilations using a bag mask and hyperventilate the patient in preparation for intubation.

27. You are dispatched on a high-priority call to a local nursing home for a patient with altered mental status. When you arrive, the staff is busy taking care of other residents, but one points you in the direction of the patient's room. You see a woman lying in bed who appears conscious. As you attempt to talk to her, a nurse comes in and states that the patient fell out of bed during the night; the patient denied any injury at the time of the fall, so they put her back to bed. This morning the patient has a decreased mental status and the following vital signs: guarded shallow respirations at a rate of 10; pulse 62/regular; and BP 100/60. Skin CTC is cyanotic, warm, and dry. The patient denies any neck or back pain, but points to her chest. You discover a bruise and tenderness on her right chest and decreased lung sounds on the right side. What actions do you take next?

a. Obtain an ECG and start an IV of normal saline.

b. Provide bag-mask ventilations and prepare to intubate.

c. Insert a nasal airway and provide bag-mask ventilations.

d. Administer high-concentration oxygen and encourage the patient to breathe deeper and faster.

28. Your unit has been dispatched to a high-rise office building for an allergic reaction to a bee sting. Security takes you and your crew up to an office on the fifth floor where a crowd of people is standing around a cubicle. You make your way through to a young woman who is sitting at her desk. She appears pale and moist, and is working hard to breathe. Her face is flushed and she has hives on her neck and arms. The company nurse reports that her respiratory rate is 28 with wheezing, pulse is 110 and regular, and her BP is 90/40. The patient has a history of allergies to bee stings and tried to use her epinephrine auto-injector shortly after being stung, but is not sure she administered it correctly. That was approximately 15 minutes ago. What is the patient's present condition?

   a. She is potentially unstable.
   b. She is in anaphylactic shock.
   c. She is experiencing hypotension as a side effect of the epinephrine.
   d. She has signs and symptoms of a possible reaction to epinephrine as well as the bee sting.

29. A woman called EMS because her aunt had passed out and fallen. Your general impression is that of a 72-year-old female who is sitting up, with no apparent signs of distress or injury, but appears confused. The niece reports that the patient was about to sit down for breakfast. She has a history of hypertension and arthritis, but she had been well prior to the loss of consciousness and fall. Your initial assessment shows that the patient is unable to talk, she has an open airway with adequate respiratory effort, clear lung sounds, and strong and regular distal pulse; skin CTC is pink, warm, and dry. What action would be appropriate next?

   a. Administer oral glucose.
   b. Perform a focused neuro exam for signs of stroke.
   c. Search the residence for medications that are associated with seizures.
   d. Perform a rapid trauma assessment, being alert to signs of physical abuse.

30. Your ambulance is dispatched to a residence for a 35-year-old male with abdominal pain. Your general impression is that of an alert patient who is in severe distress from painful muscle spasms in the abdomen. He denies any medical problems and says that he has never experienced anything like this before. He also denies difficulty breathing, chest pain, or loss of consciousness. His girlfriend is there and asks you to look at his hand; she says that he was in the attic early and was bitten by an insect, perhaps a spider. She wants to know if the muscle spasms are related to the bite. The area of the bite is red and swollen and the patient states that there is a dull ache. Which of the following insect bites or stings could produce these symptoms?

   a. wasp
   b. fire ant
   c. black widow spider
   d. brown recluse spider

Chapter 30 Answer Form

	A	B	C	D			A	B	C	D
1.	❏	❏	❏	❏		16.	❏	❏	❏	❏
2.	❏	❏	❏	❏		17.	❏	❏	❏	❏
3.	❏	❏	❏	❏		18.	❏	❏	❏	❏
4.	❏	❏	❏	❏		19.	❏	❏	❏	❏
5.	❏	❏	❏	❏		20.	❏	❏	❏	❏
6.	❏	❏	❏	❏		21.	❏	❏	❏	❏
7.	❏	❏	❏	❏		22.	❏	❏	❏	❏
8.	❏	❏	❏	❏		23.	❏	❏	❏	❏
9.	❏	❏	❏	❏		24.	❏	❏	❏	❏
10.	❏	❏	❏	❏		25.	❏	❏	❏	❏
11.	❏	❏	❏	❏		26.	❏	❏	❏	❏
12.	❏	❏	❏	❏		27.	❏	❏	❏	❏
13.	❏	❏	❏	❏		28.	❏	❏	❏	❏
14.	❏	❏	❏	❏		29.	❏	❏	❏	❏
15.	❏	❏	❏	❏		30.	❏	❏	❏	❏

Appendix A:
Answers with Rationales

Chapter 1: Foundations of EMT-Intermediate

1. d. Emergency Medical Service System.—An emergency medical service system is an organized approach to providing emergency care within a community.

2. d. a sense of complacency and the ability to not show one's feelings.—These are not appropriate attributes for an EMT-I. Complacency may be misinterpreted as being unprofessional. Professional behavior does, however, include being able to avoid showing your personal feelings in various patient care scenarios (e.g., abuse, neglect, management of seriously ill or injured children).

3. a. certification.—This is the process by which a governmental agency grants permission to an EMT-I to practice within the state, after ensuring that the individual is competent. Some states call this *licensure.*

4. b. continuing education for the EMT-I.—The medical field is dynamic and constantly improving. As a health care professional, it is essential that the EMT-I keep informed and up to date on training and current trends in care. This reassures the public and medical community that quality patient care will be delivered.

5. d. the education, certification, and licensure requirements in his or her state.—The requirements for continuing education, certification, licensure, and recertification vary from state to state. All EMT-Is should know and follow these requirements to avoid a lapse in or loss of certification.

6. d. appearance and personal hygiene.—A well-groomed provider who wears the appropriate uniform and personal protective equipment (PPE) for the job is displaying professional behavior.

7. a. being courteous to other responders on the scene —Treat other responders the way you would like to be treated. Many agencies do not permit smoking in the ambulance at any time. There are restrictions of several sorts on release of patient-related information. Wearing one's work uniform to a drinking establishment is not appropriate.

8. a. wearing his uniform in drinking establishments.— It is neither appropriate nor professional to go out in one's work clothes, especially if the destination is a restaurant or bar.

9. a. ensure her own safety and that of her coworkers.— Safety is the primary responsibility of the EMT-I. When the responder is injured because of an unsafe condition, she becomes part of the problem rather than the solution.

10. c. It will help physicians make decisions about the efficiency and effectiveness of the care we provide to patients.—You should advocate for and participate in research projects at your EMS agency to help move the profession forward into the future.

11. c. Mutual respect and understanding of each other's capabilities will lead to better patient care.—Some medical directors of EMS agencies are present in name only, and never get to know the providers who work for them. Taking the time to get to know your medical director and those who give you medical direction will ultimately lead to better patient care.

12. a. benefit of offline medical direction.—Physician development of treatment protocols, as well as input into quality assurance and training program review, are all forms of offline medical direction.

13. c. Most systems suggest that the family physician be put in touch with online medical direction to discuss the case.—This should be spelled out in your local protocols.

14. d. continuous quality improvement program.—Call review, analysis of response time intervals, and focused studies of specific types of patient complaints are all parts of a CQI program.

15. a. body substance isolation (BSI) practices.—Fever indicates infection and thus presents a risk of exposure to the EMT-I. When confronted with a patient who has a fever of unknown origin, always use BSI to minimize exposure risk.

16. a. Place an oxygen mask on the patient.—An example of airborne disease is tuberculosis; putting an oxygen mask on the patient reduces the risk of airborne transmission of the disease. The EMT-I should also consider wearing a HEPA or N-95 mask and an eye shield, and should always wear disposable gloves.

17. b. Yes, and it should be reported to the emergency department (ED) right away.—This is considered a true exposure because a needle contaminated with the patient's blood broke the skin of the crew member.

18. b. mortality.—*Mortality* refers to fatalities (deaths).

19. c. preventable injuries.—If the patient had entered the pool feet first, the injury would not have occurred.

20. d. socioeconomic impact.—This includes the costs in dollars of the injury. The high numbers associated with the costs of emergency care, rehabilitation, and life after injury should highlight the importance of injury and illness prevention, which cost significantly less.

21. c. an injury prevention activity.—Another example is a fall prevention program in senior citizen homes.

22. a. assigning crews to do citizen cardiopulmonary resuscitation (CPR) training courses—This is an illness prevention program, as members of the public may raise questions about the causes of ACS and stroke in these classes.

23. b. It helps in planning for call volume and crew safety.—Do not ignore these neighborhoods; rather, plan ahead for calls there.

24. b. Many communities have programs to help feed the homebound elderly.—Meals on Wheels, food pantries, and other outreach programs are available in many communities to help get meals to elderly persons who are homebound. The EMT-I should be aware of such services in his or her community and know how to contact them.

25. d. The number of times the patient was transported for similar complaints.—The components of negligence include: duty to act, breach of that duty, occurrence of an injury, and injury causation by the breach of duty.

26. a. an unethical act.—A "slow-code" is unfair to the patient and the family, and hence is unethical.

27. c. COBRA law.—Interhospital transfer of patients is covered by these statutory provisions, so the EMT-I should become familiar with them.

28. b. slander.—Verbally making false statements that have the potential to damage another's reputation is against the law.

29. a. implied consent.—Consent to treatment is assumed when the patient is unable to speak for himself or herself because of an altered level of consciousness.

30. a. child abuse or neglect—All states require reporting of child abuse or neglect, though the method of reporting differs from state to state.

31. c. false imprisonment.—Always obtain permission or consent to treat and transport. Also, physically forcing treatment or transport on a mentally competent adult may be considered assault and battery.

32. c. scope of practice.—This description sets the boundaries and limits for the assessment and management the EMT-I may perform.

33. b. medical direction.—In this process, a physician delegates some practice authority to the EMT-I.

34. a. tort.—Tort law covers private or public wrongs or injuries that occur due to a breach (break) of a legal duty or obligation.

35. d. a relationship between the injury and who may have caused the injury.—As the saying goes, "If it was not documented, it was not done." Documentation is extremely important both for quality patient care and for reducing legal risk to the EMT-I.

36. c. The EMT-I may be held liable for the medical supervision of other providers.—Just as the EMT-I is responsible to the physician, EMT-Bs are responsible for providing quality care under the guidance of the EMT-I.

37. d. each of the choices listed here is good advice.—Do not rely on Good Samaritan or governmental immunity clauses to keep you out of court.

38. b. the HIPAA law—A patient's privacy rights are spelled out in the Health Insurance Portability and Accountability Act.

39. d. Make sure you have a credible witness to the documented refusal, as well as to what you said to the patient.—You should make sure you have a credible witness to the refusal of medical attention (RMA), as well as to what you said to the patient. It is a good idea to involve a family member in trying to convince the patient to go to the hospital; you should always consider calling medical direction, and clearly explain the worst-case scenario of not going and have the patient sign the RMA.

40. c. abandonment.—Delegating a patient to a lower level of care when the patient needs your level of care is called *abandonment*.

41. d. in a state where it is legal for a physician to order removal for a mental health evaluation and the EMT-I has the appropriate paperwork to do so.—Make sure that the police are present and you have plenty of help.

42. d. whether the patient has signed a prehospital do not attempt resuscitation (DNAR) form—Advance directives are generally not used in the field, as they require interpretation by a physician in the hospital setting.

43. a. A young trauma victim may be a potential organ donor.—This is especially so if the trauma is isolated to one specific area of the body, such as the head.

44. c. Your PCR may be the best way to refresh your memory about the incident.—A lot of time may have passed since the call, and you will probably have gone on a lot of other calls since then, so the PCR will be helpful if it was properly completed.

45. a. legible.—If a PCR is to be an effective legal document, it should be well written, accurate, legible, and complete.

46. c. Treat all patients the way you would want your own family to be treated.—This is a good foundation for making ethical decisions.

47. b. legal decision.—The state EMS Code is a rule, regulation, or law of the state.

48. a. DNR or DNAR.—Typically, the other documents are used in the hospital setting, because they require interpretation by a physician.

49. a. prehospital DNR or DNAR form.—Most states have some form of an out-of-hospital DNAR for the EMT-I to follow.

50. a. Avoid using seat belts while off duty.—This is definitely not being a good role model for your community.

51. d. all of the above.—While the patient is in the care of the EMT-I, one of the responsibilities of the EMT-I is to serve as an advocate for that patient. Patients may include those with special needs, alternative lifestyles, and diverse cultural backgrounds.

52. d. skills will decay and you need to keep up to date.—Continuing medical education courses and programs can help you stay current and competent.

53. c. Advocate for and support research efforts in your agency.—Quality changes are often based on research findings.

54. b. taking a personal interest in and talking with elderly patients—You can learn a lot by talking to elderly patients! All the other choices are distracting and bad behaviors.

55. a. teachable moment.—When appropriate, take the time to give patients tips on injury prevention (e.g., taping down scatter rugs or removing them to eliminate trip hazards).

56. a. integrity and honesty.—The money is not yours and should be returned to the patient. This is basic honesty and integrity.

57. c. more time to sleep or watch television—This is not a wellness benefit; in fact, it may contribute to the ever-increasing waistline of Americans! Benefits of total wellness include feeling better about yourself, performing better under stress, and living longer because of appropriate weight.

58. b. Exercise regularly and watch what you eat.—This is a good way to serve as a lifestyle role model for other EMS providers. The other "strategies" listed are usually not successful (and are seldom appreciated).

59. c. wellness begins with an assessment of one's own lifestyle.—Before you can serve as a role model for wellness, you need to clean up your own act.

60. d. teaching wellness concepts in your role as an EMT-I. —Mentioning walking and sensible eating to patients is an example of teachable moments.

61. d. all of the above.—Most dying patients wish to be treated by health care providers with respect, with dignity, and as individuals.

62. c. understand her prejudices and leave them at the door.—We all have biases and prejudices. Patients do not call us to judge them based on our opinions of cultural diversity. Try to put aside your personal prejudices and give all patients the high-quality medical care they expect and deserve.

63. d. all of the above.—You can improve your well-being by maintaining proper body weight, exercising regularly, and eating properly.

64. a. respect their emotional needs.—The dying patient and his or her family members do not want you to control their lives, and they do want to be a part of any necessary decision making if possible. Also, an EMT-I should never give false hope or empty reassurance to a patient.

65. b. practice the use of personal safety precautions.—Wear gear appropriate to the level of danger; a visible vest is helpful when operating near traffic.

66. b. advocating and serving as a role model by practicing BSI.—If you do not wear the appropriate protective equipment, the other EMS providers will take your lead and get sloppy too. Do not provide false hope to the patient's family with promises like "the patient is going to be all right," especially in grave circumstances.

67. b. make prevention a personal value.—You need to believe in prevention activities yourself if you are to have a passion for its success.

68. b. personal commitment.—To make a prevention program work, both the employer and the employees need to value the program and have a passion for its success.

69. d. shows respect for the rights and feelings of patients.—This is an important quality of any good health care provider.

70. d. protecting the patient's confidentiality is very important.—Do not violate the patient's right to privacy. Leave the press conferences to the hospital personnel.

71. d. Contact medical direction to see if it is appropriate to stop the care.—If CPR has been started and you are then presented with a valid prehospital DNAR, it is best to call medical direction to obtain a termination order if there has been no return of spontaneous circulation.

72. d. all adults should seriously consider making advance directives for medical care.—Advance directives allow a person to express his or her wishes and feelings when the patient is not able to express them for himself or herself due to injury or illness.

73. d. they can reinforce the patient's autonomy in the decision-making process.—Advance directives or living wills for future medical care best serve the patient's needs and autonomy in decision making when they are prepared by the patient, physician, and surrogate together.

74. d. discuss his concerns so they are clearly understood by both parties.—If the physician orders therapy that you feel is inappropriate, discuss it before doing it.

75. c. Know your protocols and remind the physician of the standard dose.—Discuss the unusual order: perhaps there is a good reason for the irregular dose, or perhaps the physician made a mistake and will welcome the chance to correct the original order. Arguing or going ahead and giving the wrong dose serves no medical purpose, creates a potential danger to the patient, and opens the door to litigation.

Chapter 2: Overview of Human Systems

1. a. anatomy.—The terms listed refer to study of functions or abnormal body structures.

2. c. organelles, cells, tissues, organs—The ranking of levels of organization of the body, in order of simplest to most complex, is organelles, cells, tissues, organs, organ systems.

3. d. the body's ability to maintain a stable internal physiologic environment—*Homeostasis* refers to an internal physiologic environment (e.g., body temperature, the pH of blood) that remains stable under fluctuating environmental conditions.

4. a. superior.—The upper part of the body is superior to the lower part.

5. d. midshaft, medial femur.—*Medial* means toward the center or middle.

6. a. distal—The elbow is further from the body (distal) than the shoulder joint.

7. c. retroperitoneal space.—The kidneys are found in the body cavity behind (*retro*) the peritoneal space.

8. c. sagittal plane.—The other terms refer to anatomical planes that split the body differently.

9. c. right lower—The cecum and appendix are located in the right lower abdominal quadrant.

10. a. osmosis.—*Osmosis* refers to the tendency of a solvent to move from an area of low solute concentration to one of high concentration, through a semi-permeable membrane, in an effort to equalize the concentrations on both sides of the membrane.

11. b. catabolism.—Catabolism is destructive metabolism, involving energy release resulting in the breakdown of larger molecules into smaller molecules.

12. c. mitochondria; ATP.—Food that enters the body is broken down into primary sugars, amino acids, and fatty acids. These substances eventually are metabolized in the mitochondria to produce large amounts of adenosine triphosphate (ATP).

13. d. epithelial tissue.—*Epithelium* (skin) covers all the external surfaces of the human body.

14. b. epidermis.—The dermis and subcutaneous tissue lie underneath the epidermis; sebaceous glands are also located below the epidermis.

15. b. support and movement.—The human skeleton acts as a support framework, allows movement (by working with the muscles), and protects the structures of the body.

16. b. shape.—Bones are classified according to their shape (e.g., long, flat, short).

17. c. thumb.—The thumb is an example of a saddle joint. Such a joint has saddle-shaped articular surfaces.

18. b. an involuntary muscle.—Smooth muscles, such as those in blood vessels and intestines, are examples of involuntary muscle.

19. a. cardiac, and skeletal.—The three muscle types are smooth, cardiac, and skeletal.

20. b. automaticity.—The ability of the cardiac cells to generate impulses is called automaticity.

21. a. control body functions.—The nervous system does allow communication with the environment, but this is only part of its main purpose of controlling body functions.

22. b. central and peripheral divisions.—The central nervous system consists of the brain and spinal cord. The peripheral nervous system consists of the cranial nerves (except for the optic nerve), the spinal nerves, and the autonomic nervous system.

23. a. synaptic cleft.—The synaptic cleft is the space between neurons.

24. a. axons.—Projections from a nerve cell that make connections with adjacent nerve cells are called axons.

25. b. specific—Spinal and cranial nerves are part of the peripheral nervous system.

26. d. cerebral spinal—CSF (also known as cerebrospinal fluid) protects and serves as a shock absorber for the brain and spinal cord.

27. c. repolarization.—The state or process of returning the cells to their resting state, which occurs after the cell has allowed electrical activity.

28. a. brain.—The central nervous system (CNS) is comprised of the brain and spinal cord; the cerebrum is part of the brain. The peripheral nerves are part of the peripheral nervous system.

29. b. dura mater.—The name of this protective membrane comes from the Latin words *dura* (tough) and *mater* (mother).

30. d. sympathetic and parasympathetic.—The autonomic nervous system, which is part of the peripheral nervous system, comprises the sympathetic and parasympathetic nervous systems.

31. b. hormones—Hormones secreted by glands help to regulate many body functions.

32. b. insulin; glucose—The pancreas secretes insulin to help the body use glucose.

33. a. epinephrine; speed up the heart—In response to stress, the brain tells the adrenal glands to secrete epinephrine, which speeds up the heart. Norepinephrine is a counteracting chemical that slows the heart.

34. a. plasma.—Antibodies, which fight infection; hemoglobin, which transports oxygen; and red blood cells are also found in the blood.

35. a. fight infection.—Platelets assist in blood clotting; hemoglobin carries oxygen to the cells; and other cells remove the byproducts of metabolism.

36. a. platelets—Platelets form the initial clot following a vascular injury. Clotting proteins then complete the clotting process.

37. a. Cessation of bleeding; without it the person could bleed to death.—Hemostasis is the process of slowing and stopping bleeding.

38. d. center: sternum.—Most of the heart is centered in the chest, under the sternum.

39. c. pericardium.—The name comes from the Latin *peri* (around) and *cardium* (heart).

40. b. atrium; left ventricle—Blood enters the right atrium, flows through the heart, and exits by way of the left ventricle, before heading to the rest of the body.

41. a. mitral valve—Freshly oxygenated blood returns from the lungs to the left side of the heart through a vein. After the blood collects in the left atrium, it then is ejected through the mitral valve into the left ventricle of the heart before being pumped out to the rest of the body.

42. c. pulmonic; left atrium—The pulmonic valve ejects blood that has been depleted of oxygen; after reoxygenation in the lungs, the blood returns to the heart's left atrium.

43. a. closing of the aortic and pulmonic valves at the end of systole.—The "dub" or S-2 heart sound is made by closure of the aortic and pulmonic valves at the end of systole.

44. c. S-3; "da"—A soft, low-pitched heart sound that occurs about one-third of the way through diastole is the S-3 heart sound; it sounds like the syllable "da."

45. d. murmur.—An abnormal "whooshing" sound heard over the heart indicates turbulent blood flow within the heart and is called a *murmur*.

46. c. sinoatrial node; right atrium—The SA node initiates the stimulus for the heartbeat. In a healthy heart the SA node is the primary pacemaker. It is located in the right atrium.

47. a. excitability.—Excitability is the ability of cells to respond to electrical impulses.

48. d. the afterload.—The pressure in the aorta against which the left ventricle must pump blood is called the *afterload*.

49. c. cardiac output.—The amount of blood pumped through the circulatory system in one minute is the *cardiac output*.

50. d. rate and force of contraction.—The nervous system is responsible for regulating the heart's rate and force of contraction.

51. c. make it pump stronger—The beta effect causes the heart to contract more forcefully.

52. c. tunica media.—*Media* means "middle."

53. a. veins—The veins have a series of valves in them to help get the blood back to the heart.

54. d. all of the above.—The thin, semi-permeable walls of the capillaries allow diffusion of many materials from the capillaries to the cells and vice versa.

55. c. pulmonic—Blood circulation between the heart and the lungs is referred to as the *pulmonic circulation*. The blood circulation from the left ventricle through the body and back to the right atrium is called the *systemic circulation*.

56. b. vein; vena cava—Veins carry blood to the heart; arteries carry blood out of the heart. Capillaries are small vessels that infuse tissues.

57. d. all of the above—The patient's BP is influenced by blood volume, the heart rate and force, and the peripheral vascular resistance.

58. a. drop.—Blood volume is a factor with a direct relationship to blood pressure.

59. c. brain and nervous system.—The brain and nervous system regulate the blood pressure.

60. c. interstitial or extracellular fluid—Lymph fluid consists mostly of a liquid resembling blood plasma, and contains white blood cells.

61. c. inflammatory response.—An inflammatory response is a part of the immune response, in which the body releases chemicals that promote the influx of cells and other chemicals to fight the foreign challenge.

62. a. specific—Specific immunity is when the body is able to recognize, respond to, and remember a particular substance.

63. d. exchange gases at the alveolocapillary membrane.—The primary function of the respiratory system is to exchange gases; this takes place at the alveolocapillary membrane.

64. c. diaphragm; negative.—When a patient takes a normal inhalation, the diaphragm muscle contracts, creating negative pressure, which results in air being pulled into the lungs.

65. b. ventilation.—Inhalation is the process of taking in air; respiration refers to an exchange of gases. The process of moving air into and out of the lungs is called *ventilation*.

66. d. alveolocapillary junction.—Diffusion in the respiratory system occurs at the level where the alveoli and capillaries meet.

67. c. Without a functioning circulatory system, the lungs would be oxygenated but the cells of the body would not be.—The essential purpose of the circulatory system is to oxygenate the cells of the body.

68. c. carbon dioxide; increases—The chemoreceptors governing respiration would sense the high carbon dioxide level and trigger an increase in the respiratory rate to eliminate the excess CO_2 waste.

69. a. nose—The nose is a sensory organ.

70. a. mouth—Food is masticated (chewed) in the mouth by the teeth.

71. a. It stores bile, which helps to break down fatty foods.—The urinary bladder stores urine.

72. c. in the small intestine—Nutrients from food get absorbed into the body primarily in the small intestine.

73. c. intracellular fluid; 40 to 45—*Intra* means "within," so the fluid found within the individual cells is called intracellular fluid.

74. d. all of the above.—Fluid balance within the body is maintained by many factors, including the action of hormones (thyroid and diuretic) and kidney function.

75. a. osmosis.—Water moves within the human body by a process called osmosis.

76. b. nephron; dialysis—A neuron is a nerve, a component of the nervous system. Fluid infusion would exacerbate the problem in a patient with nonfunctional kidneys. The glomerulus is a capillary network that is part of the nephron. When the nephron does not function properly, the patient may need dialysis.

77. c. increased aldosterone levels.—When the tubules in the kidneys increase reabsorption of sodium from the filtrate and decrease reabsorption of potassium, water and sodium move from filtrate into the blood, and excess potassium is excreted.

78. a. Increasing the breathing rate helps to increase the pH.—Respiratory rate has a direct effect on the body's acid/base balance. Increasing the breathing rate can increase the pH by reducing the amout of carbon dioxide in the system.

79. b. buffer system.—The buffer system is one of the fastest-acting defenses for acid/base changes, providing almost immediate protection against changes in hydrogen ion concentration in the extracellular fluid.

80. d. any of the above—Some common causes of acidosis include hypoventilation from a drug overdose, COPD, or an exacerbation of asthma.

Chapter 3: Emergency Pharmacology

1. d. all of the above—Pharmacokinetics is the study of the absorption, distribution, metabolism, and excretion of a drug.

2. a. enteral—These drugs must undergo digestion and processing by the GI system, which can take a long time. Intravenous is the quickest.

3. c. distribution.—Excretion means elimination from the body; absorption refers to uptake of the drug; metabolism (in this instance) refers to use of the drug.

4. d. Harrison Narcotic Act of 1914—The Comprehensive Drug Abuse Prevention and Control Act (Controlled Substances Act of 1970) superseded the Harrison Narcotic Act.

5. c. Controlled Substances Act.—The Comprehensive Drug Abuse Prevention and Control Act (also known as the Controlled Substance Act of 1970) superseded the Harrison Narcotic Act.

6. d. chemical; generic—A drug manufacturer controls only the trade (or brand) names it gives its products.

7. d. all of the above.—Drug products are derived from many sources, both natural and synthetic.

8. c. parenteral.—The purpose of injecting most liquid drugs into the body is to bypass the gastrointestinal tract.

9. b. the *Physician's Desk Reference*—The PDR is one source for the EMT-I who wants to research a drug before administering it. Some ambulance crews carry a PDR in their unit as a reference source to look up patient meds they are not familiar with; however, there are more concise reference sources that are easier to use on the scene.

10. c. age-related liver dysfunction will extend the breakdown time of the drug. —Older people have slower metabolic processes, and age-related kidney dysfunction can extend the drug excretion time. These factors can cause toxicity due to the increased accumulation of the drug in the body.

11. c. verify with medical direction that it is safe to administer the drug to a pregnant patient.—Many medications could harm a pregnant patient or her fetus.

12. d. a smaller dose than an adult's, based on their weight.—A patient who weighs less would logically receive less of a weight-related medication.

13. b. the degree of physiologic change caused by the drug—Drug-induced physiologic changes usually affect more than one organ or tissue; the degrees of desired or undesired effects vary from drug to drug (and patient to patient). The EMT-I must know how a drug works, why it is given, and when it is given.

14. b. right dose and route.—Before administering any drug, the EMT-I should verify the (five) "rights": right time, drug, dose, route, and patient.

15. a. a side effect.—Therapeutic effect is the intended effect of the drug. Drug toxicity is an accumulation of a drug in the body to the point of being dangerous and causing poisonous effects. An anaphylactic reaction is a much more serious effect involving cardiovascular collapse.

16. d. emulsion.—An *elixir* is a mixture of the drug with water and alcohol; an *extract* is a concentration or distillate of the drug. *Spirit* usually refers to alcohol. An emulsion is a drug that is combined with water and oil.

17. c. tincture—Ointments, lozenges, and capsules are considered solid medications. A *tincture* is a medicine in an alcoholic solvent.

18. b. transdermal—Patches allow the medication to be absorbed through the skin over a period of time. *Sublingual* means under the tongue; *intramuscular* means into the muscle; *subcutaneous* means under the skin (cutaneous tissue layer).

19. d. subcutaneous—An intradermal injection goes between the layers of the skin; an intravenous injection goes into a vein; an intramuscular injection goes into a muscle. A subcutaneous injection is placed directly into the fatty layer of tissue below the skin by positioning the needle and syringe at a 45-degree angle to the skin.

20. a. increased heart rate.—The parasympathetic effect usually slows things down (e.g., heart rate). A parasympathetic blocker puts the brakes on that effect and allows the heart rate to increase.

21. b. vasoconstriction.—Stimulation of alpha-adrenergic receptors causes vasoconstriction.

22. b. increased chronotropic effect.—Medications that stimulate beta-1 adrenergic receptor sites increase inotropic, chronotropic, and dromotropic effects.

23. c. potentiation.—Potentiation occurs when two or more drugs are taken simultaneously and one drug prolongs or multiplies the effect of the other drug(s).

24. d. idiosyncratic reaction.—An idiosyncratic reaction is not the same as an allergy or a hypersensitivity reaction.

25. d. albuterol sulfate—Many regions allow EMT-Is to administer albuterol sulfate for immediate treatment of asthma.

26. d. Failure to follow procedures could cause the loss of your medical director's license.—EMT-Is who are allowed to carry and administer controlled substances *must* take the documentation and accounting procedures very seriously, because the security of controlled substances is highly regulated. If you do not follow the procedures, you could jeopardize your medical director's medical license or Drug Enforcement Agency (DEA) number.

27. c. within the temperature ranges specified by the manufacturers.—It is not appropriate to store meds in a truck for long periods of time, as ambient temperatures may become too warm or too cold. In addition, some medications are inactivated by exposure to light.

28. b. outdated.—A medication should not be administered if it is expired, outdated, or discolored, or if the vial or syringe is contaminated.

29. c. large barrel with syringe.—Dextrose 50% is usually packaged in a 50-cc barrel that attaches to a syringe for field use.

30. d. do an ongoing assessment of the patient.—The EMT-I should document the administration, as well as any changes in patient condition observed during the ongoing assessment, on the PCR.

Chapter 4: Venous Access and Medication Administration

1. d. the layers of the skin for administration of medications by injection—Many meds are given subcutaneously (SC), intramuscularly (IM), or intravenously (IV). The technique for each is different and requires knowledge of the layers of the skin and various landmarks.

2. d. how fast the bloodstream will be accessed by each route of administration—IV is the fastest administration route, and is frequently used in emergency situations.

3. d. denominator.—The number on the top of a fraction is the numerator.

4. d. slightly more (approximately 10% more) than double the size.—One kilogram equals approximately 2.2 pounds.

5. a. The 10 gtt/ml set—IV administration sets are designated by drip size (gtt) in the chamber. With a 10-gtt set, 10 drops are equal to 1 ml; the 15-gtt and 20-gtt sets would have to deliver 15 and 20 drops, respectively, to equal the same amount.

6. d. 1,000—Remember that the prefix *milli* means thousand. There are 1,000 milliliters in one liter.

7. d. one-millionth—Written another way, 1 microgram (mcg) equals 0.000001 g.

8. d. 100° Fahrenheit—100 degrees Celsius (or centigrade) is the boiling point of water; 100 degrees Kelvin is well below the freezing point of water.

9. c. To convert Fahrenheit to Celsius, subtract 48 and multiply by 4/5.—All the other equations are correct. To correctly convert Fahrenheit to Celsius, subtract 32 and then multiply by 9/5.

10. b. 250 mg—Your patient weighs 110 pounds (110/2.2 = 50 kg). She needs 5 mg per kg of the antidysrhythmic: 5 mg × 50 kg = 250 mg.

11. c. 250 mg—Your patient weighs 55 pounds (55/2.2 = 25 kg). The order is for 10 mg per kg of the medication: 10 mg × 25 kg = 250 mg.

12. b. 50 gtt/min—$\dfrac{100 \text{ ml}}{X \text{ gtt}} \times \dfrac{30 \text{ min}}{15 \text{ gtt/ml}}$
= 30/1,500 = 50 gtt/min

13. d. any of the above.—Orders for medication administration can appear in local protocols, or they can come from a medical control physician on the scene, or online by radio or telephone.

14. a. the drug that was given—Once a drug has been administered to the patient, it is the EMT-I's responsibility to document that the drug that was given, the time it was actually administered (not prepared), and exactly who administered the drug (not who was merely present).

15. d. size of syringe used.—The "rights" of drug administration are: right patient, right route, right dose, right time, and right drug administered.

16. c. If this is not done, the patient may develop a serious infection.—Nonsterile IV technique greatly increases the risk of serious infection.

17. c. antiseptic—Preparing an injection site with iodine helps to reduce the risk of infection.

18. c. disposable gloves.—The EMT-I should always wear disposable gloves, to reduce the risk of infection for both the patient and the EMT-I.

19. a. a 50-cc syringe—Typically, a 50-cc syringe is not needed for starting an IV.

20. a. flush all the air out of the line.—A patient can develop an air embolism from an IV that has air in the tubing.

21. a. upper tibia—Suitable locations for placing an IO include the upper tibia (tibial tuberosity) and the sternum.

22. c. a 3-year-old with circulatory collapse—When a 3-year-old has circulatory collapse, it is appropriate for the EMT-I to consider the administration of fluid by the IO route; it is highly unlikely that IV access can be obtained, because of collapsed veins.

23. b. albuterol—Albuterol is usually aerosolized and inhaled.

24. b. oxygen—Aerosolized medications may come premixed in saline solution, but the EMT-I will need an oxygen source for administration of the aerosol.

25. d. all of the above—Depending on the medication, oral medications can be given by teaspoon, drop, or spray.

26. b. rectal—Small children often do not like taking medicine, and will not or cannot cooperate with medication administration by the nasal, gastric, or buccal routes.

27. b. aspirin—The enteral route is by mouth into the GI tract. Aspirin is administered by mouth to patients with cardiac chest pain.

28. d. epinephrine 1:1000.—Subcutaneous injection is one example of a parenteral route. Epinephrine 1:1000 is administered subcutaneously to a patient with a severe allergic reaction.

29. d. percutaneous.—A medication given by injection is given via the percutaneous route.

30. b. sharps container—Safety first! Best practice is to have a sharps container close at hand whenever needles or other sharps are to be used.

31. d. placing it in a sharps container right away.—Proper disposal of needles is intended to avoid injury and contamination.

32. c. It helps the EMT-I understand why certain routes of administration are better than others when the body is stressed.—Understanding the pathophysiological principles of medication administration can help the EMT-I know which routes of drug administration are best with specific clinical conditions (e.g., shock or hypothermia).

33. b. exact dose of the medication.—This is imperative for preventing medication mistakes and potentially dangerous or lethal treatment.

34. b. discard it and open another one.—To prevent the possibility of infection, if you drop the IV-catheter or touch it to anything other than the injection site (e.g., your glove), you should discard it and use a new one.

35. c. deltoid.—The thigh is an alternative, but is not typically the first choice.

Chapter 5: Airway Management and Ventilation

1. a. improper seal of a bag mask.—Making a proper mask seal can be a difficult task, especially when only one rescuer is attempting to ventilate the patient. It is recommended that there be two rescuers for this, skill one to make a proper mask seal and one to squeeze the bag.

2. b. larynx.—The vocal cords (voice box) are located in the larynx, which is bounded above by the glottis and is continuous below with the trachea.

3. a. alveoli.—These small structures of the lungs provide a large surface area for exchange of oxygen and carbon dioxide between the lungs and the bloodstream.

4. a. They act as a filter to catch impurities.—The hairs in the nose physically filter out foreign particles.

5. a. nares—The alveoli, trachea, and carina are anatomical structures in the lower airway.

6. b. bronchioles.—Patients with reactive airway disease have constricted and inflamed bronchioles.

7. d. the pediatric trachea is more posterior than the adult trachea.—The pediatric airway is actually more anterior than an adult's.

8. a. approximately 6–7 cc per kg.—The normal tidal volume for an adult is approximately 6–7 cc per kg.

9. b. visible chest rise.—Visible chest rise and fall is a sign of adequate ventilation.

10. b. atelectasis.—Insufficient or ineffective ventilations can cause collapse of the alveoli.

11. a. FiO_2.—This abbreviation stands for fraction of inspired oxygen.

12. c. through the pulmonary circulation—When oxygen is inhaled into the body, the pulmonary circulation carries it to the pulmonary vein and into the left atrium and ventricle of the heart.

13. c. elevated blood pressure—Decreased oxygen concentration in the blood can be caused by: carbon monoxide poisoning, a pulmonary embolism, or a lengthy submersion. Elevated BP does not generally lower the blood oxygen concentration.

14. b. hypoventilating.—Prolonged hypoventilation fails to adequately rid the body of carbon dioxide, thus leading to increased CO_2 levels in the blood.

15. b. end-stage COPD.—Patients with end-stage chronic obstructive pulmonary disease (COPD) live in a

state of oxygen deficiency, so even a slight decrease can exacerbate the condition to a critical state.

16. b. Chemoreceptors send messages to the brain.—Chemoreceptors are plentiful in the aortic arch.

17. b. nitrogen.—Nearly 80 percent of atmospheric air is nitrogen.

18. c. fractured radius—Diabetic coma, fractured ribs, or a narcotic overdose may all alter the rate and depth of respiration.

19. b. may have a serious head injury.—Serious head injuries can alter the patient's respiratory rate and pattern.

20. c. involuntary regulation of respiration.—Involuntary regulation of the respiratory rate occurs in response to receptors' notifying the brain that there is too much carbon dioxide. The rate will increase in an attempt to blow off excess CO_2.

21. d. a combination of the above.—A patient who talks while eating large mouthfuls is unlikely to chew food adequately; alcohol blunts judgment and increases carelessness, thereby contributing to the distraction.

22. b. tongue.—The most common upper airway obstruction is the patient's own tongue.

23. d. 26–30—The normal respiratory rate for a 10-year-old child is approximately 26–30 breaths per minute.

24. d. 36–40—It is not uncommon for an infant to have a normal respiratory rate of approximately 36–40 breaths per minute.

25. b. lacerated forearm—Respiratory distress can be caused by a foreign body airway obstruction (FBAO), acute exacerbation of COPD, or a sternal fracture.

26. a. reduced oxygen in the blood.—Hypoxemia is a lack of oxygen in the blood.

27. d. oxygen deficiency to the body sufficient to cause impaired function.—An oxygen deficiency severe enough to cause impaired function is called *hypoxia*.

28. a. increased hematocrit—Hypoxemia is caused by factors such as high altitude, inadequate pulmonary ventilation, and carbon monoxide poisoning.

29. a. pulsus paradoxus.—Pulsus paradoxus is present when the systolic BP drops more than 10 mm Hg with inspiration. A change in pulse quality may also be detected during inspiration. This condition may be seen in COPD patients and patients with pericardial tamponade.

30. a. agonal gasps—Forms of modified respiration include Kussmaul's respirations, central neurogenic hyperventilation syndrome, and Cheyne-Stokes. Agonal "gasps" are dying respirations.

31. a. gag—The gag reflex is involuntary for most people, but may not be present when the patient's level of consciousness is diminished.

32. d. Using ferrous metal wrenches to change gauges and regulators.—Oxygen wrenches made of non-ferrous materials should be used for changing gauges and regulators; other types of metal tools may produce a spark when they strike metal objects (including the tank, gauge, or regulator).

33. a. allow oxygen to flow near a flame source.—This is a dangerous fire hazard.

34. d. high-pressure—The pressure in the main oxygen cylinder in the ambulance is too high to be delivered directly to a patient. A high-pressure regulator must be attached to yield a safe working pressure.

35. c. crack the tank open slightly to clean any dust out of the valve.—When changing an oxygen cylinder, the EMT-I should remove the seal that comes on the new tank, replace the washer on the regulator (if required), and "burp" the tank to clean any dust out of the valve. Only then is the regulator placed on the new tank.

36. c. non-rebreather mask; 12—High-concentration oxygen administration is indicated for a male patient who has severe chest pain. Nasal cannulas at lower flows will not deliver sufficient oxygen.

37. d. end-stage emphysema.—High-concentration oxygen is contraindicated in end-stage emphysema because of the hypoxic drive associated with this condition. High-concentration oxygen should never be withheld from a COPD patient who is in moderate to severe respiratory distress.

38. b. bag mask to assist ventilations.—Assisted ventilations, using a bag mask with supplementary oxygen, are indicated for patients in severe respiratory distress and with altered mental status.

39. c. Oxygen tends to dry out the mucous membranes.—It is appropriate to consider using an oxygen humidifier for a patient during a lengthy interhospital transport because oxygen tends to dry out the mucous membranes.

40. a. stoma.—*Stoma* is the name for a surgical opening; in a patient who has had a laryngectomy, it is in the neck.

41. d. to prevent fluid droplets from entering your mouth or eyes—Wear a mask and eye shield during any airway or ventilation procedures, to prevent contamination from fluid droplets and other substances.

42. d. perform the Sellick maneuver on a patient who does not have an advanced airway in place.—Some believe that this technique helps prevent gastric distension and reduces the risk of vomiting and aspiration.

43. b. sufficient volume to achieve visible chest rise—When ventilating an adult patient using a bag mask, the EMT-I should ensure a good mask seal, sufficient volume to achieve visible chest rise, and no more than 1 ventilation every 6 seconds.

44. a. hypoventilation—The EMT-I should avoid ventilating too slow or too fast, overinflation, and underinflation.

45. c. gastric distension.—This increases the risk of vomiting and aspiration.

46. b. providing excessive ventilations with the device.—Excessive ventilations can increase the risk of complications such as vomiting and aspiration.

47. b. Sellick maneuver.—Another name for this technique is cricoid pressure.

48. b. increase the rate per the resuscitation standards.—The ventilatory rate should be age appropriate.

49. d. try using a pediatric mask to seal around the opening.—There are special masks designed to be used with stomas, but if such a mask is not available, try sealing a pediatric mask around the opening.

50. d. complete airway obstruction.—A patient with a partial airway obstruction may still be able to speak or cough.

51. c. experiencing a completely blocked airway.—When a patient has poor air exchange, the EMT-I should provide immediate assistance.

52. c. encourage the patient to cough, but not intervene just yet.—A patient with good air exchange may be able to clear the airway on his own.

53. a. verify that the patient cannot speak.—If the EMT-I suspects a complete airway obstruction in a conscious adult patient, the EMT-I should verify that the patient cannot speak, verify that the patient is choking, and deliver a series of abdominal thrusts.

54. d. Attempt a direct laryngoscopy and remove the obstruction with forceps.—If manual maneuvers have proven ineffective, the EMT-I can consider a direct laryngoscopy to remove a foreign body airway obstruction (FBAO).

55. c. suction the patient with a rigid-tip Yankauer.—The airway should be suctioned rapidly to prevent aspiration. A rigid-tip catheter is the appropriate device in this case.

56. d. through a tube such as an endotracheal tube.—A soft catheter has no form and cannot be directed as easily as a rigid-tip catheter.

57. d. inserting the catheter into the nose if you suspect a skull fracture—The reason is to avoid placing the catheter into an opening in the skull.

58. b. bulb syringes—Suction units commonly used on adult patients include the manual unit, the oxygen-powered unit, and the battery-powered suction unit. Small pediatric patients, such as newly borns and small infants, cannot tolerate the high suction levels produced by these devices.

59. b. ensure that the patient continues to be adequately oxygenated.—Best practices when suctioning the upper airway include limiting suction time, ensuring adequate oxygenation, and avoiding stimulation of the gag reflex.

60. d. watch for a decrease in the pulse rate due to vagal stimuli.—Suctioning can stimulate a vagal response that causes a decrease in heart rate. This is especially true in children.

61. b. tracheobronchial suctioning in an intubated patient.—"Deep suctioning" or sterile suctioning is the technique used to suction through the endotracheal tube.

62. d. Combitube™ in place.—Advanced airway can mean a Combitube™, an endotracheal tube, or a Laryngeal-Mask Airway (LMA™).

63. a. LMA™—The least effective advanced airway for a patient with a full stomach and the possibility of gastric regurgitation is the LMA™, which is designed for a patient with an empty stomach. This device is not designed to protect the airway from aspiration.

64. b. nasogastric tube.—A nasogastric tube relieves the pressure in the stomach that may be restricting the excursion of the diaphragm.

65. d. place the pillow behind the patient's shoulder rather than behind her head.—This position helps to open the airway.

66. c. the jaw-thrust maneuver.—The jaw-thrust maneuver minimizes movement of the patient's neck.

67. c. if you need to access the oropharynx in a patient with clenched teeth.—An NPA should be used whenever: you might consider using an oropharyngeal airway (OPA), you need to access the oropharynx in a patient with clenched teeth, or you must insert a catheter for suctioning the patient.

68. d. endotracheal intubation—When properly inserted, an endotracheal tube (ET) provides direct ventilation of the lungs and prevents aspiration of blood, vomitus, and other secretions.

69. d. all of the above—A misplaced ET tube, if unrecognized, will not properly ventilate the patient, and may cause serious harm or death.

70. b. It requires frequent retraining and practice to stay proficient.—Without frequent practice, proficiency in ET tube insertion can deteriorate quickly.

71. c. It helps isolate the trachea and can limit aspiration into the lungs.—When the tube is properly inserted, endotracheal intubation helps to isolate the trachea and can limit aspiration into the lungs.

72. c. Place a pillow behind the patient's upper back and ventilate him with a bag mask.—Positioning is key when placing an endotracheal tube. On large patients, obtaining an airway is often difficult. The best approach is to place a pillow behind the upper back, ventilate the patient with a bag mask, and then attempt intubation; this position helps to align airway structures for the best visualization. After each unsuccessful attempt, resume ventilation with a bag mask to prevent hypoxia.

73. b. vallecula.—Doing so lifts the vallecula and allows visualization of the vocal cords.

74. d. all of the above—Once the endotracheal tube has gone through the vocal cords, it is appropriate to apply an EID, listen over both lung fields, and check both the pulse oximeter and the $EtCO_2$ readings as an alternate means of confirming tube placement.

75. b. suction unit—Removal of an advanced airway adjunct causes vomiting in many patients. Be prepared and have suction ready.

76. c. larger—Each tube, pilot balloon, and syringe of the Combitube™ is labeled as either "one" or "two." The larger bulb, labeled "one," is inflated first.

77. a. dual-lumen—The Combitube™ has two tubes and thus is also called a dual-lumen airway.

78. d. unconscious adult patients without a gag reflex.—Contraindications for the use of a Combitube™ include: height (too short or too tall), a positive gag reflex, known ingestion of a caustic substance, and esophageal varices.

79. d. all of the above—Contraindications for the use of a Combitube™ include: height (too short or too tall), a positive gag reflex, known ingestion of a caustic substance, and esophageal varices.

80. b. Carefully position the head, as the occiput is large.—It may be necessary to place a pad behind the shoulders of a small child.

Chapter 6: History Taking

1. b. ineffective listening skills—Professional demeanor, good eye contact, and positive body language all improve the EMT-I's communication abilities.

2. a. measuring the $EtCO_2$—The $EtCO_2$ measurement yields diagnostic information rather than history. Diagnostics (e.g., SpO_2, ECG, blood glucose, and $EtCO_2$) are obtained as part of the physical examination.

3. d. when the EMT-I would like the patient to describe his or her symptoms in detail—An example of an open-ended question is: "Why did you call us here today?"

4. c. when it is necessary to speed up the information gathering—Examples of situations in which it would be important to use closed-ended questions are unsafe surroundings or a serious patient condition requiring quick transport.

5. d. asking the patient to describe his last incidence of chest pain—An open-ended question asks for more than a one- or two-word answer.

6. b. clarification.—An example of clarification is asking for more detailed information about a hypertensive medication. Some of these medications (beta blockers) are used to control heart rate as well as blood pressure.

7. d. interpretation.—The EMT-I uses all available information to analyze the patient's problem and begin the appropriate treatment.

8. a. facilitation.—The EMT-I uses facilitation to build a good rapport with the patient. This in turn helps the EMT-I to make a better interpretation of the patient's problem and to provide the best care.

9. d. empathetic response.—Empathy is a form of facilitation and is used to make a better interpretation of the patient's problem, so that the EMT-I can provide the best care.

10. a. health history.—Obtaining a health history takes time. EMT-Is commonly try to establish a relationship with the patient during this phase, so as to draw upon the pertinent information about the patient's medical history.

11. c. which hospital the patient would like to be taken to today.—An adult patient's history should include preliminary data, current health status, a review of the body systems, and a general physical exam. It does not include the specific facility where the patient might want to be taken.

12. a. the skin and gastrointestinal tract.—The review of body systems should include assessment of the skin; head, eyes, ears, nose, and throat (HEENT); and gastrointestinal tract.

13. d. all of the above—It is often difficult to gather reliable information (or any information at all) from these patients.

14. b. shouting at the patient so she can hear you clearly—If a patient has a hearing problem, it is

appropriate to position yourself in front of the patient so he can see your lips, speak to the patient's best ear, and speak slowly in a low-pitched voice. Shouting can distort sounds and intimidate or frighten the patient.

15. d. be patient and accept the crying as a natural venting of emotions.—This approach allows patients to express their feelings. Showing patience with the patient, when time permits, helps to build rapport and possibly a better understanding of the patient's problem.

Chapter 7: Techniques of Physical Examination

1. a. palpation—Using the sense of touch, as in feeling the abdomen for tenderness or rigidity, is called *palpation.*

2. d. auscultation.—Listening for the sounds of an underlying organ, such as the lungs or stomach, or for BP sounds with a stethoscope is referred to as *auscultation.*

3. c. percussion.—Tapping on the outer surface of the body, in an attempt to determine the size and location of a solid mass or hollow area beneath, is called *percussion.*

4. a. inspection.—Inspection includes comparisons of left and right areas.

5. c. Hold the wrist and count first the pulse, then breaths, for 15 seconds each.—A patient who knows you are attempting to count respirations may change his or her breathing pattern. One way to obtain an accurate respiratory rate while the patient is watching is to combine that count with a pulse check; the patient will not know which measurement is being taken when.

6. a. palpation—A blood pressure taken by palpation is not an exact measurement, but it provides a close measure of the systolic pressure.

7. c. hypertensive.—An adult BP of 150/100 mm Hg or higher is considered hypertensive.

8. c. 100 or more; tachycardia—*Tachycardia* refers to an abnormally fast heart rate of more than 100 beats per minute.

9. b. verbal—If the patient was confused after the collision, he would be rated "V" for verbal; he probably would not score an "A" for alert unless he knows his name, the place where he is now, and the day of the week.

10. d. A patient who is not alert may have a serious head injury.—A patient who is not alert may have a serious head injury or medical problem, such as hypoglycemia.

11. d. The generalized survey can yield subtle findings that may relate to the chief complaint.—A generalized survey helps the EMT-I refine the assessment and can help identify findings consistent with the chief complaint.

12. d. all of the above.—The EMT-I should note the patient's skin color, temperature, and condition (skin CTC).

13. b. The patient may be dehydrated.—Tenting of the skin is a sign associated with dehydration. If you suspect dehydration, look for other signs to confirm your suspicions, such as a dry, furrowed tongue, hypotension, or altered mental status.

14. a. clubbing; smokers—Clubbing, which may be present in the nails of the hands and/or feet, is a sign often associated with smoking and COPD.

15. a. tenting.—Tenting of the skin is a sign associated with dehydration. If you suspect dehydration, look for other signs to confirm your suspicions, such as a dry, furrowed tongue, hypotension, or altered mental status.

16. d. all of the above.—The EMT-I should suspect that a patient with these signs is contagious and should take the proper precautions.

17. b. Battle's sign—This finding is associated with a basilar skull fracture.

18. a. epistaxis—Blood in the nostrils is most likely from a nosebleed (epistaxis).

19. a. "H"—The six cardinal positions of gaze refer to the primary extraocular movements (EOMs), or movements of the eyeball. This simple test is used to evaluate cranial nerves III, IV, and VI to detect midbrain and pontine dysfunction. Checking EOMs is the best single method for measuring brain stem integrity. In the "H" pattern, the patient is directed to look up and down, left and right, and diagonally.

20. d. shining a light into both eyes at the same time.— When examining a patient's eyes, the EMT-I should assess for size of each pupil, reaction to light, and ability to follow the motion of a finger. Shining a light into both eyes is uncomfortable, blinding, and unnecessary.

21. d. There is no significance if the patient is looking into the sunlight.—A constricted pupil can mean a number of things, but it may also not be significant. The pupils of both eyes will normally constrict when exposed to bright light.

22. d. Do you have contact lenses in at the moment?—Contact lenses can irritate the eyes and alter the color of the eyes, in addition to affecting vision; all these can distort the assessment of the eyes.

23. c. The patient may have a basilar skull fracture.—Fractures may allow the escape of blood and fluid that are normally contained within the skull.

24. d. cerebrospinal fluid—CSF is clear, but is often present with blood from a traumatic injury to the head.

25. d. an explosion within a confined space—The mechanism of this type of injury is typically the blast effect from an explosion within a confined space or close proximity to the blast out of a confined space.

26. c. The patient may have inhaled superheated fumes at a fire scene.—The nose hairs could have been singed during inhalation; the cough that produces dark sputum most likely is clearing inhaled ash and debris from the lungs.

27. d. A nasal airway may not slide easily into one of the nostrils.—Knowing that a patient has a deviated septum is useful in case you must choose to place a nasal airway adjunct.

28. d. patient's mouth for broken teeth and bleeding.—This is the "A" in assessment of the ABCs; a mouthful of blood and/or broken teeth can easily obstruct the patient's airway.

29. c. relationship of the structures to the midline.—Vital structures in the neck (e.g., trachea, carotid artery, internal and external jugular veins) should be assessed. Typically, part of the assessment of these structures determines their relationship to the midline of the neck.

30. d. She may have fractured her larynx.—A raspy voice with low volume can be caused by a blow to the neck. A fracture of the larynx will produce a raspy voice and progressively worsening dyspnea.

31. d. all of the above—If the mechanism of injury (MOI) leads you to suspect that a patient may have a cervical spine injury, you should open the airway with a jaw thrust (if the patient is unconscious), apply a rigid collar, and fully immobilize the entire spine on a long backboard.

32. d. a segment of ribs that is unstable, with a feeling of crepitus—Upon palpation of the chest wall, you would expect to feel a segment of fractured ribs broken in two or more places and possibly crepitus (grating of the bones). Subcutaneous emphysema (bubble-wrap sensation) may also be palpated in some cases if lung has been punctured.

33. b. a dull sound compared to the rest of the lung fields—Pneumonia or a tumor in the lungs will cause a dull sound upon percussion over the affected area.

34. b. Kussmaul's respirations in the diabetic patient—Decreased ventilation volume may be caused by a flail chest, a pneumothorax, or a drug overdose.

35. d. injuries to both the anterior and posterior chest.—During the physical exam on a trauma patient, the EMT-I should check for injuries to both the anterior (front) and posterior (back) of the chest. Searching for other items is not part of the physical exam.

36. d. excursion or movement of the diaphragm.—Normally, the location of the sounds will change as the patient breathes in and out.

37. a. rales.—Rales are also called crackles.

38. c. a wheeze.—The musical tones that can be heard when listening to a patient's chest when the patient's bronchioles are constricted is wheezing.

39. d. pleural rub.—This coarse, grating sound is very different from any other lung sounds. It is associated with a lack of fluid or inflammation of the membranes that surround the lung.

40. d. rate, regularity, and strength.—Assessment of the rate, regularity of the rhythm, and strength of the arterial pulses provides information about the patient's perfusion status.

41. d. semi-Fowler's—The semi-Fowler's position places the patient at a 45-degree angle. Neck veins will normally be distended when a patient is supine and mostly flat when he or she is sitting upright. Distention when the patient is in the semi-Fowler's position is abnormal and should be noted.

42. a. distended neck veins.—Any injury that limits the flow of blood can cause distention of the neck veins from blood backing up from the heart.

43. d. point of maximal impulse (PMI)—The normal place to see or feel the PMI is on the chest, where the left ventricle of the heart is. If the PMI is out of place, there may be a problem with the heart (e.g., hypertrophy, tension pneumothorax).

44. b. movement of the valves.—The "lub" and "dub" sounds heard upon auscultation of the heart are caused by the opening and closing of the valves.

45. b. abnormal, and may indicate a problem.—Galloping heart sounds are abnormal and may indicate a problem.

46. d. pleural rub if it can be heard upon inhalation or exhalation.—This coarse, grating sound, which is heard when the patient inhales or exhales, is very different from any other lung sounds. Pleural rub is associated with a lack of fluid or inflammation of the membranes that surround the lung.

47. a. all four quadrants.—The abdominal cavity is large and contains many organs. For assessment purposes, it is divided into four quadrants. The EMT-I should know the underlying structures in each quadrant and know how to assess each quadrant.

48. a. normal.—A soft and supple abdomen is normal.

49. c. if the EMT-I suspects that labor is causing crowning—The EMT-I would need to examine a female patient's external genitalia if he thinks that delivery is imminent.

50. d. all of the above—The EMT-I should examine the male external genitalia if it is likely that the patient sustained injury in that area.

51. c. full range of motion—When a patient has a suspected fracture of an extremity, you should assess for distal pulses, distal motor function, and distal sensation. Assessing for full range of motion may cause further injury.

52. d. both arms for equal strength, at the same time.—While assessing both sides at the same time, you assess for a deficit on one side.

53. d. Deep palpation is usually done on the abdomen of a patient who is in the hospital.—Deep palpation is used, for example, to assess the size and location of the liver.

54. d. the elasticity of the skin—*Skin turgor* refers to the elasticity of the skin.

55. d. peripheral vascular system.—Phlebitis is infection of a vein and thus affects the peripheral vascular system.

56. b. assessment of the cranial nerves.—A nervous system exam should include assessment of the cranial nerves, the strength in the extremities, and the patient's mental status.

57. d. Korotkoff's sounds.—The sounds heard through the stethoscope while taking a BP are called *Korotkoff's sounds*.

58. d. poor skin turgor, due to deterioration of connective tissue.—In elderly patients, the loss of connective tissue causes the skin to become loose and hang.

59. d. in the midaxillary line at the fourth to sixth intercostal spaces—The apical pulse may be heard or felt over the heart. An apical pulse is frequently assessed in infants.

60. b. properly document the findings on the PCR.—All exam findings should be carefully documented on the PCR. This information becomes part of the patient's permanent record.

Chapter 8: Patient Assessment

1. c. it is night time and the porch light has not been turned on.—The EMT-I should suspect a potential hazard when things appear out of place or irregular, such as lights have not been turned on at night, there is screaming coming from the house, or the front door has broken glass.

2. c. a 12-inch-high marble statue—A statue or other ornament in a typical living room or family room can be knocked over while the EMT-I is working in that area. Such items may also be used purposely to hurt the EMT-I. Be careful!

3. c. an improperly vented fireplace that is leaking carbon monoxide—Exposure to a low-oxygen environment, such as a room filled with carbon monoxide from an improperly vented fireplace, poses a greater potential hazard than any item that might be used in an intentional act of violence.

4. c. discreetly notify the police and do not touch anything.—The cookers in a homemade laboratory can easily explode if improperly handled.

5. d. all of the above.—Their clothing, or "colors," are very important to gang members, who often carry weapons. You must respect these patients and their property or you may be seriously injured or killed.

6. d. the traffic flow.—Always watch out for passing cars and other vehicles; inattentive drivers can drive right into the accident scene and you.

7. a. send police to the scene for traffic control and investigation.—The fire department is dispatched when a hazard is reported or extrication is needed. A second ambulance is usually sent with the first ambulance, though on low priority, until the actual number of patients is determined.

8. a. up-and-over—A frontal collision tends to eject the patient up and over the steering wheel and/or dashboard into the windshield, producing injuries to the head and neck.

9. c. recent upper respiratory infection.—An upper respiratory infection can exacerbate respiratory problems in a patient who has emphysema and is on home oxygen.

10. a. It can help predict injury patterns.—An EMT-I who recognizes and appreciates the MOI can predict probable injuries the patient may have sustained. This helps the EMT-I prepare to care for specific injuries that might otherwise go unnoticed initially and potentially lead to a life-threatening condition.

11. c. identify the total number of patients and call for any additional needed help.—Additional help should be summoned as soon as possible, as it takes them time to respond and get to the scene.

12. b. conducting an initial assessment of the patient—The initial assessment is not part of the scene size-up. The scene size-up does include determining if there are any hazards to you and your crew, taking BSI precautions, and ensuring that you have appropriate help on the way.

13. d. all of the above—These rationales all relate to the basics of the EMT-I job: ensuring safety and rendering timely, appropriate assistance to patients.

14. a. patient priority—The general impression of the patient includes the patient's approximate age, degree of distress, and sex.

15. d. verbally responsive—A patient who is conscious but confused after striking his head is most likely verbally responsive.

16. a. alert—If the patient knows his name, where he is, and the day of the week, he is classified as alert.

17. b. the patient's baseline mental status as discovered on the scene—The initial mental status could indicate a head injury that might be missed if you do not give report about it.

18. d. unresponsive—A patient who is unconscious and does not react to painful stimuli is classified as unresponsive.

19. a. withdraw from the pain source.—When pain is applied to a patient who is not alert, in an effort to determine the patient's mental status, an "appropriate" response is to withdraw from the pain source.

20. d. maintain manual head/neck stabilization if you suspect trauma.—When an unconscious patient is discovered, the cervical spine should be managed with special care until a mechanism of injury can be determined.

21. d. attempt insertion of an oropharyngeal airway.—The loss of a gag reflex indicates that the patient cannot protect his own airway; the EMT-I must do this for him with an OPA.

22. d. jaw thrust with head stabilization.—This technique is used to open the airway without compromising the cervical spine.

23. c. spinal precautions are—When assessing a scene, one of the first things the EMT-I should determine is if spinal precautions are needed. Delaying this choice could compromise the patient's spinal cord.

24. c. check the patient for breathing.—Follow the ABCs: airway, breathing, and circulation.

25. d. breathing may not be adequate.—Rib fractures make every breath painful, and the patient tends to guard and hypoventilate because of the pain.

26. a. look for chest rise.—An assessment of patient breathing always includes looking for chest rise, listening for air exchange, and feeling for air coming out of the mouth and nose.

27. b. increase the respiratory rate—Tachypnea (increased respiratory rate) is normal with a chest wall injury.

28. c. quickly check for external bleeding.—Follow the ABCs: airway, breathing, circulation. Checking for external bleeding is part of the assessment of circulation.

29. d. control the bleeding in the arm and proceed with the initial assessment.—After the airway and breathing are managed, serious bleeding should be controlled, as part of the "C" (circulation) step of the ABCs.

30. d. color, temperature, and condition.—Skin CTC is part of the assessment of circulation.

31. a. cyanosis; hypoxia—Blue skin coloring is called cyanosis. Likely causes are hypoxia or exposure to cold.

32. d. a fever or infection.—Fever and chills indicate the presence of an infection. Take the proper precautions!

33. d. indicates that you should actually measure the body temperature with a thermometer.—An abnormal finding of cold, dry skin should prompt you to make more precise measurements.

34. b. dehydrated.—Tenting of the skin is usually caused by dehydration, and may occur in patients of any age.

35. a. made a decision as to transport priority.—During the initial assessment, the EMT-I decides on the transport destination and priority, and reassesses or reconsiders the MOI.

36. c. a patient who may have sustained an injury to the lower back from a fall—Patients with cardiac chest pain, respiratory depression, and complicated childbirth are critical, with high priority for immediate transport.

37. a. a 37-year-old female with a suspected ectopic pregnancy—Even if you have the resources to provide appropriate treatment on the scene, the patient with the possible ectopic pregnancy has the highest priority for transport.

38. d. only if you have to convince the patient to go to the hospital—Assessment of orthostatic vital signs can be dangerous for the patient, so these signs should be assessed only when the EMT-I has to persuade a trauma victim who is vehemently refusing to go to the ED.

39. c. focused—The EMT-I performs a focused exam based on the patient's chief complaint and findings from the initial assessment.

40. a. a rapid trauma exam.—The rapid physical exam is similar to the rapid trauma exam performed on trauma patients.

41. a. do a focused neuro exam.—The Cincinnati and Los Angeles stroke exams are two examples of mini neuro assessments used in the prehospital setting for the patient with a suspected stroke.

42. d. you want to be sure that no significant trauma was involved—Many MOIs have predictable injury patterns that can help responders anticipate specific injuries. When the forces a patient has suffered can be mentally visualized, so can the potential for injury.

43. d. the patient who has a minor laceration or sprained ankle—These injuries are minor and isolated to one region of the body. A focused trauma exam of that specific body region is appropriate.

44. c. mouth.—The rapid trauma exam includes the head, posterior, and pelvis, but not the mouth, which is part of the detailed physical exam (DPE).

45. d. treat it as if found during the initial assessment and begin to stabilize.—A flail chest is a significant injury affecting breathing (the "B" of the ABCs) and must be managed immediately.

46. d. all of the above.—The ongoing assessment includes repeating the initial assessment as needed, reassessing the vital signs, and reassessing the interventions.

47. d. the patient who is unconscious from serious head trauma—A DPE is performed on patients with a significant MOI. Typically it is performed en route to the hospital, manpower and time permitting.

48. b. to reassess life threats and treat them quickly—Emergency care is dynamic and the patient's status can change suddenly.

49. d. a much more detailed look at the head.—The DPE includes a detailed examination of the nose, mouth, ears, and eyes.

50. c. blood or leaking fluid.—Hearing is assessed as part of a comprehensive exam, which takes a lot more time and is rarely done in the field.

51. c. the presence of a Medic Alert® bracelet.—This piece of jewelry alerts responders to specific medical conditions such as diabetes, heart problems, or hypertension.

52. c. Trending can help the EMT-I determine if the patient's condition is changing—It is important to trend vital signs so you will know whether the patient's condition is changing (improving or deteriorating).

53. d. reassessment of the vital signs—Reassessment is a component of the ongoing assessment, which is done en route to the ED. The SAMPLE history, DCAP-BTLS, and OPQRST are parts of the FHPE, RTE/RPE, and elaboration of the chief complaint.

54. c. severity—The "S" in OPQRST stands for severity.

55. b. abrasions—The "A" in DCAP-BTLS stands for abrasions.

Chapter 9: Clinical Decision Making

1. a. a relatively controlled environment in the hospital.—Care in the field is heavily influenced by environmental factors such as weather, hazards, time constraints, limited personnel and resources, extrication, and access. Other differences in the out-of-hospital setting include the need for ongoing adaptability and thinking on the fly.

2. a. not life-threatening.—A call for assistance in lifting and moving a wheelchair-restricted patient is an additional example of non-life-threatening situations.

3. b. Protocols often omit patients with multisystem failure.—Each of the other choices is an advantage of using protocols and standing orders.

4. c. Standing orders are typically not helpful for patients with vague symptoms or when the patient has complaints associated with multiple systems or disease processes.—Each of the other choices is a disadvantage of using protocols and standing orders.

5. d. all of the above.—Each of the answers gives an essential concept of clinical decision making for the EMT-I.

6. c. both positively and negatively.—Hormonal responses may result in improved reflexes and muscular strength, enhanced visual and auditory acuity, diminished concentration and assessment abilities, and impaired critical-thinking skills.

7. d. using a radical plan of action—There is a short list of mental preparation tricks to fall back on when critical things becomes clouded. Stay calm and take a look at the situation; stop and think before acting. This will help to avoid panic. Anticipate and plan for the worst. This will help you follow a systematic and controlled plan of action. Reassess frequently and facilitate a dynamic course of management using a system approach. Pause and take a deep breath when experiencing a sensory overload; rely on the priority MS-ABC plan.

8. b. review.—Review of performance is the final "R"; this suggests that EMT-Is should discuss and analyze their actions after the call.

9. a. mechanism of injury—Reading the scene includes evaluating the MOI, the environmental conditions, and the immediate surroundings.

10. b. Look up the correct dose in your protocol reference.—We all have memory lapses from time to time. When it comes to treatment, especially with drugs, do not guess; take a moment and look it up or ask someone. Even doctors carry pocket references and look things up. It is unethical and unprofessional to guess.

11. a. documenting medical ambiguity—Identifying and managing medical ambiguity, rather than documenting it, is a fundamental element of critical thinking.

12. a. Ask the patient questions.—Critical thinking integrates both objective and subjective data. Always ask "Why?" and encourage the patient to actively participate in the process (e.g., by providing explanations and using teaching moments).

13. a. maintaining a systematic assessment pattern.—Anticipate and plan for the worst. This will help you follow and maintain a systematic and controlled plan of action.

14. c. collecting information and formulating concepts.—The framework and flow of the critical-thinking process should follow a logical plan that resembles the following: collect information and formulate concepts; interpret and process information; provide treatment and manage the patient; reevaluate and reflect.

15. b. Ask your partner to reassess the blood pressure.—Verify assessment data that is significantly out of the normal range. When you get an abnormal reading, double-check it or ask a partner to check it.

Chapter 10: Communications

1. b. the physician can assist the EMT-I with treatment orders.—Communication is an essential component of emergency medical services. The EMT-I is an extension of the in-hospital team and must effectively communicate patient assessment and management to the ED physician so that the physician can assist with treatment orders and the staff can prepare for the patient's arrival.

2. d. verbal, written, and electronic—The EMT-I must use verbal communication to receive, respond to, assess, manage, transport, and turn over a patient to the ED. Documentation is an essential skill for completing the prehospital care report (PCR). Electronic devices are integrated through all phases of patient management (radios, monitors, meters, telephones, and the like).

3. c. Emergency medical dispatch (EMD) receives a call for help and dispatches an ambulance.—The phases of a communication for a typical EMS call include: occurrence, detection, notification, response, treatment, preparation for transport, and preparation for the next call.

4. d. special codes increase the possibility of multiple interpretations.—Proper verbal communication helps to prevent confusion. Special codes add an unnecessary level of complexity, especially during hazmat incidents and multiple-casualty incidents (MCIs).

5. d. television shows about EMS—Fancy jargon sounds good on television, but adds an unnecessary level of complexity during EMS events. The trend in EMS has been to use plain English, especially during large events (e.g., MCIs) where more than one agency is involved.

6. c. using technical terminology—Two factors that tend to impede verbal communications are use of technical terminology and semantics. EMT-Is should select their words and phrases with the audience in mind. Use technical terms with peers or other health care providers and use plain English with patients.

7. b. Use terms that are easy to understand and avoid mumbling.—Speaking clearly enhances verbal communication. Open your mouth, don't mumble words, and use terms that are easy to understand.

8. a. it is the written and legal record of the incident.—In medicine, the saying goes, "If you didn't write it down, you didn't do it!" This is how important documentation is to patient care.

9. a. documenting opinionated information—When documenting, always try to use objective language and not make judgments. Be specific and concrete by documenting exactly what you see, hear, feel, or smell. Avoid adding your interpretation of the reasons why the patient exhibited specific behavior.

10. b. Document patient statements on a PCR using exact quotations.—The EMT-I should document the patient's own words by using quotes in the PCR (e.g., "I only had two beers.").

11. a. to a third party for billing purposes is legal.—The release of patient information requires written

permission from the patient or legal guardian in all situations, except the following: when the law requires mandatory reporting, in response to a subpoena, to health care providers with a need to know so that they can provide care to the patient, and when a third party requires the information for billing.

12. b. interpreting body language—Body language constitutes nearly 97 percent of nonverbal communication.

13. c. obtain a court order or search warrant.—Depending on the circumstances and type of information desired, a search warrant or a court order is needed for legal access to electronic communications, either stored or during transmission.

14. a. Radio transmissions are public and open for all to hear.—Assume that radio transmissions are open for all to hear. Never say anything over the radio, including the patient's name, that you would be uncomfortable saying during a news conference.

15. b. duplex communication.—This type of equipment involves two frequencies, both of which have the capability to transmit and receive (e.g., telephone).

16. c. A public safety access point—Most communities access the PSAP through 9-1-1. Other means of access include highway call boxes, citizen band radio, and amateur radio.

17. b. regulating all aspects of the communication industry.—The FCC's primary goals include promoting competition in communication, protecting consumers, and supporting access by every American to existing and advanced telecommunication services.

18. a. providing prearrival instructions.—A trained EMD may give prearrival instructions to a caller, telling the caller specific skills to perform (e.g., how to control bleeding or perform cardiac compressions).

19. d. What is the patient's past medical history?—The fourth key question is: "What is the patient's age?"

20. a. queue—This is the time between receipt of the call and the time the call is given to the unit to respond.

21. b. second—A first-party caller is the patient; a third-party caller is someone who is calling for the patient but is not in direct contact with the patient.

22. c. based on a format that is standard, but varies slightly in each community.—The format is standard, but there may be some local variances based on your hospital's needs and your medical director's wishes.

23. c. give the staff time to prepare for the patient.—A verbal report over the radio or telephone helps prepare the ED for the arrival of the patient. Sometimes they will need to clear a bed or locate a specialty physician or complete other time-consuming activities before the patient arrives.

24. d. ensure that the message was received and understood correctly.—Echoing should always be done, particularly when confirming a medication order, to ensure that the EMT-I received and interpreted the message correctly.

25. b. sender decodes the message—The basic model of communication has six steps: the sender has a message, the sender encodes the message, the sender sends the message, the receiver receives the message, the receiver decodes the message, and the receiver gives feedback to the sender.

26. b. telemetry.—One example of telemetry is the transmission of a patient's ECG to the ED by the EMT-I in the field.

27. b. very high—The VHF spectrum is further divided into high and low bands.

28. d. all of the above—Sometimes buzzing or 60-cycle interference can occur when the radio is too close to these objects.

29. a. analog.—Analog is a voice transmission. This is old technology, and there are a limited number of radio frequencies available for analog technology. Therefore, many analog systems are switching to digital communication.

30. b. determine which unit to send to a call.—Specialized versions of CAD use devices placed in each emergency vehicle that constantly send messages to the dispatcher's computer screen, to give the EMD the exact location of the vehicle.

Chapter 11: Documentation

1. a. Poor documentation is an indication of a poor assessment.—Documentation is a very important component of patient care. In medicine, the saying is that if you didn't write it down, you didn't do it. Whether or not the EMT-I's patient care was optimal, poor documentation is hard to explain or defend, and a difficult legal hurdle to overcome.

2. b. infarct—The definition is provided in the question.

3. d. saturation of partial pressure of oxygen.—The abbreviation SpO_2 represents oxygen saturation (more specifically, the partial pressure of oxygen or PO_2) as measured by pulse oximetry.

4. a. run times—PCRs typically include administrative information such as address, patient's date of birth, telephone number, and run times.

5. a. cefalad—The correct spelling is *cephalad*. The term means toward the head.

6. d. third-party payer—The patient's insurance company is often referred to as the third-party payer.

7. d. The patient was calm and cooperative during the transport.—Expressions and terms used on a PCR must be professional and standardized. Avoid judgments, biases, stereotyping, derogatory terms, or reference to an EMS system-abuse call.

8. d. The patient stated that he vomited twice this morning.—It is important to use objective, concrete language. Document only what you see, hear, feel, or smell. When a patient, family, or bystander gives you specific information, use quotes or say that "the patient stated" or "the spouse stated."

9. c. the patient's response to the drug—The information that the EMT-I should document regarding a medication administration includes: name of the drug; the person administering the drug; the dose, route, and time of administration; and the patient's response to the medication.

10. d. mm Hg—*Millimeters of mercury* refers to the units of a blood pressure gauge.

11. d. PCRs that are used for quality improvement or educational purposes should not include the patient's name.—Federal legislation requires health care providers to maintain the privacy of certain confidential health care information, known as protected health information or PHI.

12. c. may indicate that the EMT-I did not provide proper patient care.—Incomplete, inaccurate, or illegible information on a PCR can create problems where none really exists, because the presumption often is that the EMT-I either did not provide the proper care or had something to hide.

13. a. triage tags.—At an MCI, triage is done on all patients to ensure that the patients with the most serious conditions are treated and transported first. Triage tags are often used as the first line of documentation at an MCI.

14. b. narrative.—The narrative gives a written-out report of the call, unlike other sections of the PCR that are fill-in or check-the-box style.

15. d. SOAP and CHEATED—The SOAP narrative format is Subjective (what the patient tells you), Objective (what you observe), Assessment (examination findings), and Plan (action of management and treatment). The CHEATED narrative is Chief Complaint, History of present illness (also past medical history), Examination, Assessment, Treatment, Evaluation of treatments, and Disposition (health care provider turned over to).

16. d. refusal of medical attention—The RMA is written by the EMT-I on the scene. Some agencies document the RMA on the PCR; others also complete a special addendum designed especially for this type of call.

17. c. auscultation of bilateral breath sounds—All of the information listed in the question choices should be recorded in the PCR; however, the *vital* findings to be recorded include the auscultation of bilateral breath sounds, auscultation of the epigastrium, and at least two other methods for confirming tube placement (e.g., visualization of the tube passing through the vocal cords, use of an esophageal intubation detection device (EID), or capnography).

18. d. The PCR contains complete and accurate information regarding the patient's needs and the care provided.—The record should provide a portrait of the patient's needs and the care given in a clear, legible, and concise fashion.

19. a. no shortness of breath—Cardiac-type chest pain with no shortness of breath is a pertinent negative, because dyspnea is frequently associated with acute cardiac syndromes.

20. c. Document the information on an addendum and distribute copies of the addendum.—Once copies have been distributed, it is not good practice to add information to only one copy. Typically, additional or omitted information is documented on an addendum and the copies are distributed the same as the original PCR. Follow local protocol or check with your medical director for guidance on this matter.

21. d. doing the right thing if she initials the changes.—The appropriate way to make changes on a PCR before copies are distributed is to draw a line through the error (do not erase or block out), initial the change, and make the correction.

22. c. an emergency vehicle collision en route to a call—Each of the examples provided is typically recorded on the PCR as well as a special incident report, except for an incident in which no patient is involved as yet.

23. d. The use of standard abbreviations is acceptable in many EMS systems.—If you are not sure about an abbreviation, look it up in the dictionary or refer to your local protocols. Many EMS systems have a list of acceptable and unacceptable abbreviations.

24. c. standardized.—A simple rule to remember about the language used in a PCR is to keep it professional and standardized; avoid judgmental biases, stereotyping, and derogatory terms.

25. b. document the patient's statements in the narrative using quotation marks.—When the patient makes statements for which there is no designated space on the PCR (e.g., dying statement, threat of suicide, or "I drank two six-packs"), the EMT-I should document the statement using the patient's exact words and quotation marks.

Chapter 12: Trauma Systems and Mechanism of Injury

1. a. hospice care.—The components of a trauma system are injury prevention programs, prehospital care (triage, treatment, and transport), ED care (with interfacility transport if necessary), definitive care, critical trauma care, rehabilitation, and data collection (trauma registry).

2. b. resources and programs available at the facility.—Each community has different needs and resources, so trauma centers have been classified into four levels based on the resources and programs available at each facility.

3. a. in your local protocols.—These criteria are based on the structure of the region's trauma care system and thus can vary from region to region. An intermediate training text may offer general information, and more information specific to the region can usually be found in local protocols.

4. a. critical burn patient—One criterion for air-medical transport is the need for access to specialized critical care personnel or specialty units in certain hospitals (e.g., burn center, neonatal intensive care unit, reimplantation center).

5. c. mechanism of injury.—The type of force, its intensity, its direction, and the body area(s) affected are all part of the MOI. The forces that cause injury must be considered when the EMT-I tries to predict certain types of injuries.

6. a. speed the object was traveling is significant.—The formula for kinetic energy is $KE = mass/2 \times velocity^2$. This means that the more speed (motion) there is, the more energy there is. The way kinetic energy relates to the MOI is summed up in the concept that "speed kills."

7. b. cavitation.—Cavitation is a good example of an energy exchange. As the bullet enters the body, the tissues are forced apart momentarily, accelerating away from the track of the projectile and thereby creating a cavity. This cavity can be temporary or permanent depending on the amount of energy transferred and the density of the object struck.

8. a. coup—Coup injuries develop from directly beneath the point of impact. Contrecoup injuries develop on the side opposite the point of impact.

9. c. the loss of consciousness—The EMT-I must consider that any change in mental status resulting from a traumatic event may indicate possible brain injury; this makes the patient unreliable. If the patient is unreliable, and you suspect a significant or questionable MOI for the spinal injury, it is essential that spinal immobilization be done.

10. a. rotation—This is the movement of the head to the left or right from the midline. In a collision, the victim typically sees (even if only for a split second) the direction from which the force is coming. Excessive rotation beyond the normal range, caused by acceleration forces (collision), may cause flexion-rotation dislocation, as well as fracture or dislocation of the vertebrae. A rupture of the supporting ligaments may also occur. The cervical spine is the most common region for this type of injury.

11. c. airbag deployment—When an airbag is deployed in a crash, the bag fills rapidly. Often the sudden impact of the filling bag, together with the rapid deceleration, cause minor injuries such as facial and forearm abrasions. If the vehicle occupant is wearing glasses, the frames can leave a mark or small laceration on the face. The cornstarch in which the airbag is stored creates a cloud that often causes the occupant to choke in the first few seconds after impact. Tenderness and bruising of the sternum are also common.

12. d. velocity.—Speed kills! The units for kinetic energy yield a significant increase of 52,500 units with just 10 additional mph. In contrast, an increase of 50 pounds yields an increase of only 22,500.

13. a. Both types of injuries can be lethal.—Penetrating trauma is usually easier to recognize than blunt trauma, which creates a temporary cavity but does not penetrate body tissues.

14. c. tertiary—In the tertiary phase, injuries result from the patient becoming a flying object and striking other objects.

15. d. create a large entry point and more tissue damage.—Tumbling bullets create greater tissue damage because the side of the bullet, rather than the smaller leading edge, enters the body, thus creating a larger entry point.

Chapter 13: Hemorrhage and Shock

1. a. severity of bleeding.—The severity of bleeding, the treatment provided for the patient, and the patient's previous health each have an impact on the patient's mortality from hemorrhage and shock.

2. c. decompensatory—As bleeding continues uncontrolled, the body, in an effort for self-preservation, will shunt blood from nonvital organs (such as the skin and intestines) and redirect the blood to the brain, heart, and lungs.

3. d. consider occult gastrointestinal (GI) bleeding as the cause.—The EMT-I must consider intraabdominal bleeding as the cause of shock in a patient who presents with signs and symptoms of hypovolemia but no external cause.

4. c. hematochezia.—The passage of bright red blood in stools is called *hematochezia*.

5. b. apply direct pressure and elevation.—The steps for bleeding control are the same for any injury: direct pressure with a bandage, elevation, application of a pressure bandage, and compression of a pressure point. When a possible fracture is involved, consider laying the patient supine until the extremity can be splinted and then elevate the extremity.

6. d. All of the above.—The application of a cold pack or ice is helpful for all of the reasons listed.

7. c. Apply direct pressure on the popliteal artery.—The nearest pressure point for controlling bleeding in the lower leg is the popliteal artery.

8. d. none of the above.—Typically, the bleeding from a gunshot wound will remain uncontrolled in the prehospital setting. Even when the patient's vital signs appear normal, the EMT-I should suspect internal bleeding and treat for shock.

9. c. volume expansion.—The primary role of IV fluid replacement in the management of hemorrhage is volume expansion. The fluid controversy is ongoing, and answers as to what type of fluid to use, and how much, will vary in different areas of the country. For trauma, the accepted approach is fluid therapy using normal saline, despite a few studies that have disputed this. Follow your local protocol.

10. a. increase the arterial pressure.—When the body senses a decrease in systolic pressure, the body compensates in several ways: by vasoconstriction of the peripheral vessels, by stimulation of the vasomotor center to increase the arterial pressure, by stimulation from the sympathetic nervous system to release of epinephrine and norepinephrine. Insulin secretion is diminished by the release of epinephrine, and hormones that regulate water retention are activated.

11. b. is experiencing early hypovolemic shock.—A narrowing pulse pressure is an early sign of hypovolemic shock. The systolic pressure drops slightly (due to volume loss) and the diastolic pressure increases (representing vasoconstriction as a compensatory mechanism).

12. a. Baroreceptors sense decreased arterial blood flow.—As the arterial pressure decreases, because of blood loss (internal or external) or the loss of vasomotor tone, the baroreceptors in the carotid sinuses and aortic arch sense the decrease. They then activate the vasomotor center, which in turn causes vasoconstriction of the peripheral vessels.

13. b. minimal blood flow to the capillaries—The cells switch from aerobic to anaerobic metabolism in response to minimal blood flow to the capillaries. Anaerobic metabolism is less efficient and produces many acids.

14. d. the cells switch from aerobic to anaerobic metabolism.—In the ischemic phase, there is minimal blood flow to the capillaries, so the cells switch from aerobic to anaerobic metabolism.

15. a. ischemic, stagnation, and washout—During decreased perfusion states, the cells go through three distinct phases: the ischemic phase, the stagnation phase, and the washout phase.

16. c. cardiogenic—The myocardial depressant factor(s) that are released during cellular changes lead to cardiogenic shock.

17. d. the amount of blood ejected from the left ventricle with each contraction.—In an adult, the stroke volume is approximately 70 ml of blood per beat, or 4,900 ml per minute.

18. b. the transport of blood.—To have perfusion, there must be blood (fluid), vessels (the pipes), and a working heart (the pump).

19. a. one—A person can go into stage one shock by donating a pint of blood; that is why it is recommended that donors rest for half an hour and avoid drinking alcohol or doing strenuous activity.

20. b. isotonic solutions—Normal saline or Ringer's lactate have the same tonicity (osmolarity) as plasma.

21. c. a large gaping wound in the upper arm—Sources of bleeding that the EMT-I should not pack in the prehospital setting include vagina, rectum, mouth, and ears.

22. a. bleeding is coming from the lungs or upper GI.—Bright red blood indicates active arterial bleeding, usually from a laceration, of the lungs or esophagus.

23. d. decreased mental status.—A significant decrease in mental status is a sign of the late or decompensated phase of hypovolemic shock.

24. c. cardiogenic.—Cardiogenic shock occurs with a loss of 40 percent or more of the functioning ventricular myocardium, regardless of the reason for the loss. Cardiogenic shock is differentiated from hypovolemic shock by one or more of the following: chief complaint of dyspnea, chest pain, tachycardia, bradycardia, and signs of congestive heart failure (JVD, rales, and dysrhythmias).

25. b. obstructive—Obstructive shock occurs with blockage to the heart or great vessels. It can be differentiated from hypovolemic shock by the presence of distended neck veins and a narrowing pulse pressure.

26. a. distributive—Anaphylactic shock is a form of distributive shock in which there is increased venous capacitance and low resistance, or vasoconstriction. Distributive shock can occur with spinal injury, and septic shock also fits in this category of shock.

27. a. lay her down—Dizziness following a syncopal event suggests hypotension from volume depletion until proven otherwise. Lay the patient down before she falls down (again), then administer oxygen and obtain a blood pressure, ECG, and glucose level.

28. d. intravascular volume depletion.—Dizziness or syncope in a patient who is sitting or standing during your assessment suggests significant intravascular volume depletion. If this condition occurs when the patient moves quickly from the supine to a sitting or standing position, it is known as *orthostatic* or *postural hypotension.*

29. c. bleeding from the stomach.—Vomiting of a substance that resembles coffee grounds can result from a mix of upper GI bleeding and the digestive substances from the stomach. Coffee-ground vomitus is also associated with other substances that were recently eaten and aggravated the stomach, such as chocolate or too much spicy food.

30. a. a serious condition.—Patients can bleed to death from rectal bleeding, so this condition should always be taken seriously.

31. a. distributive—Distributive shock occurs with a mechanism that causes vasodilation, such as spinal cord injury, drug overdose, sepsis, or anaphylaxis.

32. b. loss of vasomotor tone.—Vasodilation from spinal cord injury, drug overdose, sepsis, or anaphylaxis, when unrecognized or untreated, can cause the progression of shock to death.

33. b. two.—This stage or phase is also referred to as *compensated shock*. In stage two, the cardiac output is maintained by arteriolar constriction and a reflex tachycardia.

34. d. increased blood pressure and organ perfusion.—A hot topic for debate is the mechanism by which PASGs work. Originally, it was thought that the garment increased the blood pressure by acting as an "autotransfusion" of up to two units of blood. Several studies have suggested that its primary action is really increasing the system vascular resistance (SVR) or constricting the blood vessels and tamponading bleeding vessels.

35. b. pelvic fractures.—Many EMS systems have restricted the use of PASGs to the stabilization of pelvic and femur fractures. Contraindications for the use of a PASG include pulmonary edema, CHF, pregnancy, cardiogenic shock, penetrating chest trauma, and chest injuries.

36. a. Septic—Sepsis is a toxic condition resulting from the spread of infection through the blood. The blood vessels dilate, causing the blood to pool. This is a form of distributive shock.

37. c. hypovolemic shock—Persistent and uncontrolled hemorrhage can progress to hypovolemic shock.

38. d. intravascular space.—About one-third of the fluid infused stays in the intravascular space. It does not carry hemoglobin like a transfusion of whole blood would.

39. d. interstitial space.—The infused IV fluid moves from the blood in the intravascular space into the interstitial fluid.

40. c. psychogenic—The patient faints because of a common nervous system reaction, in which a sudden dilation of the blood vessels occurs in response to a strong emotion (or the sight of blood) and the proper blood flow to the brain is momentarily interrupted. It is a temporary condition and self-correcting.

Chapter 14: Burns

1. a. an eschar formation.—*Eschar* is the thick, nonelastic scab or scar that forms on the skin following a burn. If large enough, it may impair circulation or respiration.

2. a. 10:00 a.m. to 2:00 p.m.—The sun's ultraviolet (UV) rays are the strongest during this time of day.

3. b. the heart—Preexisting problems with the kidneys, lungs, or heart may make it difficult for the patient to handle the tremendous movement of body fluids that occurs with a burn injury. Trauma also makes it difficult for the patient to recover from a burn.

4. c. chemical—The types of chemicals that commonly cause burns are acids, bases (alkalis), dry chemicals, and phenols.

5. c. full-thickness.—This burn involves all layers of the skin and may include underlying muscle and soft tissues (e.g., fascia) below the skin layer. The *fascia* is the layer of connective tissue covering other body structures.

6. d. use the surface area of the patient's palm to correspond to 1 percent of the patient's BSA.—Though this is a rough estimate, the surface area of the patient's palm (minus the digits) can be considered to correspond to approximately 1 percent of the patient's body surface area.

7. c. 18 percent—Using the rule of nines, an infant's head accounts for 18 percent of the infant's BSA.

8. b. The severity of a burn for a child involves less BSA than for an adult.—A severe burn for an adult is 30 percent BSA; for children, it is 15 percent BSA.

9. d. malignant melanoma—Malignant melanocytic tumors may present in a pigmented area of the skin, mucous membranes, eyes, or CNS. Sun exposure is a risk and the incidence is rising rapidly: there are about 25,000 new cases yearly and 6,000 deaths.

10. a. age—For patients over the age of 50, the rule is that the older the patient, the lower the percentage of total BSA burn he or she can tolerate. Infants and toddlers also do not tolerate serious burns well.

11. a. hot tar—The temperature of hot tar ranges from 400° to 500°F. Tar also sticks to the skin, creating a longer exposure time.

12. d. airway compromise from inhaling superheated gases—In most cases, victims found unconscious in structure fires have succumbed to inhalation injuries. The EMT-I should suspect airway and respiratory compromise from superheated and/or poisonous gases.

13. b. airway maintenance.—When singed nasal hairs and blood soot in the sputum are present, the EMT-I must be alert for any alteration in the volume and tone of the patient's voice, wheezing, or stridor. Assess the need for ventilation and intubation.

14. a. skin.—The skin is the largest organ of the body, accounting for nearly 15 percent of body weight in adults. It is a massive protective barrier for the body, but is itself exposed.

15. a. The eschar does not allow the chest to expand for ventilation.—Eschar is thick and nonelastic. When eschar is circumferential on the thorax or an extremity, it may impair respiration or circulation.

16. b. hypothermia.—The skin plays a primary role in heat regulation, insulates the body, and also serves as a protective barrier against infection and foreign elements. When it is damaged, the patient can become hypothermic and develop serious infections.

17. c. sweat ducts—A partial-thickness burn involves the dermis. The dermis contains sweat ducts, hair follicles, blood vessels, nerves, and sebaceous glands.

18. b. stop the burning.—First, stop the burning process and move the patient away from the burning environment, if that has not already been done. Then provide high-concentration oxygen, keep the patient warm, treat for shock, and provide emotional support.

19. d. covering the burn area with a dry burn dressing. —Dress a burn wound with a dry dressing unless the burn covers a very small BSA percentage or is a minor injury. Follow your local protocol.

20. d. partial-thickness—This burn involves the epidermis and dermis. In addition to the reddening, blistering, and peeling skin, the patient will have intense pain and will develop swelling.

21. d. microwave—Nonionizing radiation comes from sources such as light, radio waves, microwaves, and radar. It generally does not cause tissue damage.

22. c. carbon monoxide—Hyperbaric oxygen therapy for carbon monoxide inhalation is beneficial because it helps decrease the time it takes for the hemoglobin to become saturated with oxygen.

23. c. chemical—Chemical inhalation injury occurs more frequently than other types of inhalation burns. Chemical inhalation injuries are associated with toxic inhalation, smoke inhalation, carbon monoxide poisoning, and thiocyanate intoxication.

24. a. stridor—*Stridor*, or inspiratory wheezing, indicates that there is swelling in the airway due to an inhalation injury. Singed facial hair or soot on the face are clues that should prompt the EMT-I to be alert for possible inhalation injury.

25. d. amyl nitrate and thiosulfate—A cyanide antidote kit includes amyl nitrate and thiosulfate.

26. a. There is nothing you can do.—No treatment the EMT-I can provide will prevent airway swelling. The EMT-I should assess the need for assisted ventilation and intubation and provide what is necessary for the patient before the swelling becomes a complete airway obstruction. When the patient is conscious, sedation is often necessary. Call for the additional resources needed and follow local protocol.

27. a. primary—The primary phase of a blast creates a pressure wave that can cause major effects on the

lungs and GI tract. This is accompanied by a heat wave that affects the eyes and skin, and can burn any exposed areas of the body.

28. a. steam—Superheated gases will cause injuries to the upper airway (e.g., nose, mouth, and throat).

29. a. Ionizing radiation can cause injury by inhalation.—Ionizing radiation can be dangerous when taken internally, whether by inhalation or ingestion.

30. b. Remove the lenses or assist the patient to remove them.—Contact lenses should be removed as soon as possible when a patient has an eye injury or burn from a chemical agent. Leaving the lenses in could keep the chemical in the eye and keep the burning process going.

31. c. an industrial setting.—Many chemicals used in manufacturing processes are highly corrosive to the skin.

32. c. Sponge it off with a dry towel.—When the spray is still wet, carefully sponge it off and do not spread it around. Consider using water only to flush the eyes and for gargling.

33. b. phenol—If available, use alcohol to rinse off phenol (carbolic acid). Then irrigate the area with water to remove both the alcohol and any remaining phenol.

34. b. Inhalation injuries are often associated with chemical burns to the eyes.—The proximity of the chemical exposure to the airway creates a high risk for inhalation of chemical vapors.

35. a. Flush the affected area with a lot of water. —Flushing the affected area with copious amounts of water will dilute the chemical, cleanse the area, and cool the burn.

36. a. Assist the patient to a well-ventilated area.—Safety first for you, your crew, and the patient.

37. a. continued irrigation of both eyes—The patient is alert, his ABCs are protected, and his vital signs are adequate. Both eyes should be continuously irrigated for at least 20 minutes. This can be done en route to the hospital.

38. b. the body consists primarily of water.—Water is a great conductor of electricity, and 50 to 70 percent of a person's total body weight is fluid.

39. a. low-frequency AC—Low-frequency current of 50 to 60 Hz (cycles/second), which are commonly used, are more dangerous than high-frequency currents, and are 3 to 5 times more dangerous than direct current (DC) of the same voltage and amperage.

40. a. Lightning rarely produces an exit wound.— Lightning usually flashes over the patient, rather than striking the patient directly, so it seldom causes either entry or exit wounds.

41. d. hands—Current most commonly enters via the hands; next most common is the head. The most common exit point is the foot.

42. c. calloused palm—Well-keratinized, intact skin can alter resistance considerably. A thickly calloused palm or sole of the foot may have a resistance of 2 to 3 million ohms/cm^2. Wet, moist, or broken skin has a much lower resistance.

43. b. Anything between the two locations may be injured.—When evaluating an electrical burn, look for two burn locations. If present, the electricity may have traveled through the body.

44. b. singed nasal hair.—This is associated with thermal burns and is not a physiologic dysfunction.

45. d. identify the source of the electricity before approaching the patient.—Personal safety first! Be sure you know what the source of the electrical injury was, and if it is still a live source, before approaching the patient.

46. a. cannot be seen, heard, or felt.—Ionizing radiation cannot be seen, heard, or felt, so the history of the event and the type of location are the EMT-I's best clues to suspect radiation exposure. Be especially careful if there is a fire in a medical office that has sources of radiation (e.g., nuclear medicine facility or research laboratory).

47. a. radiation absorbed dose.—RAD stands for radiation absorbed dose.

48. d. any of the above.—Radiation sickness can occur as a result of any of the mechanisms described in the question.

49. d. patient is contaminated and is an exposure hazard for rescuers.—In a dirty accident, the patient continues to be a secondary exposure hazard to the EMT-I; therefore, the patient should be monitored with a Geiger counter and decontaminated by appropriately trained personnel.

50. a. Many signs and symptoms are the same as those seen with radiation therapy for cancer.—The patient may complain of any of the following symptoms: nausea, vomiting, diarrhea, skin burns, weakness, fatigue, syncope, dehydration, inflammation, hair loss, ulceration of the oral mucosa, hematemesis, bloody stool, bruising, open sores, sloughing of skin, and/or bleeding from the nose, mouth, gums, and rectum.

51. d. White blood cells—White blood cells are very sensitive to radiation. The higher the absorbed dose, the more depressed the WBC count will be.

52. a. finding and correcting life-threatening injuries. —First, protect yourself from exposure; then focus on the patient's life threats and injuries. With the appropriately trained personnel, remove the patient

from the source of exposure as soon as possible. Monitor with a Geiger counter and decontaminate both patient and rescuers.

53. d. the age and physical condition of the rescuer—Factors that EMT-Is should consider for protecting themselves from exposure include time spent near the source, distance from the source, the actual amount of radioactive material constituting the source, and the type of barrier to use as a shield.

54. b. He must ensure that no embers or smoldering portions can burn the patient further.—One of the first actions the EMT-I must take with a burn patient is to stop the burning. Next, remove all clothing and jewelry quickly.

55. a. when the history is inconsistent with the injuries—When a child's injuries or pattern of injuries do not appear to be consistent with the patient's, parent's, or caregiver's history of the MOI, the EMT-I should consider the possibility of abuse.

Chapter 15: Thoracic Trauma

1. b. second—Head injuries are the leading cause.

2. c. mediastinum.—The mediastinum also contains all the great vessels of the chest, except the lungs and pleurae.

3. b. pneumothorax.—This is called the "paper bag" injury: the MOI is just like blowing up a paper bag, closing the opening, and then popping the bag by hitting it. This is a predictable injury based on the MOI.

4. d. any of the above—Chest trauma may impair cardiac output because of overall blood loss (e.g., an intercostal artery bleeds at 50 ml/min), increased intrapleural pressure (pneumothorax), blood accumulation in the pericardial sac (tamponade), myocardial valve damage, or vascular disruption.

5. d. chemoreceptors—Chemoreceptors located in the aortic arch and the carotid sinus constantly monitor and measure CO_2 levels in the blood. Respiratory centers in the brain adjust the rate and depth of breathing to maintain normal CO_2 concentration.

6. b. 2,000–3,000—The adult chest cavity can hold 2 to 3 liters of blood.

7. d. lung or chest wall problem.—Chest pain that increases with breathing, movement, or palpation is more likely due to a problem with the chest or lung (e.g., fractures, pleurisy, pneumonia, costochondritis, or muscle strain) than a cardiac problem.

8. a. atelectasis.—Alveoli are not part of the chest wall, although the collapse of alveoli (*atelectasis*) may be associated with traumatic injury as well as disease processes.

9. b. 4 to 9.—Ribs 4 to 9 are the most often fractured because they are thin and poorly protected.

10. b. minimal when the flail segment is small, because of muscle spasm.—A flail segment is a very serious chest injury. The EMT-I must remove the patient's clothing and look, listen, and feel to find the injury. When the flail segment is small, the paradoxical movement is minimized by muscle spasm. Large segments can have a very serious effect by compromising ventilation.

11. c. of the associated injuries that occur to the organs under the sternum.—The sternum is a thick bone. If the chest receives enough force to fracture the sternum, the EMT-I must assume that the same force was transmitted to the heart, great vessels, lungs, and diaphragm.

12. c. cover the wound with your gloved hand.—Once she discovers an open wound to the chest cavity, the EMT-I must cover the opening. Using a gloved hand is the fastest way to stop a sucking chest wound and is a life-saving measure.

13. d. tension pneumothorax.—When a defect in the airway allows pressure to build up the chest, air becomes trapped in the pleural space. The pressure causes the lung to collapse on the affected (injured) side, with mediastinal shift to the opposite side. The increased pressure compresses the great vessels and decreases preload, which leads to shock and death.

14. a. hemothorax—In the patient with a suspected hemothorax, expect to find the signs and symptoms of shock, decreased breath sounds, respiratory distress, and a chest that is dull on percussion.

15. d. Assist ventilations with a bag mask.—High-flow oxygen has not improved the patient's condition, so the EMT-I must assist the patient's ventilations. Positive pressure may be helpful to reexpand the injured lung, which in turn may help reduce the bleeding. Consider and evaluate the need for intubation.

16. b. is associated with severe thoracic injuries.—Patients with pulmonary contusions also tend to have other severe thoracic and abdominal injuries. In this situation, always assume that multiple potential injuries are present.

17. a. cellular injury.—The contusion causes a hemorrhage with edema and fragmentation of myocardial fibers. There is cellular injury and vascular damage may also occur.

18. c. hypotension with distended neck veins—Assessment findings with pericardial tamponade include: tachycardia, narrow pulse pressure, pulsus paradoxus, ECG changes, dyspnea, cyanosis, jugular vein distention, and muffled or distant heart sounds.

19. a. IV fluid challenge.—Prehospital care by the EMT-I includes airway and ventilation control with high-flow oxygen, positive pressure ventilation or intubation, IV fluid challenge, early notification to the ED, and rapid transport to a facility capable of pericardiocentesis (most EDs) and preferably surgical repair (trauma center).

20. a. early notification to the ED.—For the patient with a suspected pericardial tamponade, an emergency pericardiocentesis can be life-saving. The removal of as little as 20 ml of blood can drastically improve the patient's cardiac output. Call ahead so that a physician can be waiting at the doorway to do a pericardiocentesis as soon as you arrive. (Most patients still require surgery thereafter to repair the myocardial bleeding.) Transport the patient to the closest appropriate facility.

21. a. dissection or rupture.—An aortic dissection or rupture is a shearing injury involving a separation of the aortic intima and media. The blood enters the media through a small intima tear.

22. b. The expansion compresses the great vessels.—Expanding hematomas in the chest cavity may cause the compression of any of the following structures: vena cava, trachea, esophagus, great vessels, or the heart.

23. a. rapid but gentle transport to the nearest hospital.—Treatment includes airway management and ventilation, IV fluids (do not overhydrate), ECG monitoring (if available), gentle handling, and rapid transport to a hospital that can treat this type of injury.

24. c. the chest and abdomen.—Diaphragmatic injuries are associated with a high-pressure compression to the abdomen with a resultant intraabdominal pressure increase. The injury can cause a mediastinal shift with the resultant cardiac and respiratory compromise.

25. b. diaphragmatic—Bowel sounds in the chest indicate that a portion of the bowel has moved up through the diaphragm into the thoracic cavity. This can produce very subtle signs and symptoms, such as bowel obstruction and strangulation. Lung expansion is restricted, resulting in hypoventilation and hypoxia.

26. a. Trendelenburg position—Do not place the patient in the Trendelenburg position, because it may make the patient's respiratory distress much worse. If positive pressure is necessary, use it with caution because it may worsen the injury. Be alert for vomiting.

27. d. tracheobronchial laceration—Tracheobronchial injuries are rare. When they are present, they cause rapid movement of air into the pleural space. Often the tension pneumothorax is refractory to a needle decompression. There is a continuous flow of air from the needle in a decompressed chest.

28. b. tension pneumothorax—Tracheobronchial injuries produce rapid movement of air into the pleural space, which can rapidly progress to tension pneumothorax. Often the tension pneumothorax is refractory to a needle decompression. There is a continuous flow of air from the needle in a decompressed chest. This patient has severe hypoxia and will be difficult to manage even in the ED.

29. a. IV fluid challenge.—Emergency care includes airway management and ventilation with high-concentration oxygen. When the patient is hypotensive, administer fluids and transport to the closest appropriate facility.

30. d. traumatic asphyxia.—This injury occurs when chest movement is impaired to the point that the patient is unable to breathe effectively. The most common cause is a crush injury.

31. c. associated injuries to the surrounding organs.—Penetrating trauma is the most common MOI of this type of injury. Intrathoracic perforation may cause tracheobronchial injury, mediastinal injury, and more. Any of these can be life-threatening.

32. a. blunt trauma.—Blunt trauma is a rare MOI of esophageal injury. Penetrating trauma is the most frequent cause.

33. d. traumatic asphyxia—This injury occurs when chest movement is impaired to the point that the patient is unable to breathe effectively. The most common cause is a crush injury.

34. c. airway management.—The priority of emergency care is the same for any patient. Airway management comes first: ventilatory support with high-concentration oxygen, and treatment for hypotension.

35. c. the jugular veins engorge.—When the chest is unable to expand to create an inflow of air, blood backs up into the head and neck, distending the neck veins.

36. c. 1,000–1,500 ml—Bleeding from a pulmonary contusion generally causes 1,000 to 1,500 ml of blood loss.

37. a. pediatric—Because children are continuously growing, incomplete calcification of bones makes bones softer and less likely to fracture than adult

bones. Rib fractures are rare because of this softness, but when fractures are present, the risk of mortality is increased.

38. d. any of the above—With the MOI and the initial presentation and chief complaints, this patient could have any or a combination of the injuries suggested in the question.

39. b. perform a focused exam of the chest.—The EMT-I should assess the chest for DCAP-BTLS, crepitation, symmetry, and paradoxical motion, and should reassess breath sounds.

40. c. the impact of the mediastinum striking the chest wall—The first collision occurs when the car strikes an object; the second collision is when the body strikes the car's steering wheel or windshield; the third collision occurs when internal organs strike against the body parts surrounding them.

41. a. primary—In the primary phase of the blast effect, there is a pressure wave that can cause major effects on the lungs and GI tract. This is accompanied by a heat wave that affects the eyes and skin, and can burn exposed areas of the body.

42. d. cracked steering wheel—This is the most obvious finding for a potential chest injury in an MVC. The other findings (suggesting possible head, extremity, and pelvic injury, respectively) may also be associated with a chest injury.

43. c. hypoventilation—Pain from an injury to the chest, such as a rib fracture, causes the patient to guard the breathing and take slow and shallow respirations (hypoventilate) to minimize the movement and consequent pain.

44. c. Encourage the patient to breathe deeper.—To prevent further desaturation and the development of atelectasis, the patient should be encouraged to frequently take deeper breaths and cough. This can be challenging because it is painful for the patient.

45. a. esophagus—Esophageal injuries may occur when the throat or upper chest is perforated (e.g., by a knife, bullet, or missile).

Chapter 16: Respiratory Emergencies

1. c. pulmonary capillary.—Normally, each healthy alveolus is surrounded by a functioning pulmonary capillary, from which carbon dioxide passes out of the blood to be eliminated by breathing.

2. d. Ventilation and oxygenation are not always interrelated.—When a patient hypoventilates (e.g., from a narcotic overdose), hypoxia occurs because of the slow respiratory rate. Another example is a patient with a pulmonary embolus who hyperventilates, but has a low partial pressure of oxygen (PO_2). Patients with diabetic ketoacidosis also hyperventilate to compensate; most have normal PO_2 levels.

3. d. pulmonary embolism—Any condition that disrupts the pulmonary circulation or the alveoli (e.g., asthma, pulmonary edema, trauma) can cause a mismatch of blood flow to alveolar gas flow.

4. d. She has developed an upper respiratory infection.—An upper respiratory infection (URI) is an acute, usually self-limiting infection of any part of the upper respiratory tract. Most commonly, the mouth, throat, and ears are affected by a URI.

5. a. Administer oxygen by non-rebreather mask.—Anxiety-hyperventilation syndrome results in tachypnea without a physiologic demand for increased oxygen, leading to respiratory alkalosis. Many disease states (asthma, COPD, MI, PE, stroke, fever, spontaneous pneumothorax, meningitis) cause hyperventilation; therefore, oxygen should never be withheld from a patient who is hyperventilating.

6. d. who has a good respiratory effort.—The use of a NRB is indicated whenever a patient needs oxygen, has a good respiratory effort, and is not apneic.

7. c. aerosolized albuterol and subcutaneous epinephrine—The EMT-I may administer a few emergency medications under local protocol and medication direction. For the patient experiencing a severe asthma attack, the appropriate pharmacologic therapy is a bronchodilator (albuterol) and SC epinephrine to relax smooth muscle.

8. b. SpO_2 and ECG—The patient's symptoms and initial presentation are enough to start treatment (e.g., high-flow oxygen and bronchodilator). Diagnostic information that is helpful for continued care includes SpO_2 (pulse oximetry) and, if local protocol permits, an ECG to confirm suspicions of cardiac irregularity.

9. c. creating airway pressures that keep the alveoli open.—Pursed-lip breathing causes resistance to exhalation at the mouth. This leads to a backup of airway pressure into the lungs. The pressure forces previously collapsed alveoli to open and improves oxygenation.

10. c. chronic bronchitis.—Excess mucus production causes the patient to experience a productive cough. When this condition persists or recurs for weeks or months within the same year, and recurs for two or more consecutive years, chronic bronchitis is the typical diagnosis.

11. a. resistance to expiratory airflow.—The loss of normal alveolar structure leads to a decrease in the elastic recoil, which creates resistance to expiratory airflow. Air is trapped within the lungs, resulting in poor air exchange.

12. a. The patient with pneumonia is contagious.—Pneumonia is an acute inflammatory condition of the lungs, usually caused by either bacterial or viral infection. Personal safety must be the first consideration for the EMT-I who is managing a patient with pneumonia.

13. c. right-sided heart failure—The patient could have any of the conditions suggested. However, the findings of JVD, peripheral edema, pulmonary edema, and ascites are the most common manifestations of right-sided congestive heart failure, whatever the underlying cause.

14. c. spontaneous pneumothorax—The signs and symptoms of spontaneous pneumothorax include sudden onset of unilateral chest pain, shortness of breath, decreased breath sounds on the affected side, increased respiratory rate, anxiety, and sometimes coughing. Young, tall, thin male smokers are most likely to develop pneumothorax from the rupture of a congenital bleb. The patient's profile and history of a recent cold with coughing may help differentiate this episode from a pulmonary embolism, which has similar signs and symptoms.

15. c. IV medications.—IV medications do not cause pulmonary emboli, but the administration technique may. If large air bubbles are administered with the medication, the air can move through the circulation to the lungs.

16. d. an overly aggressive intubation attempt—A frequent cause of laryngeal spasm is trauma from an intubation attempt. It may also occur following extubation, in drowning, and in anaphylaxis.

17. d. help you visualize the vocal cords.—When intubating supine medical patients, place a folded hand towel behind the head to approximate the sniffing position.

18. a. respiratory arrest—Apnea is a contraindication because the tube is passed blindly and advanced as you hear the sounds of air moving through the glottic opening and vocal cords. If the patient is in respiratory arrest, there is no air movement to hear.

19. b. capnograph—A capnograph provides continuous EtCO$_2$ readings in both number and graph forms. The capnometer provides only a numeric reading and the colorimetric device changes color during exhalation.

20. b. water-soluble; it is less irritating to airway tissues—Vaseline and other hydrocarbon-based products are not biodegradable and can actually break down the plastic, latex, or rubber in the airway device, as well as cause lung tissue damage (chemical aspiration pneumonia).

Chapter 17: Cardiovascular Emergencies

1. d. have improved because of improvements in treatments.—Significant advances in the treatment of cardiovascular disease have reduced morbidity and mortality, and extended lives and the quality of lives so much that cancer has now become the number one cause of death in the United States.

2. a. sinoatrial node.—Specialized cells called pacemaker cells, found only in the heart, establish a regular rate of contraction. The fastest pacemaker sets the heart rate. Under normal conditions, the fastest pacemakers are located in the sinoatrial (SA) node.

3. a. reducing sodium intake.—Studies confirm that reducing the amount of sodium (salt) in the diet reduces the risk of cardiovascular disease.

4. c. cigarette smoking—A few additional risk factors for cardiac disease include hypertension, diabetes, family history of cardiac disease, obesity, high cholesterol, and hyperlipidemia.

5. a. obtaining a focused history, vital signs, ECG, and blood samples.—The components of assessment of a patient with suspected cardiac compromise include obtaining a focused history and physical exam, obtaining blood samples while starting an IV, obtaining a 12-lead ECG (if possible), and performing serial reassessments of the initial assessment, vital signs, ECG, and level of distress.

6. b. impulse through the atria into the AV node.—The P-R interval represents the time from the beginning of the P wave to the beginning of the QRS, and correlates to the impulse through the atria into the AV node and through the bundles of His to the ventricles.

7. a. heart is not adequately filling the ventricles.—When the electrical stimuli of the heart cause the rate to race at a sustained, rapid tachycardia, the patient will develop symptoms (e.g., dizziness, dyspnea, chest pain). How soon the patient develops symptoms will depend on the patient's age, physical condition, and medical history.

8. a. rhythm should be regular.—There is more than one way to calculate the heart rate from an ECG

recording. Any of these methods works well when the rhythm is regular.

9. a. pulse deficit.—Certain dysrhythmias, such as atrial fibrillation or ectopic beats, can cause pulse deficit. The patient's distal pulse will be less than the heart rate on the ECG, which represents the apical pulse. This is why a pulse must be palpated on every patient, rather than relying on the ECG for the heart rate.

10. a. assessing the R-R interval.—The R wave is the tallest positive wave in the ECG recording. You can quickly determine the regularity of an ECG recording by measuring the distance between each R wave.

11. a. 0.2—The ECG recording is a grid composed of boxes, lines, and markings. The large boxes represent 0.2 seconds each. Within each large box are five small boxes that represent 0.04 seconds each.

12. b. ventricular tachycardia.—The clinical indications for defibrillation are a patient who is not breathing and has no pulse with one of two rhythms: V-fib or V-tach.

13. a. Start an IV and administer a fluid bolus.—For many EMT-Is, the preferred treatment options (e.g., pacing, atropine) for this patient require on-line medical direction. While obtaining medical direction, the EMT-I should keep the patient supine, administer high-flow oxygen, start an IV, give fluids (following local protocols), and be prepared for the patient's condition to worsen.

14. c. The person has heart disease that causes irregular pacemaker activity.—Internal defibrillators are placed in patients who are at high risk of or actually have irregular pacemaker activity that causes the heart rhythm to change to ventricular tachycardia or ventricular fibrillation.

15. a. stable angina.—Chest pain that predictably occurs with exercise or exertion, and is quickly relieved with rest or nitroglycerin, is referred to as *stable angina*.

16. d. any of the above—Because so many different conditions—some life-threatening—can cause chest pain, the EMT-I should treat the patient as having a cardiac problem until proven otherwise.

17. d. occlusion of a coronary artery from a thrombus—Myocardial infarction is the death of heart muscle from a lack of oxygen. A clot or thrombus is the most common mechanism by which an MI occurs. The best chance of recovering from an MI is for the patient to quickly (within 4 hours) get to a facility capable of providing thrombolytic therapy.

18. c. pulmonary embolism—Pulmonary embolism (PE) can cause an MI, but when a patient is experiencing an MI, it is uncommon for a PE to develop during transport to the hospital. Cardiac arrest is common within the first hour of the onset of symptoms, as is CHF. When a patient experiences a massive heart attack, cardiogenic shock may also result.

19. b. It is one of three components used to make a cardiac diagnosis.—The three primary components used for diagnosis of an AMI include the patient's history (OPQRST and SAMPLE), abnormal ECG or ECG changes, and cardiac enzyme analysis. Even with this data, it is sometimes difficult to exclude or fully diagnose an AMI.

20. d. all of the above—The elderly (especially women) and diabetic patients are prone to altered pain sensation. These patients may experience atypical symptoms from myocardial ischemia, which may include syncope, shortness of breath, weakness or fatigue, confusion, or epigastric pain.

21. b. The patient is experiencing cardiac ischemia.—The patient has a cardiac history and takes nitroglycerin, so the EMT-I must first consider and treat the patient for cardiac ischemia until an MI can be ruled out. Old or expired nitroglycerin and the development of unstable angina should also be considered.

22. a. nitrates and aspirin—The current EMT-I curriculum allows EMT-Is to administer nitroglycerin for chest pain. The administration of aspirin for chest pain has become standard under medical direction (follow local protocols).

23. a. discreetly prepare for the possibility that the patient may go into cardiac arrest.—This patient is at high risk of sudden cardiac arrest. The EMT-I must consider the possibility of cardiac arrest and be prepared to manage it.

24. b. blood backs up in the venous system.—The condition in which cardiac pumping is insufficient to meet the circulatory demand of the body is called *cardiac* or *heart failure*. In cardiac failure, cardiac output decreases and blood backs up in the venous system, causing inadequate circulation and inadequate tissue oxygenation.

25. d. exacerbation of paroxysmal nocturnal dyspnea—PND usually indicates significant congestive heart failure.

26. c. an exacerbation of COPD.—Sometimes it is really difficult to differentiate between APE and acute COPD. Both conditions may present as a sudden shortness of breath with wet-sounding lungs. The patient may have one or both of these conditions at the same time.

27. d. blood pools in the lungs and causes pulmonary congestion.—PND usually indicates significant congestive heart failure. Patients with advanced heart failure will usually sleep sitting up in a

recliner or propped up with pillows in bed to avoid such attacks.

28. d. brain, heart, and kidneys.—The high pressures sustained during a hypertensive crisis put the brain at risk of bleeding or stroke, the heart at risk of an MI, and the kidneys at risk of failure.

29. d. can lead to serious, irreversible, end-organ damage. —If left untreated, severely high blood pressure can cause organ damage.

30. c. preeclampsia—This is an example of a hypertensive emergency. The patient's signs and symptoms suggest preeclampsia from pregnancy-induced hypertension.

31. d. starting an IV, and reassessing the patient every 5 minutes.—The patient is unstable and may progress to eclampsia with seizures. The EMT-I's management plan for this patient should include: close airway observation, because the patient has vomited already and may vomit again; administration of high-flow oxygen; administration of an IV that runs to keep a vein open (KVO); monitoring of the ECG (per protocol); and reassessment of the patient every 5 minutes if possible.

32. a. She is having a massive MI.—The assessment findings and witnessed report of the event all indicate that the patient is having a massive heart attack (inferior MI) with cardiogenic shock.

33. b. Administer a fluid bolus and treat for shock.—This patient is in shock, most likely because of an inferior-wall MI. The EMT-I must manage the airway and breathing as needed and treat for shock (e.g., Trendelenburg position, warmth, IV access, and fluids per local protocol or medical direction).

34. b. cardiogenic shock.—Cardiogenic shock, the most severe form of heart failure, results from inadequate cardiac output because of left ventricular malfunction.

35. c. cardiac arrest.—*Cardiac arrest* is defined as the sudden stopping of the heartbeat and therefore of the pumping action of the heart.

36. c. Rapidly assess the patient for signs of irreversible death.—With no witness, the time of death is unknown. Before beginning resuscitative measures, the EMT-I should rapidly assess the patient for signs of irreversible death (e.g., lividity, rigidity).

37. c. Continue resuscitation efforts while you contact medical control and request an order to secure the patient.—In general, once advance directives are provided, the EMT-I should make an effort to comply with the patient's wishes. How you do this will depend on local protocol. Typically, once resuscitation has begun, it is continued until medical control gives an order to secure the patient or the patient has been transported to the ED.

38. a. perfect CPR.—The latest evidence shows that perfect CPR (specifically, good-quality compressions) is the single most effective treatment for sudden cardiac arrest until an AED can be attached.

39. b. Give nothing by mouth, because people with myocardial ischemia often have nausea.—As a general rule, acutely ill or injured patients receive nothing by mouth. Drink or food can cause or worsen nausea and stimulate vomiting. When a patient has to go to the OR, any contents in the stomach create a risk of vomiting and aspiration.

40. d. epinephrine, atropine, and an antidysrhythmic by IV or ET—Administering medications by IV or ET is a skill that the EMT-I is trained to do, and is within the scope of practice. Which medications an EMT-I may administer, and the circumstances under which they are administered, is determined by the medical director and local protocol. It is common for the EMT-I to assist with medication administration, under medical control, for a cardiac arrest.

41. b. ventricular fibrillation—V-fib is a chaotic, disorganized rhythm that does not produce a pulse.

42. d. patient is able to receive therapy within 4 hours.— The sooner treatment is received, the better the chance of survival for a greater number of cardiac cells. Most experts agree that earlier is always better, but the accepted "window of opportunity" ranges from 4 to 6 hours in most situations.

43. b. ventricular fibrillation—The MOI of being struck in the chest followed by sudden death has occurred with many young athletes. The blow to the chest causes the heart to go into V-fib. If an AED is not made available to the patient within a few minutes, sudden death becomes irreversible. This rare and often fatal phenomenon is called *commotio cordis*.

   This was the cause of Louis Acumpura's death, an incident that led to passage of a New York state law requiring AEDs to be placed in all grade schools and high schools.

44. d. Obtaining an ECG does not take priority over care for life-threatening injuries.—An ECG should be obtained on any patient when the EMT-I feels that she needs the data to confirm suspicions of cardiac irregularity (e.g., palpitations from V-tach). However, it is very important that the ECG not take priority over caring for life-threatening injuries, such as a compromised airway or uncontrolled bleeding.

45. c. dilates blood vessels that increase blood flow to the head.—Nitroglycerin relaxes vascular smooth muscle, resulting in peripheral vasodilation. In addition to increasing blood flow to the heart through dilation of the coronary arteries, nitro increases blood flow to the head. This causes many patients to experience a headache.

Chapter 18: Diabetic Emergencies

1. c. decrease in the secretion of insulin.—People with diabetes either do not produce enough insulin to regulate the blood sugar level (Type 1) or are relatively resistant to whatever insulin is produced (Type II).

2. c. moving sugar molecules from the blood into the cells.—Insulin moves sugar molecules from the blood into the cells for storage. In addition, insulin prevents the breakdown of fat tissue in the body.

3. d. cell starvation.—When a person's insulin supply is inadequate, sugar and other substances (e.g., free fatty acids, amino acids) fail to enter the cells properly, causing the cells to become starved. The hungry cells will turn to secondary food sources, such as fat and then muscle, for nutrients.

4. b. altered mental status.—When the blood sugar level decreases significantly, the patient's mental state will be altered. Prolonged hypoglycemia may lead to seizures, coma, permanent brain cell damage, and death.

5. b. treat the patient for hypoglycemia until a blood sugar level reading is obtained.—At times, it is difficult to decide whether a patient's symptoms indicate hypoglycemia, normal blood sugar levels, or hyperglycemia. The immediate problem of the brain not receiving an adequate amount of sugar occurs rapidly in hypoglycemia. Treat the patient for hypoglycemia until proven otherwise!

6. b. it disrupts the acid-base balance in the body.—Anyone who becomes malnourished can experience the production of ketones, as the body metabolizes fat in an effort to nourish the cells. The difference with diabetes is that the counterregulatory hormones are affected. Excess ketone accumulation upsets the acid-base balance in the body and acidosis develops.

7. c. decreased blood sugar level.—When the body has too much insulin, such as when an insulin shot has been administered but the person does not eat following the injection, the effects include a drop in the blood sugar level. This scenario can lead to hypoglycemia in the diabetic patient.

8. c. abnormally high blood sugar.—Hyperglycemia is an elevation of the blood sugar level above normal. The most common cause of hyperglycemia is diabetes.

9. c. A patient with hyperglycemia may have no immediate symptoms.—Hyperglycemia by itself may be asymptomatic. When symptoms are present, they may include weakness, headache, frequent urination, increased thirst, and weight loss or gain.

10. a. correct dehydration.—The most important immediate problem in hyperglycemia is dehydration. This must be corrected as soon as possible.

11. b. Conduct the initial assessment and determine the patient's priority.—The approach with any patient is to complete the initial assessment, manage the ABCs as needed, and determine the patient's priority. This is especially important with the patient who has an altered mental status and vomiting.

12. d. encourage the patient to consume a drink with lots of sugar and eat carbohydrates.—This patient is conscious, and is able to speak and protect his own airway. It is appropriate to encourage the patient to drink a beverage with plenty of sugar in it. To keep the blood sugar level from dropping again, get the patient to eat food containing carbohydrates.

13. c. Administer high-flow oxygen and obtain a blood sugar level reading.—When a patient has a new onset of altered mental status, the EMT-I must quickly rule out hypoxia (administer high-flow oxygen) and hypoglycemia. The signs and symptoms of hypoglycemia can mimic those of a stroke.

14. c. IV, D50 (per local protocol), or oral glucose.—The patient has a low blood sugar level and significant signs and symptoms of hypoglycemia, as well as an elevated temperature. Even if the patient is not a diabetic, an infection may have depleted his blood sugar reserves, causing a hypoglycemic episode. An IV is appropriate, as is administration of D50 or oral glucose when your local protocol permits.

15. c. hyperglycemia with diabetic ketoacidosis—DKA is a metabolic condition consisting of hyperglycemia, dehydration, and excess ketones and ketoacids in the body. When ketone levels get high enough, acidosis develops. One of the ways in which the body rids itself of the acidosis is to blow off the acid with deep, rapid respirations (Kussmaul's respirations). The most common reason a diabetic patient develops DKA is because of infection.

16. b. Administer oxygen, IV, and fluid bolus (per local protocol).—The management plan for the patient with suspected or known hyperglycemia, with or without DKA, is airway and breathing support as needed, high-flow oxygen, and an IV and fluid bolus (following local protocol).

17. c. abdominal pain—In some patients with (e.g., children, the elderly) new-onset diabetes mellitus, abdominal pain may be your only clue to a diabetic problem.

18. c. Insert an airway adjunct and assist the patient's ventilations.—The first step in the care of a patient

with known or suspected hypoglycemia, or altered mental status, is to control the airway and assist breathing as necessary. Patients with an altered mental status may have partial airway obstruction.

19. b. Contact medical control for instructions.—The patient is in critical condition. He needs glucose quickly; his airway, breathing, and circulation require support; and he is cold (hypothermic). Talking directly with medical control is appropriate

with any critical patient, especially when a specific treatment option is not available. Determining if glucagon is available in the residence is a good idea, but many EMT-Is will need to get approval from medical control to administer it.

20. d. 25 grams of dextrose diluted in 50 cc—The standard first dose of one ampule of D50 by IV push is 25 grams of dextrose diluted in 50 cc.

Chapter 19: Allergic Reactions

1. b. antigen.—When an antigen (foreign body) enters the body, the immune response detects the antigen and produces antibodies, which in a normal response will destroy the antigen.

2. d. an allergic reaction.—*Autoimmunity* is when a person's antibodies attack the person's own tissues, causing tissue damage and organ dysfunction. An *allergen* is a substance that induces an allergy; *anaphylaxis* is the most severe form of allergic reaction.

3. c. an immune response.—An *immune response* is a bodily response that occurs when a foreign substance tries to invade the body. *Immunity* is a state of protection that enables the body to resist foreign substances. Adrenalin (epinephrine) insufficiency is not relevant to this question.

4. b. anaphylaxis.—*Histamine* is a mediator that is released when an antigen reacts with an antibody. *Immunity* is a state of protection that enables the body to resist foreign substances. An antibody is a protein substance but not a protein response.

5. a. allergen.—An allergen is a foreign substance that enters the body by ingestion, injection, inhalation, or exposure through the skin and triggers an allergic reaction.

6. b. anaphylaxis.—An immune response occurs when a foreign substance tries to invade the body. *Urticaria* is a medical term for hives, and *isoimmunity* is the formation of antibodies directed against antigens of another person's cells.

7. b. injection—An insect sting is an injection similar to a needlestick.

8. c. ingestion—Many antibiotics are combination sulfa drugs. The most common route of exposure is ingestion of an prescription oral antibiotic.

9. a. He is having an allergic reaction to latex.—Latex is in nearly every medical product used today (e.g., stethoscopes, gloves, ECG leads, tourniquets, bandages). Assume that any patient is potentially allergic to latex and carry appropriate latex-free equipment.

10. b. due to a sting or injection.—Allergens can enter the body by ingestion, injection, inhalation, or topical exposure. Any of these routes of exposure can cause an allergic reaction that includes hives (urticaria).

11. d. antibiotics, insect stings, blood products, and foods.—The most common antigens that cause anaphylaxis are medications, and the medications that most commonly cause anaphylaxis are antibiotics. The two major antigen types associated with blood are A and B. Foods and insect stings are the other common antigens.

12. b. GI tract; abdominal pain—The majority of mediators released from mast cells are found in the skin and the respiratory and GI tracts.

13. b. vascular dilation and plasma loss into tissues.—The body's response to any substance to which the body is abnormally sensitive creates a variety of reactions. In anaphylactic shock, the body experiences vascular dilation, plasma escape into the tissues (causing hives and angioedema), and fluid escape from the alveoli (causing pulmonary edema).

14. b. The patient is progressing to anaphylaxis and is potentially unstable.—The patient has experienced a major antigen exposure. Even though he is not allergic to bee stings, he has already developed dyspnea and chest tightness; his skin is pale and he is tachycardic. He is unstable and you should expect progressive anaphylaxis. This patient needs epinephrine.

15. c. She has signs and symptoms of an allergic reaction and appears stable.—The patient has mild signs and symptoms of histamine release with no respiratory symptoms. She is currently stable.

16. b. high-flow oxygen, position of comfort, reassurance, and supportive care.—Allergies should be managed to rule out progressive hives or anaphylaxis. Consult medical control if the patient wants to refuse care; otherwise, provide oxygen, a position of comfort, reassurance, and supportive care.

17. d. diphenhydramine—Diphenhydramine (Benadryl) is the antihistamine most commonly used in pre-hospital emergency care. It can be taken orally, injected intramuscularly, or injected intravenously.

18. d. epinephrine—Epinephrine is the bronchodilator most commonly used; it also decreases vascular permeability (it is a vasoconstrictor).

19. c. dysrhythmias and cardiogenic shock.—Acquired immunity develops over the course of one's lifetime. GI symptoms occur with some allergic reactions, and vascular dilation ultimately causes shock.

20. d. Antihistamines do not block all of the mediators released in an immune response, so this treatment could potentially be fatal.—Epinephrine is the drug of choice for ongoing anaphylactic reactions. Once the cascade of events is triggered, all anaphylactic reactions have the potential to progress to anaphylactic shock. The use of antihistamines alone does not block all the released mediators, and thus is potentially fatal.

21. c. Yes; use IV epinephrine because subcutaneous epinephrine may be ineffective.—If the patient is in cardiovascular collapse, and an IV has been started, administer epinephrine IV. The peripheral circulation may be so poor that an SQ injection will be ineffective.

22. a. obstruction due to swelling—Swelling in the upper airway can cause obstruction and reduce the amount of air getting into the lungs. Pulmonary edema and wheezing occur in the lower airways, and urticaria is not observed in the upper airway.

23. a. manage the airway. The ALS management of anaphylaxis includes management of the airway, with positioning, oxygen, assisted ventilations, and ET tube placement as needed; management of circulation; and pharmacological intervention with epinephrine, antihistamines, steroids, and vasopressors for hypotension that is not responsive to fluids alone.

24. c. The patient is potentially unstable, and you should assume that she may progress to anaphylaxis as she has in the past.—Many peanut allergies are severe. Once a patient has experienced anaphylaxis, the EMT-I can presume that the patient will have a similar reaction when exposed to the same allergen. Palpitations are normal following a dose of epinephrine. The patient is potentially unstable and requires close monitoring and transport to the ED for evaluation.

25. b. oxygen, supportive care, and antihistamines—The patient is having a local reaction with no respiratory symptoms. However, the area involved is close to the airway and has the potential to progress to anaphylaxis. Supportive care and the administration of Benadryl (either IM or IV) is appropriate.

Chapter 20: Poisoning/Overdose Emergencies

1. c. gloves and eye protection for the EMT-I, to prevent exposure to the patient's body substances—At a minimum, the rescuer should wear gloves and eye protection to prevent possible exposure to vomitus and excrement that may be on the patient, and to prevent possible exposure in the event that the patient continues to vomit or is incontinent during the move and transport.

2. c. when the substance has been identified, even if the patient has no symptoms—If the EMT-I suspects that the patient has been poisoned, the EMT-I should try to get the container or name of the suspected poison. When first-aid instructions are available from the package, follow those at the same time (if possible) while you call POISON HELP at 1-800-222-1222 right away. Always follow local protocol!

3. c. inhalation—Signs and symptoms of poisoning will vary depending on the substance and route of exposure. Shortness of breath and coughing are commonly associated with inhalation exposure.

4. a. providing information about treating poisonings. —A poison center is an emergency telephone service that is always available; anyone can call to get information or ask questions about poisons. The caller will speak with specially trained nurses, pharmacists, and doctors, and all services are free and confidential.

5. c. which toxic substances are specific to your region. —The AAPCC is associated with the Toxic Exposure Surveillance System (TESS), the only comprehensive poisoning surveillance database in the United States. This database contains detailed toxicological information on more than 31 million poison exposures reported (as of 2002) to U.S. poison centers.

6. b. Advise dispatch to send the fire department and the police.—Safety first! The patient appears confused in the middle of the night. There may be more patients (family). This could be a crime scene or a hazmat (carbon monoxide poisoning), so it is appropriate to call for help at this point.

7. a. cleaning the site with soap and water.—Emergency care for snakebite includes keeping the patient calm, cleaning the wound with soap and water, removing any tight clothing and jewelry from the extremities, transporting, and treating for shock. Constricting bands and cold packs should not be applied unless you are directed to do so by the poison control center or medical direction. Always follow local protocols!

8. b. removing any contaminated clothing and flushing all exposed areas with water.—The emergency care for poisoning by absorption includes removing all contaminated clothing, jewelry, socks, and shoes; flushing the affected area with water; and, if possible, washing the affected area with soap. You can contact the poison control center or medical direction for further instructions.

9. a. aspirin.—Early toxicity of aspirin has a respiratory stimulant effect, and later progresses to metabolic acidosis with deep, rapid respirations. Ringing in the ears (tinnitus) is a unique characteristic of aspirin overdose. Other assessment findings may include GI distress, GI bleeding, altered mental status, pulmonary edema, acute renal failure, fever, and dehydration.

10. d. administration of activated charcoal.—The cornerstone of management of the poisoned patient is maintenance of airway, breathing, and circulation. Activated charcoal has been shown to absorb many different ingested toxins from the stomach. In EMS systems that permit the use of activated charcoal, the patient must be alert enough to drink the slurry. Additional management depends on the severity of the patient's condition, and may include the administration of sodium bicarbonate, glucose, antiseizure medications, and cooling.

11. d. acetaminophen.—The most common poisonings by overdose are from nonprescription pain medications (e.g., acetaminophen and nonsteroidal anti-inflammatory agents) and prescription drugs (e.g., antidepressants and antibiotics).

12. b. ensuring that he has an open airway and assisting ventilations—The cardinal principles of management of the poisoned patient are: maintenance of airway, breathing, and circulation; consideration of specific antidotes, as provided in local protocols (e.g., naloxone, an antagonistic to narcotics), and transport in a timely fashion to the nearest appropriate facility.

13. c. wearing the appropriate PPE during removal of the transdermal patches and continuing care of the patient—As with any patient, the first priorities are to ensure your own safety and maintain the ABCs of the patient.

14. c. drug dependence.—Drug dependence is a psychological problem, not a physical one. True addiction is both a psychological and physical craving for a substance, and drug or substance abuse is the use of a drug for a nontherapeutic effect, especially one for which the drug was not prescribed or intended.

15. a. get everyone out of the residence.—The first step in the care of any patient with a suspected poisoning by inhalation is to move the patient into fresh air. In this case, you would move everyone out of the residence until the fire department gets a CO reading and determines that the residence is safe.

Chapter 21: Neurological Emergencies

1. b. an artery in the brain ruptures.—A stroke or cerebrovascular accident (CVA) occurs when an artery in the brain becomes blocked (thrombus) or ruptures, causing blood and oxygen to be cut off from the brain cells.

2. b. that a TIA has no lasting effect.—A mini-stroke or transient ischemic attack (TIA) is a temporary occlusion of an artery to the brain caused by a blood clot. Although they have no lasting effect, TIAs are a strong predictor of stroke risk and may occur days, weeks, or months before a stroke.

3. b. Meningitis—Meningitis is an inflammation of the tissues that surround the brain and spinal cord. This condition may temporarily or permanently affect neurological function. Bacterial meningitis is most common, and is highly contagious. It may cause severe complications or death. None of the other choices involves infection.

4. b. substernal chest pain—Substernal chest pain is associated with cardiac, esophageal, and leaking thoracic aortic aneurysm. An outbreak of shingles, an infectious neurological disorder, can present with chest pain, but will follow nerve pathways on the torso or chest that radiate around to the back, rather than causing substernal pain.

5. a. starting two IVs—The best chance of survival for a stroke patient is early recognition of signs and symptoms of a stroke (less than 3 hours). Stroke symptoms can mimic hypoglycemia, so it is appropriate to obtain a glucose reading to rule out hypoglycemia. The patient must then be transported quickly to the nearest facility that can do fibrinolytic

therapy. En route, complete a thrombolytic checklist, obtain an ECG to help rule out cardiac conditions. If time permits, establish two IVs in different arms; one for "clot buster" access and one for parenteral therapy, but avoid multiple needle punctures.

6. b. the onset of symptoms is gradual.—The onset of stroke is more gradual if caused by a thrombus. Thrombolytic strokes typically occur during sleep. The patient falls asleep with no problems and then awakens with a neurological deficit. Hemorrhagic or embolic strokes are more abrupt, usually occurring when the patient is awake.

7. b. the same as for a patient with a suspected cerebrovascular attack (CVA).—The risk factors and signs and symptoms of TIA and CVA are the same. Every suspected TIA or CVA must be treated as a life-threatening emergency. For the patient to receive clot-buster therapy, the diagnosis of stroke must be made and treatment begun within 3 hours of the onset of symptoms.

8. c. rising intracranial pressure—The three signs of rising intracranial pressure are rising blood pressure, decreasing heart rate, and changes in respiratory pattern. These three findings combined are a clear, but late, sign of rising ICP called Cushing's triad.

9. d. epinephrine auto-injector—The epinephrine auto-injector, used in the treatment of severe allergic reaction, is not typically associated with syncope. Common prescription medications that are include beta blockers, diuretics, antihypertensives, narcotics, antiarrhythmics, nitrates, digitalis, ACE blockers, and psychiatric medications.

10. a. speech, pronator drift, and grimace—The Cincinnati and Los Angeles stroke scores assess three primary factors: speech deficits, pronator drift/grip strength, and facial symmetry.

11. d. open the airway; if that is not possible, insert an NPA—A patient who is seizing requires special attention to the airway and breathing. The mouth may be clenched shut and there may be bleeding from tongue biting. Seizing patients are also prone to brief periods of apnea. Begin the assessment by opening the airway and looking for injury, then suction as needed. An OPA may be attempted if the airway can be opened. The NPA is an excellent airway adjunct for the seizing patient, especially when the teeth are clenched. It can be used on patients with or without a gag reflex, and you can suction through one.

12. a. hypoxia and hypoglycemia—Each of the items listed will have to be considered as part of the complete assessment. Regardless of a patient's history, the first two possible causes of altered mental status (AMS) to consider and rule out in any patient are hypoxia (administer oxygen) and hypoglycemia (obtain a blood glucose reading). The brain requires a constant source of oxygen and glucose; without them, brain cells will begin to die.

13. b. children and adolescents—Seizures occur in patients of all ages, though the causes of seizures vary slightly with each age group. Idiopathic (epileptic) seizures occur most frequently in the child and adolescent age groups.

14. c. confusion—Syncope often comes without warning and the patient does not remember passing out. It is natural and very common for a patient to awaken confused.

15. d. lost the ability to speak, because of a defect in or loss of language function.—Damage to any part of a specialized area of the cerebral cortex will interfere with language functions, including speech, writing, and sensory information.

Chapter 22: Nontraumatic Abdominal Emergencies

1. b. digesting blood in the stomach.—Vomitus of material that looks like coffee grounds suggests digested blood. This can come from bleeding in the upper airway (e.g., nosebleed or mouth) that has been swallowed. The blood in the stomach causes nausea and may cause vomiting.

2. d. gallbladder disease—Eating fatty foods causes the gallbladder to contract and release bile. For people with preexisting gallbladder disease, contraction of the gallbladder causes distention and is accompanied by pain. Fatty foods may also cause an attack of acute cholecystitis (inflammation of the gallbladder).

3. b. gastroenteritis—*Gastroenteritis* is a general term for inflammation of any part of the small or large bowel due to infection. The most common infection is viral and is usually self-limiting.

4. b. hepatitis—Hepatitis is an inflammation of the liver, an organ located in the upper left quadrant of the abdomen.

5. b. appendicitis—Common causes of abdominal pain in the right lower quadrant of a male patient include appendicitis, diverticulitis, and kidney stones. The patient with a kidney stone will usually be writhing with the most severe pain he has ever experienced. This is accompanied by associated symptoms of nausea and vomiting.

6. d. Lay her supine on the floor and elevate her legs.— A cardiac problem and GI bleeding must be considered quickly in a patient with unexplained hypotension. Place the patient in a supine position before she falls down. Then administer oxygen, obtain vital signs, SpO_2, and a glucose level.

7. a. An ectopic pregnancy can rupture, creating life-threatening bleeding.—Any woman with an ectopic pregnancy is at risk of rupture. A ruptured ectopic pregnancy carries a high mortality rate due to hemorrhagic shock, but it is one of the most frequently missed diagnoses.

8. d. abdominal aortic aneurysm.—An *aneurysm* is a bulging sac in the wall of a blood vessel due to a localized weakness; an abdominal aortic aneurysm is an aneurysm on the abdominal aorta. As the bulge of the sac continues to grow, the pressure it exerts on other structures often causes symptoms such as abdominal or back pain. When the sac leaks or bursts, the patient may complain of thigh pain and/or difficulty breathing.

9. b. rebound tenderness.—Rebound tenderness occurs when gentle pressure elicits less pain on palpation than the release of pressure from palpation. The presence of rebound tenderness indicates peritoneal irritation. Any movement that jars the inflamed peritoneal cavity should result in rebound tenderness; this includes jarring the stretcher when moving the patient to the ambulance and bumping in the road during transportation.

10. b. somatic.—Somatic pain is caused by a stimulation of nerve fibers in the inflamed parietal peritoneum. The patient usually lies quietly, with the thighs flexed to relax the peritoneum. The patient will guard the abdomen and not allow palpation.

11. c. visceral.—Visceral pain is caused by the sudden stretching or distention of a hollow organ (viscus).

This type of pain is usually associated with a crampy, gas-like, and often intermittent pain. The patient may experience nausea, vomiting, diaphoresis, and dysrhythmias.

12. a. an orthostatic exam.—The tilt test measures orthostatic BP and pulse changes, and is useful in determining whether significant intravascular volume depletion has occurred. A positive tilt means that the BP decreased, the pulse increased, or both, after changing from a supine to a sitting or from a sitting to a standing position. In this case, the patient has no distal pulses while supine, a significant finding that suggests severe hypotension. Moving him to an upright position may cause a loss of consciousness and possible injury.

13. a. treating for shock.—Prehospital care for a suspected GI bleed is the same regardless of the cause. Initial treatment starts with administration of high-flow oxygen. Beware of vomiting and bleeding in these cases. An IV should be established and a fluid bolus given per your local protocol. The use of MAST/PASG may be appropriate if authorized in your local protocol. Keep the patient warm and elevate the legs. If this patient's breathing is not worsened by lying supine, you should try that as well.

14. d. an infectious disease—Many people are not aware when they become infected with hepatitis, for example, because symptoms do not develop immediately. When symptoms become apparent, they include nausea, vomiting, fever, night sweats, loss of appetite, weight loss, dark-colored urine, clay-colored stool, weakness, extreme fatigue, yellow eyes or skin (jaundice), and upper right quadrant tenderness. Most forms of hepatitis are infectious.

15. c. yellow eyes or skin—Many people are not aware they are infected with hepatitis, because symptoms do not develop immediately. When symptoms become apparent, they usually include nausea, vomiting, fever, night sweats, loss of appetite, weight loss, dark-colored urine, clay-colored stool, weakness, extreme fatigue, yellow eyes or skin (jaundice), and upper right quadrant tenderness.

Chapter 23: Environmental Emergencies

1. d. medical condition exacerbated by below-average temperatures.—An *environmental emergency* is a medical condition caused or exacerbated by weather, terrain, atmospheric pressure, or other local factors. Age, health, and medications are risk factors that predispose patients to environmental emergencies.

2. d. all of the above—Risk factors that predispose patients to environmental emergencies include extreme ages (e.g., very young or very old); serious medical conditions (e.g., heart failure, cancer, diabetes); certain medications, both prescription and over-the-counter; and fatigue. When people are tired, they may not exercise appropriate judgment

in potentially dangerous environmental situations (e.g., staying out too long in the heat).

3. a. mild hypothermia.—The patient has been lying on the floor for several hours, possibly all night, and her body has been conducting heat to the floor the whole time. Even in a warm house, a body on a floor can lose a significant amount of heat. Wetness (urinary incontinence) will speed up the heat loss, and the age of this patient is a predisposing risk factor for an environmental emergency.

4. d. all of the above.—Inaccessibility due to the location and terrain, and inclement weather, especially when unexpected, can all impede treatment and delay transport.

5. c. pressurization illnesses, and localized injuries.—Pressurization illnesses relate to atmospheric pressure and altitude (such as diving illness and high-altitude illness). Localized injuries include frostbite or sunburn.

6. a. 30°C/86°F.—Critically low body temperature (those below 30°C/86°F), with signs and symptoms of severe hypothermia, is described as severe hypothermia. Severe hypothermia mimics clinical death. Therefore, a reliable CBT reading must be obtained and the patient warmed before resuscitation is terminated. Patients who have been pronounced dead of hypothermia have actually awakened in the morgue.

7. b. rectal—CBT is measured most accurately with a rectal thermometer. To assess the temperature of a patient who is suspected of being hypothermic, a special thermometer that covers lower temperatures than most normal thermometers is used.

8. d. four—Heat is gained or dissipated from the body by conduction, convection, radiation, and evaporation.

9. b. muscular activity.—Body heat is generated as a side effect of normal metabolic processes and by muscular activity (shivering).

10. d. hypothermia.—Frostnip and frostbite are less common. Shivering is a method by which the body attempts to produce heat and is not a disorder. Heat cramps and heat exhaustion are common heat problems.

11. d. thyroid disease—Thyroid disease causes both excessive and abnormally low sensitivity to heat and cold.

12. a. antihistamines.—Many OTC medications have anticholinergic side effects that predispose patients to heat disorders. These include antihistamines, cold remedies, and allergy preparations.

13. d. the body's inability to adequately dissipate heat.—*Heat illness* is defined as an increased CBT due to inadequate thermolysis (the body's normal means of shedding heat).

14. d. an excessive loss of salt and water in the sweat.—Heat cramps occur with overexertion and dehydration in a hot environment.

15. c. an altered level of consciousness.—Suspect heat stroke (a true emergency) in any patient who develops an altered LOC in a hot environment. An altered LOC is the key finding indicating that a heat or cold emergency is extreme.

16. b. drinking regardless of thirst.—Thirst is a poor indicatory of dehydration, especially in the elderly. The color of urine is a better indication of one's hydration status. The darker yellow the urine (more concentrated), the more dehydrated one is.

17. d. The patient with heat exhaustion will have a normal or slightly elevated temperature.—Signs and symptoms of heat exhaustion include pale skin, profuse sweating, hypotension, orthostatic changes, headache, weakness, fatigue, thirst, and a normal or slightly elevated temperature.

18. a. Both fever and heat stroke may cause an altered mental status.—Differentiating between fever and heat stroke may be difficult because both fever and heat stroke may cause this sign.

19. c. often decreases the pain from heat cramps.—Other than mild cases of heat illness, patients who are dehydrated will benefit from IV fluid therapy. A bolus of 500–1,000 ml of normal saline (0.9 percent saline) will help correct dehydration and often decreases the pain from heat cramps as salt is replaced.

20. c. removing some of the patient's clothing.—The treatment plan for a patient with heat illness is to maintain the ABCs and to begin cooling by removing the patient's clothing and moving him to a cooler environment.

21. b. He is dehydrated.—The patient has signs and symptoms of heat exhaustion. The primary problem is dehydration combined with overexertion. When a person is ill, as in this case, or has an infection, that person is more susceptible to heat illness. OTC cold medications may dry the patient out too much.

22. c. decreased production of heat.—Generalized hypothermia is a condition in which the CBT is less than 35°C or 95°F, when the lowered temperature is caused by either decreased production of heat or increased heat loss from the body.

23. d. any elderly person living alone with a chronic disease—Any elderly person who lives alone, especially a person with a chronic disease or who has suffered a stroke, is at risk of developing hypothermia.

24. c. alcohol and tobacco use—People participating in outdoor activities in cool temperatures should anticipate the possibility of hypothermia and prepare accordingly by planning to wear the proper clothing in layers. Alcohol use can cloud judgment, and tobacco use constricts blood vessels, thereby accelerating cooling of the body.

25. b. the core body temperature.—The severity of hypothermia is determined by the presence of signs and symptoms and the CBT. Mild hypothermia is defined as a CBT of less than 86°F.

26. b. chronic—This common occurrence is an example of urban hypothermia. It occurs to people who are inside but lack appropriate thermoregulation.

27. d. loss of fine motor control—There is no reliable correlation between signs and symptoms and a specific CBT. Common signs and symptoms begin with diminished coordination and psychomotor function. As hypothermia progresses, coordination and movement become slower, altered mental status progresses to a loss of consciousness. Severe hypothermia can mimic death.

28. a. core body temperature—There is no reliable correlation between signs and symptoms and specific CBT. Always obtain a reliable CBT reading. This may not be possible in the field; therefore, the patient must be transported for evaluation in the ED to obtain a CBT.

29. a. use normal chest compressions and ventilation.—Perform CPR as necessary. Check the pulse for 30–45 seconds before beginning chest compressions and use normal chest compressions and ventilation. Apply the AED as per local protocol.

30. a. splinting only.—The affected area should be handled gently. Protect the area by covering it. When the affected area is an extremity, splint it to prevent the patient from using it.

31. c. a submersion episode with at least transient recovery.—Near-drowning occurs when the process of drowning is interrupted or reversed.

32. c. Upon initial assessment, the patient may appear normal.—This is why it is important that the patient always be transported for evaluation. Signs and symptoms that may develop include progressively worsening dyspnea, abnormal lung sounds,

tachycardia, chest pain, AMS, and respiratory or cardiac arrest.

33. a. Cold may decrease cerebral metabolism.—Hypothermia in a near-drowning victim may decrease cerebral metabolism and thereby prolong survival.

34. d. time to the first spontaneous breath.—The shorter period of time until the first spontaneous gasp, the better the neurological prognosis.

35. d. assessing lung sounds and quality of the pulse.—The initial assessment of a near-drowning victim is the same as with any other patient. Assess the mental status and ABCs.

36. a. normal saline at a rate to keep the vein open.—Treatment of near-drowning victims includes high-flow oxygen, warmth, and IV fluids of normal saline. Follow local protocol for positioning and use of the Heimlich maneuver.

37. b. contract.—As a diver descends, the gases in her lungs and tank contract; the deeper the diver goes, the quicker the gases in the tank are used up. As the diver ascends, the gases expand. The diver must remember to exhale continuously while ascending to prevent injury to the lungs from overpressurization.

38. c. occur because of the body's abnormal response to hypoxia at altitude.—High-altitude sickness occurs as a result of decreased atmospheric pressure and the resulting hypoxia.

39. b. Complete a neuro exam, including the prehospital stroke score.—The patient is presenting with stroke symptoms that may or may not be associated with a recent diving trip. Complete a focused neurological examination and include a prehospital stroke score, either Cincinnati or Los Angeles (e.g., speech, pronator drift, and facial symmetry).

40. b. Consult medical control about hyperbaric therapy.—The sudden, unilateral loss of sensation or motion following scuba diving (even 10 days or more after the dive) suggests decompression sickness; specifically, air embolism in the brain. Hyperbaric therapy is beneficial even in late cases where patient waited to seek help, hoping that the symptoms would resolve. Consult medical control or follow local protocol regarding hyperbaric therapy. The Diver's Alert Network (DAN) is another resource.

Chapter 24: Behavioral Emergencies

1. c. that person's reaction to a crisis.—The reaction to a crisis will vary from person to person. When people feel that they have lost control, the world appears to crash in on them, triggering the emergency. The patient may become depressed,

violent to himself or herself, or violent toward others.

2. c. Multiple factors cause both behavioral and psychiatric disorders.—The pathophysiology of both disorders is multifactoral and includes genetics, a

person's surroundings and circumstances, organic illness, and chemical imbalances.

3. a. limiting interruptions when listening to the patient.—Therapeutic interviewing techniques include avoiding threatening actions, statements, and questions; focusing your questions on the immediate problem; being supportive and empathetic; engaging in active listening; and limiting interruptions.

4. a. Surround the patient with plenty of people.—The general techniques for physical assessment of a patient with a behavioral emergency include being alert for potential danger by watching for overt behavior; respecting the patient's personal space; limiting the number of people around the patient; asking the patient to permit you to obtain vital signs; limiting contact to only absolutely necessary evaluations; approaching slowly but purposefully; and avoiding threatening actions, questions, and statements.

5. b. being honest with the patient.—Keeping safety in mind at all times, attempt to establish a good rapport with the patient. Be honest; use a calm, even voice; and express a willingness to listen.

6. a. male less than 19 years of age.—Statistics have shown that these gender and age factors increase the risk that a person will become suicidal.

7. d. allow the relatives to stay only when the patient will not cooperate otherwise.—The general theory about removing relatives or bystanders from the patient in a behavioral emergency is that the provider will be able to provide better care when relatives and bystanders are not in the way. When the patient will not calm down or cooperate, it may be necessary to allow another individual to be present (e.g., family member or caretaker).

8. b. psychiatric diagnosis.—The EMT-I is not legally or ethically responsible for making or knowing the patient's exact psychiatric diagnosis.

9. b. a person with altered mental status—Patients must be transported against their will in any situation in which the patients are a danger to themselves or others.

10. c. leather restraints—Soft restraints made of leather or Velcro for the wrists and ankles are considered humane restraints.

11. a. have enough personnel to complete the task.—Before you physically restrain and move any patient, be sure that you understand and are following your local protocols. Use medical direction and law enforcement whenever possible and as indicated by your local protocols. You must ensure safety for yourself, your crew, and the patient, so do not attempt to restrain a patient unless you have sufficient personnel to do the job.

12. c. psychosis—Psychosis is when the patient has no concept of reality. However, the person truly believes that his situation or condition is real and often hears voices. The psychotic person often also develops hyperactive and dangerous behavior, but can be calmed by the "talk-down" method. Such a patient needs reassurance.

13. b. pacing back and forth—Clues that a patient may become violent include pacing, inability to sit still for more than a couple of seconds, excessive body language, anger in the voice, acting out, and bragging about how tough he is. Any domestic violence situation and any drug or alcohol intoxication situation carries a risk of violence; also, males are more likely than females to exhibit violent behavior.

14. a. a phobia.—Phobias are irrational, intense, and obsessive fears of specific things, such as an object or a physical situation. These fears can affect both personal and societal relationships.

15. b. suicidal gesture—A suicidal gesture is something a person does to ask (indirectly) for help, rather than to die. The person performs the act in a potentially reversible way, such as taking a small handful of pills. This patient must be treated as the same as a poisoning patient, as well as being treated for the behavioral emergency. Remember, sometimes gestures turn into true suicides, and the patients manage to kill themselves.

Chapter 25: Gynecological Emergencies

1. a. estrogen—Estrogens stimulate bone and muscle growth and induce the development of female sexual characteristics. Progesterone helps to restore and prepare the uterus for pregnancy after menses.

2. c. abdomen.—The components of the physical exam of a patient with a gynecological complaint include initial assessment, vital signs, focused exam of the abdomen (guarding, tenderness, masses, and distention), and assessment for discharge (amount, type, and odor).

3. c. abdominal pain.—Typically, gynecological emergencies (infection, sexually transmitted diseases or STDs, ovarian torsion, renal stones, ruptured ovarian cysts, sexual assault, and ectopic pregnancy) are associated with acute abdominal pain.

4. a. to suspect and treat for shock.—In the prehospital setting, all abdominal complaints, especially in females of childbearing age, are managed alike, with supportive treatment and care for shock. Ruptured ectopic pregnancy is a potentially life-threatening condition that must be rapidly ruled out in the ED. Getting a good history is paramount so that medical personnel can begin to rule out life-threatening or potentially life-threatening conditions.

5. d. pelvic inflammatory disease (PID).—PID is an infection in the female reproductive and surroundings organs that can lead to complications, including sepsis and infertility.

6. b. fluids from the rupture irritating the peritoneum.—Ovarian cysts often cause no symptoms, but when they rupture the patient will have sudden, sharp pain, which is caused by the fluids from the rupture irritating the peritoneum and causing peritonitis.

7. b. ectopic pregnancy—All female patients of childbearing age are considered pregnant until pregnancy is ruled out (e.g., by a serum pregnancy test at the ED). Ruptured ectopic pregnancy is a potentially life-threatening condition that must be rapidly acted upon in the ED. Consider and treat for ectopic pregnancy first!

8. b. supine position, IV access, and transport to the appropriate facility.—In the prehospital setting, all abdominal complaints, especially in female patients of childbearing age, are managed alike, with supportive treatment and care for shock. This patient had a syncopal event, is tachycardic, and is pale and moist. Signs of shock with an unexplained source are considered and managed as intraabdominal bleeding until the true cause is found.

9. d. any of the above.—Physical signs of abuse include bruising of the mons pubis, labia, or perineum, and vaginal or rectal tears. If the patient struggled, there will most likely be other associated injuries

as well, such as defensive wounds on the extremities, back, head, or neck.

10. c. directed toward providing emotional support.—After life-threatening injuries have been managed, emotional support is crucial. Respond to the victim's physical and emotional needs while preserving evidence from the crime scene and providing a safe environment for the patient.

11. a. Protect her privacy and modesty.—Sexual assault is a crime of violence with serious physical and psychological implications. You must be prepared to respond to the victim's physical and emotional needs. First, try to help the patient feel safe by providing a safe environment (e.g., your ambulance). In the ambulance you can protect her privacy and modesty. If there is a female crew member, police officer, or crisis worker at the scene, allow the patient the choice of having another female with her during care and transport.

12. b. Handle the victim's clothing as little as possible.—Methods of preserving evidence from the patient include taking the victim's clothing to the ED, handling the clothing as little as possible; avoiding the use of plastic bags (paper bags are good) for blood-stained articles, because plastics degrade the evidence; bagging each item separately; not cleaning wounds; and asking the patient to avoid changing clothes or bathing.

13. d. an elderly patient with signs and symptoms of an STD—STDs in the very young or very old may indicate sexual abuse.

14. d. chlamydia.—Chlamydial infection is currently the most common of all bacterial STDs in both men and women. Because many people (especially men) experience no symptoms, they may not know they have it.

15. c. menstrual cycle.—The normal menstrual cycle is 28 days long, and can be divided into three phases: menses, the proliferative phase, and the secretory phase.

Chapter 26: Obstetrical Emergencies

1. d. implantation of the fertilized egg in the endometrium.—The development of the placenta is initiated when the fertilized egg (zygote) contacts the endometrial wall, erodes the epithelium, and buries itself in the endometrium.

2. b. The blood pressure increases during the second trimester.—Normal changes during pregnancy include increased heart rate (by 10–20 bpm), increased cardiac output, decreased BP during the second trimester with a return to normal in the third

trimester, and increased circulating blood volume (by nearly 50 percent).

3. c. consider the normal changes in vital signs that occur during pregnancy.—Certain normal physical changes occur during pregnancy, such as increased heart rate and BP changes. These may obscure the clinical picture of the patient if the changes are not recognized as normal.

4. a. 1—Stage 1 begins with contractions and ends with the crowning of the baby's head at the vaginal

opening. It is during this stage that the cervix dilates in preparation for delivery.

5. c. the baby's buttocks pass through the cervix first —A delivery is abnormal when any body part other than the head passes through the cervix first (e.g., breech, limb presentation, or umbilical cord presentation).

6. a. hypertension—A new onset of hypertension (140/90 or greater) during pregnancy is an indication of possible toxemia. Preexisting hypertension requires close monitoring. Unrecognized or untreated hypertension during pregnancy places the patient at high risk of stroke, acute pulmonary edema, renal failure, and eclampsia.

7. b. abruptio placenta—*Abruptio placenta* is the partial or complete separation of the placenta from the uterine wall after 20 weeks' gestation. The mother experiences constant pain and increased fetal movement, and may have contractions. The separation causes blood loss that is life-threatening to the fetus. The bleeding is not always apparent because it may be trapped behind the placenta.

8. c. bowel movement during a contraction—The urge to push out the baby or to have a bowel movement during a contraction occurs close to delivery of the baby. Contractions and ruptured membranes indicate that delivery is imminent, but not immediate. Labor can last for several hours.

9. b. the possibility of inducing supine hypotension syndrome.—When a sizeable fetus lies on the mother's vena cava and compresses it, such as when the mother lies on her back, the pressure can cause a decrease in the blood return to the heart. The mother may experience syncope or near-syncope as a result of the decreased blood return. The condition is easily corrected by tilting the backboard slightly to the left, allowing the fetus to move off of the vena cava. A pillow, blankets, or towels placed under right side of the backboard can be used to keep it tilted during transport.

10. d. telling the mother to push with the contractions and breathe deeply in between.—Prepare the mother for delivery by having her lie down on your stretcher. Provide privacy and have your partner or the patient's coach (e.g., spouse, relative, or friend) encourage the patient to push with the contractions and breathe deeply in between contractions.

11. b. place both hands on the baby's head to keep it from exploding out of the vaginal opening.—Perineal tearing is common, especially with a first delivery. The EMT-I should assist with the delivery of the baby by gently placing both hands on the baby's head to keep it from coming out of the vaginal opening too fast.

12. c. look for a cord wrapped around the baby's neck. —A nuchal cord (umbilical cord wrapped around the neck) is common during delivery. Once the baby's head is delivered, the EMT-I must look for nuchal cord. If a nuchal cord is present, gently lift the cord over the head; if you are unable to do so, quickly clamp and cut the cord. The cord must be handled gently because it can tear.

13. b. hypotension in the baby.—If the cord is not cut immediately, the baby should be placed at a level lower than the placenta to prevent placental transfusion. Think of an IV bag and how gravity works with the fluid. When you raise the IV bag above the patient's heart, the fluid flows into the patient. When you lower the IV bag, the patient's blood drains into the line. The baby's blood will drain with incorrect positioning.

14. b. The clamp attached to the cord near the placenta should not be removed.—Removal of the clamp prior to complete delivery of the placenta will cause unnecessary and potentially excessive bleeding.

15. b. allow the baby to suckle the mother's breast. —Uterine massage after delivery of the placenta (not before) will slow vaginal bleeding. If the mother and baby are both willing, encourage the mother to let the baby suckle the breast; this also slows bleeding.

16. a. typically requires a cesarean section.—Limb presentation is a complicated delivery, and management includes gentle and rapid transport to the hospital. Do not attempt to deliver a baby in this position. Administer high-flow oxygen to the mother and start an IV en route.

17. a. 2—The information gathering about prior pregnancies includes asking how many pregnancies the patient has had (i.e., gravida) and the number of births (i.e., para, parity).

18. d. pulmonary embolism—Pulmonary embolism results from a blood clot in the pelvic circulation. This can occur during pregnancy, labor, or the postpartum phase. This condition occurs frequently and has a high mortality rate, so it must be considered right away. Also consider AMI when a pregnant patient suddenly develops dyspnea and chest pain.

19. d. has experienced or is experiencing fetal distress. —The presence of meconium-stained amniotic fluid indicates fetal distress until proven otherwise. The baby's airway must be suctioned quickly before the baby is stimulated to breathe. Complications such as aspiration pneumonia arise when the baby aspirates the thick green meconium.

20. c. maternal use of tobacco—Maternal use of drugs, alcohol, and tobacco are all avoidable risk factors for premature birth and low birth weight.

21. b. 2—The mother and the baby you are helping to deliver are the two patients who will require your attention. Consider calling for additional help to assist in the care of your two patients and the other children present at the scene.

22. a. eye protection and a gown—Childbirth is messy, and the OB kit does not typically include sufficient PPE for you and any others assisting. At a minimum, you should have gloves, eye protection, and a gown for yourself and any crew members who are assisting.

23. a. protect the patient's modesty and privacy.—One role of the EMT-I is to value and maintain the patient's modesty and privacy, during both assessment and management. This is one way of demonstrating compassion and consideration for the pregnant patient.

24. c. Coach your partner and explain the management steps in the delivery.—The EMT-I should serve a role model for other EMS providers. Mentor the inexperienced EMS provider by reviewing the steps of the delivery and coaching him or her through it. Reassure the mother and explain everything that is happening to her.

25. d. the weight of the fetus will be off the mother's vena cava, allowing adequate blood return to her heart.—The left lateral recumbent position is the optimal position for avoiding supine hypotension syndrome. In this position, the weight of the fetus is shifted off the vena cava, thereby allowing normal blood return to the heart.

Chapter 27: Neonatal Resuscitation

1. a. neonate.—A baby is considered a newborn or newly born for the first few hours of life and a neonate until 6 weeks of age.

2. b. intrapartum.—*Antepartum* refers to the mother before the onset of labor. *Extrauterine* means outside the uterus, and *pre-embryonic* describes the period (weeks 1 and 2 of pregnancy) during which fertilization and implantation of the embryo into the endometrium occur.

3. c. Diabetes and hypertension syndromes are two antepartum factors that can affect childbirth.—There are factors that are avoidable (e.g., drug and alcohol use), and factors that are not avoidable (e.g., multiple fetuses, placenta previa).

4. a. placenta previa.—The danger of placenta previa is hemorrhaging from the placenta, which can result in significant blood loss. The patient typically experiences no pain, unlike abruptio placenta.

5. c. skin color.—Skin color is assessed for perfusion. At 1 minute and 5 minutes after birth, the Apgar score is used to assess appearance, pulse, grimace, activity, and reflex. Each sign in the chart is rated a number (0, 1, or 2). Ten is the highest score, 7 to 10 is a good to excellent score, and 4 to 6 is fair. An Apgar score of less than 4 is poor and indicates the need to begin aggressive assisted ventilations.

6. b. airway and ventilation equipment.—Resuscitative efforts are directed at airway management and ventilation. The inverted pyramid for newborns is the accepted standard for resuscitation steps. Proceed from simple BLS interventions (such as airway, ventilation, oxygenation, and chest compression) to ALS management.

7. d. at 1 minute and 5 minutes after birth.—Each sign in the chart is rated a number (0, 1, or 2). Ten is the highest score, 7 to 10 is a good to excellent score, and 4 to 6 is fair. An Apgar score of less than 4 is poor and indicates the need to begin aggressive assisted ventilations.

8. c. 9.—A pulse greater than 100 = 2 points; crying = 2 points; coughing or sneezing = 2 points; moving = 2 points; pink body and blue extremities = 1 point. The total is 9 points.

9. d. all of the above.—Signs of respiratory distress can occur within minutes or hours of birth. Any of the signs listed indicates respiratory distress in the neonate.

10. d. cuffed endotracheal tube.—Uncuffed endotracheal tubes are more appropriate for the size and position of the vocal cords in the neonate. The vocal cords are parallel and make a natural seal around the tube.

11. d. when the heart rate falls below 60 bpm despite adequate assisted ventilations for 30 seconds—The neonate's adequacy of respirations is determined by the heart rate. If the heart rate falls below or remains below 60 bpm despite adequate assisted ventilations for 30 seconds, you must provide chest compressions.

12. a. the same for BLS and ALS providers.—The current American Heart Association (AHA) guidelines do not distinguish between BLS and ALS for compression/ventilation ratio for a newborn.

13. b. increased heart rate—The adequacy of respirations is judged by the heart rate and the newborn's response to stimulation. An increasing heart rate is a good sign.

14. a. Provide blow-by oxygen.—The baby should be kept warm and placed on its back with a towel under the shoulders. Reassess the respiratory rate and effort. If the baby is responding slowly, provide blow-by oxygen, continue to observe closely, and be ready to assist with ventilations.

15. a. Let oxygen blow by the face, rather than placing a mask on the face.—Oxygen tubing is placed near the mouth and nose to allow the oxygen to blow by the baby's face.

16. c. slowly decrease the rate and pressure of the ventilations.—If the baby improves with positive pressure ventilations, slowly decrease the rate and pressure. Watch for signs of adequate perfusion and respiratory effort before stopping altogether.

17. a. intubation.—The steps for neonatal resuscitation begin with simple BLS interventions (e.g., suction, warm, dry, stimulate, oxygenate, and assist ventilations with a bag mask). ALS interventions are begun only after BLS airway, ventilation, and oxygenation steps are done.

18. d. has a heart rate above 160 bpm.—The neonate's adequacy of respirations is determined by the heart rate. A heart rate of 160 bpm in a neonate is a good rate.

19. c. when the baby's heart rate is 80 bpm after drying and warming.—The normal heart rate range of a newborn is 140–160. A slow heart rate indicates a problem that must be corrected quickly. Assess the respiratory effort and response to stimulation while upgrading your transportation considerations.

20. c. not recognizing the presence of meconium.— Meconium aspiration accounts for a significant number of neonatal deaths. Recognizing the presence of meconium and managing the airway accordingly when a baby is distressed will reduce the risk of aspiration of meconium.

21. d. small airway obstruction and aspiration pneumonia.—Meconium staining and aspiration occur in 9–16 percent of all births. In 20 percent of these cases, further complications, such as pneumonia or pneumothorax, develop.

22. a. fetal distress.—Meconium is the baby's first bowel movement. If it occurs while the fetus is still in utero, it is considered a sign of fetal distress. Meconium staining and aspiration occur primarily in postterm gestation.

23. c. with an ET tube and meconium aspirator.—A bulb syringe or French catheter is not very effective for suctioning because the meconium is very thick and sticky. The ET tube is inserted for deep suction rather than ventilation purposes. Repeat the suction, using a new ET tube each time, until no meconium appears in or on the ET tube.

24. a. primary apnea.—If the condition is allowed to continue without intervention, the baby progresses to secondary apnea, continued bradycardia, unresponsiveness, and finally death.

25. a. bradycardia—Assessment of the fetal heart rate is the standard of care in the clinical setting to determine if the fetus is in any distress. In the field, listening for a fetal heartbeat can be difficult because of loud ambient noises and the lack of sensitive listening equipment.

26. b. 60 bpm.—If the heart rate falls below or remains below 60 bpm despite adequate assisted ventilations for 30 seconds, provide chest compressions.

27. b. 1—A heart rate greater than 100 is given a score of 2 points; less than 100 is given 1 point; and no heart rate is scored 0.

28. a. Surfactant—At birth, some premature babies lack enough surfactant, a chemical that prevents the alveoli from collapsing when the baby exhales. Surfactant is not present in adequate quantities until after 34 weeks' gestation.

29. b. immature respiratory muscles.—Poorly developed lungs, along with immature respiratory muscles and drive, increase the need to provide assisted ventilations.

30. d. decreased lung capacity.—The effect of a distended abdomen in a baby is decreased lung capacity. In babies, full stomachs and vomiting go together, so the EMT-I should watch the airway and ensure adequate oxygenation during management of a distended abdomen.

31. c. a misplaced tube.—Barotrauma and pneumothorax are always potential complications of positive pressure ventilation. Uncuffed tubes are recommended for children less than 8 years of age, but the uncuffed tube does allow air to blow back up and into the esophagus, causing gastric distention. Therefore, a gastric tube should be inserted anytime a neonate is intubated.

32. c. have a large body surface area in relation to their weight.—They also have much smaller amounts of subcutaneous fat to keep them warm, and their temperature regulation mechanisms are immature.

33. c. quickly drying the baby and removing wet linens.—Newborns do not do well when they get cold. Quickly dry the newborn, remove wet clothing, wrap the baby using warm blankets, and turn up the heat in the ambulance.

34. c. ambient temperature is cool.—Heat loss can occur even in a reasonably warm room if the baby is still wet. Check to see that the baby's clothing is dry; be sure to remove wet clothing quickly and dry the baby thoroughly.

35. c. assess for and manage hypoxia and hypoglycemia. —The oxygen demand increases with stress due to cold, so tissue hypoxia may result with hypothermia. The neonate does not have a lot of glycogen reserve and burns up sugar and calories quickly. The newborn should be monitored for respiratory depression, apnea, and hypoglycemia.

36. a. respiratory arrest.—Unlike adults, most neonates, infants, and children suffer cardiac arrest as a result of respiratory events and hypoxia.

37. d. after aggressive assisted ventilations are begun. —Resuscitative efforts are directed at airway management and ventilation. If the baby does not improve after 30 seconds, provide chest compressions.

38. c. Dry, warm, suction, and stimulate.—BLS care is listed in the first level of care for neonatal resuscitation.

39. a. warmth and oxygenation.—A cold and/or hypoxic baby will not do well. Follow local protocols and medical direction for additional interventions.

40. d. answering a telephone while meeting with the family—This action implies that the phone call is more important than the patient's critical condition or death.

41. d. Any of the above.—If she does not learn and use the child's name in conversation with the family, the EMT-I's behavior could be misconstrued. The family may be offended and believe that the EMT-I did not value the patient as an individual.

42. d. Designate a provider to stay with the family to explain and answer questions.—It is most appropriate to assign someone to stay with the family and provide ongoing support. Abruptly leaving without doing this may make the family feel abandoned.

43. b. The EMT-I introduces himself or herself to the parents right away.—When EMT-Is do not introduce themselves, the family may not understand their role and are less likely to trust them.

44. c. Be supportive and reassuring while caring for the baby.—This is an example of having empathy for the parents. Having empathy in emergency medicine means identifying with and understanding the feelings, situations, and motives of your patients, their families, and other health care providers. Sympathy is less effective and involves actually taking on the patient's pain.

45. a. hypoxia.—Additional causes include drug or alcohol withdrawal and (less commonly) genetic or metabolic disorders.

Chapter 28: Pediatrics

1. c. wearing a helmet when riding—Most pediatric bicycle-related deaths are due to head trauma. Wearing helmets significantly reduces the number of deaths and serious head injuries.

2. d. immature abdominal muscles.—Lordosis or curved spine with a protruding belly is common in young children because of immature abdominal muscles.

3. a. Tell her it will hurt.—Tell the truth rather than risking the loss of her trust and cooperation. Distraction is another technique that works well with children. Use a parent, or a flashlight, or a favorite toy to distract the child while you do what you need to do.

4. b. managing emotionally distressed parents.—Plan on assigning a team member to inform and deal with the parents or caregivers of the patient. When a child sees a parent who is upset, the child is likely to become upset. Try to avoid this.

5. a. Maintain a calm approach.—When a child sees that her parents are upset, she will become upset too. A calm approach helps to keep both the child and the family calm.

6. a. increase.—The normal range of blood pressure increases with each older age group.

7. b. the patient's general appearance.—A child's general appearance is usually a very reliable indicator of how ill the child really is. Your evaluation of the child's general appearance should take only a few seconds as you first approach the patient.

8. b. 30—The normal respiratory rate range for a 5-year-old is 20–30 breaths per minute. When a sick or injured 5-year-old has a respiratory rate that persists at a minimum of 30 or more, consider the need for ventilatory assistance.

9. b. cause a falsely low reading.—To get an accurate assessment, you must use the right equipment for the right patient. Do not try to force adult equipment to fit children.

10. a. socially.—*Human lifespan development* refers collectively to all physiological, psychological (mental and emotional), and sociological changes that a person normally undergoes from infancy to late adulthood.

11. b. nasopharyngeal airway—The NPA is an excellent airway adjunct for a seizing patient. It does not require visualization of the airway or absence of a gag reflex, and it can be placed when the patient's teeth are clenched, which is common during seizures.

12. a. hypoxia—An airway adjunct that is used incorrectly can cause bleeding of the soft tissues and/or airway obstruction, but most significantly it can cause or worsen hypoxia.

13. a. a bag mask.—Use the proper size bag mask for the size of the patient. High-pressure ventilatory devices can actually do more harm than good in children. Injuries such as pneumothorax and tension pneumothorax can result from the high pressures.

14. c. Their breathing rate increases.—In an effort to correct hypoxia, the child initially responds with an increased respiratory rate (tachypnea).

15. a. also have one size smaller and one size larger available.—This is a good approach to use in case the first size you select does not fit the child. Having two additional sizes ready to go can help avoid further hypoxia.

16. a. gastric distention.—A special consideration when intubating the pediatric patient is the problem of an extended abdomen because of air trapped in the stomach. This causes the diaphragm to press up against the lungs, limiting respiratory excursion. Placing an orogastric or nasogastric tube to decompress the stomach allows improved ventilation.

17. d. A poor general appearance is a good indication of respiratory distress.—A child who appears distressed is distressed. Regardless of the cause, early signs of respiratory distress usually cause noticeable changes in the child's general appearance.

18. d. maintain adequate O_2 and CO_2 levels in the blood to meet the body's needs.—This is the definition of pediatric respiratory failure. When respiratory distress goes unrecognized or untreated, and the child can no longer compensate, he will deteriorate to respiratory failure.

19. c. respiratory arrest.—In infants and children, respiratory arrest often precedes cardiac arrest. If the EMT-I recognizes respiratory arrest early and treats the patient appropriately, cardiac arrest can be prevented.

20. d. respiratory distress—Respiratory distress is the leading medical complaint in pediatric calls, though the causes of distress vary (e.g., asthma, respiratory infections, foreign body airway obstructions).

21. d. even minor swelling in the airway can cause a complete obstruction.—The smaller openings are prone to obstruction from secretions, head position, and foreign bodies.

22. d. an aspirated foreign body—The EMT-I must suspect and assess for a foreign body airway obstruction (FBAO) when the onset of respiratory distress or stridor is sudden. FBAO is especially prevalent in children aged 1 to 3.

23. d. any of the above—Handle the child gently and avoid aggressive maneuvers that may startle the child, agitate her, or make her cry.

24. d. endotracheal intubation—Uncuffed tubes are often used in the out-of-hospital setting for children less than 8 years of age. The uncuffed tube allows air to blow back up and into the esophagus, distending the abdomen. Therefore, a gastric tube should be considered whenever an endotracheal tube is inserted into a small child.

25. a. croup—Croup is caused by viral or other infections and may result in swelling of the tissues of the upper airway.

26. a. viral—Fever in children is usually caused by a viral infection (e.g., bronchiolitis, croup, ear infection, pneumonia, and other respiratory infection).

27. d. tissue under the epiglottis—Croup typically occurs in children in the 3-month to 3-year age group. The patient may have a seal-like, barking cough due to swelling in the airway that affects the trachea, vocal cords, and/or tissue under the epiglottis.

28. a. croup—Croup is associated with a recent upper respiratory infection, including ear infection, and often progresses into difficulty breathing. Symptoms typically worsen at night.

29. c. calming him so he will be more comfortable.—An upset child's condition can rapidly worsen. It is very important to get the child calm and comfortable as soon as possible. Let the child sit up, or have the parents or caregiver hold him for comfort.

30. b. mucus—Mucus is a primary cause of foreign body obstruction in the neonate, newborn, and infant. This is because at this age, the child breathes primarily through the nose, and mucus can plug up the airway.

31. a. tissue swelling.—Transportation to the ED is recommended following a choking, because of the possibility of airway swelling and the potential for internal injuries caused by chest thrusts or back blows.

32. d. unresponsiveness—Stridor, drooling, and wheezing may be present with a partial airway obstruction, but not a complete obstruction.

33. b. 12 months and older—Back blows and chest thrusts are used to relieve a FBAO in a child less than 1 year old.

34. c. Epiglottitis is relatively rare, but is potentially life-threatening.—The infection causes a severely inflamed and swollen epiglottis that has the potential to completely obstruct the airway.

35. d. bacterial infection.—Typically, the child has a history of mild flu-like symptoms, but within 1 to 2 hours develops severe respiratory distress.

36. b. epiglottitis—This is a rare but potentially life-threatening infection that causes a severely inflamed and swollen epiglottis. Signs and symptoms include difficulty swallowing, sore throat, profound drooling, and difficulty breathing.

37. c. provide humidified oxygenation and keep the child calm.—Avoid alarming the child by slamming the ambulance doors or using the siren.

38. c. pneumonia—Consolidation in one or more lobes is associated with pneumonia.

39. a. asthma—Allergies differentiate asthma from croup, epiglottitis, and foreign body airway obstruction.

40. a. 2; winter and spring—Bronchiolitis is associated with respiratory infections and typically occurs in children less than 2 years of age during the winter and spring seasons.

41. c. bronchiolitis.—Bronchiolitis is an infection of the bronchioles that causes a swelling of the lower airways, which in turn causes tachypnea, retractions, and cyanosis.

42. d. of sharp localized pain associated with movement.—The patient may have sharp chest pain that is increased by coughing and deep breathing.

43. a. 1 to 3 days.—A mask, gloves, and handwashing after patient contact are sufficient precautions for a newly diagnosed case of pneumonia.

44. a. keeping the child calm and providing high-concentration oxygen.—These measures are the most important out-of-hospital treatment the EMT-I can provide.

45. c. increasing the rate and effort of breathing.—In the early stages of an asthma attack, the child is able to inhale, but has great difficulty exhaling, resulting in trapping of the residual air in the lungs. The child compensates by increasing the rate and effort of breathing.

46. b. drowning.—In the United States, drowning is the third leading preventable cause of pediatric deaths.

47. a. inhaling vomitus.—Aspiration pneumonia is a serious respiratory infection caused by inhaling vomitus, blood, meconium, or any foreign fluid or substance.

48. c. sudden onset of unilateral wheezing—When a child has a rapid onset of a respiratory problem, the EMT-I must consider the possibility of FBAO immediately. Sudden unilateral wheezing may indicate that a foreign body has been aspirated into the lower airway.

49. c. submersion—Drowning and near-drowning occur most commonly in children under 3 years of age. Freshwater drownings (pools, bathtubs, lakes, toilets, buckets) are more common than saltwater.

50. a. SIDS.—*Sudden infant death syndrome* is the unexpected death of an infant from an unexplained etiology.

51. a. mental status.—Sick kids look sick and act sick. The general impression and mental status are the initial, key clues to the severity of shock in a child.

52. a. children have less blood volume.—The total blood volume of a child is less to begin with, so even a seemingly small amount of blood loss is significant for an infant or child.

53. d. increasing their heart and respiratory rates.—Infants initially compensate for shock with an increase in both heart rate and respiratory rate.

54. a. shock.—Skin signs are very reliable in children because they have good circulation. Cool extremities in warm ambient temperature suggests loss of distal circulation, a sign of shock in a small child.

55. c. begin rapid transport—Vascular access and fluids are needed in this case, but may take time to achieve. Begin transport and attempt vascular access en route.

56. d. epinephrine.—The first drug of choice in cardiac arrest is epinephrine.

57. d. defibrillation.—The treatment of V-fib and pulseless V-tach requires good CPR and defibrillation.

58. c. recognize when the patient is stable or unstable.—The EMT-I must be able to recognize when a child is unstable, assess the rhythm, and identify and treat either the underlying cause or the rhythm itself.

59. d. 2 J per kilogram.—The initial dose for ventricular fibrillation in a child is 2 J per kilogram.

60. d. inadequate tissue oxygenation—When an infant can no longer maintain adequate tissue oxygenation, the heart rate will begin to slow (bradycardia). This is a grave sign.

61. d. capillary refill of more than 2 seconds—Capillary refill that takes longer than 2 seconds in a child is considered abnormal (absent cold ambient temperatures) and a sign of poor perfusion.

62. a. wide QRS complex—A wide QRS complex may be caused by ventricular tachycardia, a potentially lethal rhythm.

63. a. sepsis.—Many things can cause tachycardia, including fever, infection, dehydration, hypovolemia, trauma, and toxic ingestion. The coupling with poor perfusion is a clue to suspect sepsis.

64. a. hypoxia.—Hypoxia leads to acidosis and suppression of the SA node, causing bradycardia.

65. b. bradycardia.—Infants and young children with bradycardia can become unstable quickly because their cardiac output depends largely on the heart rate.

66. a. beta blocker ingestion—The most obvious clues (e.g., missing medication; unresponsive, abnormal breathing; and slow pulse) point to an overdose of the heart medication (a beta blocker).

67. a. Ventilate with high-concentration oxygen.—Failure to rapidly provide adequate ventilation and oxygenation will cause the patient to progress to cardiopulmonary arrest.

68. a. heart rate—Children do not tolerate bradycardias well. The most common cause of bradycardia is hypoxia, so ensure adequate ventilation and oxygenation. In this case, beta blocker overdose is the likely cause and must be addressed after the ABCs.

69. a. deterioration to asystole.—Bradycardia is an ominous sign in an infant and child. If it is not quickly recognized and corrected, cardiac arrest is imminent.

70. b. A ratio of 5:1 provides more ventilations per minute than a ratio of 15:2.—For infants more ventilations are more appropriate because these patients are often hypoxic.

71. d. all of the above.—Each of these factors is significant in providing adequate CPR to an infant, child, or adult.

72. a. Treatment is based on weight or size.—Pediatric patients come in many ages, weights, and sizes; fortunately, there are many reference resources available about caring for a child.

73. b. 3 months to 3 years—Febrile seizures are a common cause of seizures and are most common in children between the ages of 3 months and 3 years. Infection and trauma are two other frequent causes of seizures in this age group.

74. b. a sudden, rapid rise in body temperature.—Febrile seizures are associated with a rapid rise in body temperature, usually above 102°F (39°C).

75. c. febrile seizure—Febrile seizures are caused by high fevers and are common in children between 6 months and 6 years of age. Typically, another condition is also present, such as a cold, ear or respiratory infection, which causes the fever. Most febrile seizures are generalized and last only a few moments.

76. c. Suction the airway and remove excess clothing. —Management is supportive, with attention to the airway and removal of any excess clothing to cool the child.

77. a. a hypoglycemic event.—Hypoglycemia is the most dangerous complication of diabetes mellitus at any age.

78. c. giving too much insulin.—Hypoglycemia may be caused by taking too much insulin without adequate food intake, or by increased physical stress.

79. b. 80–120—The normal blood glucose range is the same for all patients.

80. c. dextrose 25 percent/25 grams.—Children are given half the adult concentration; newly borns and neonates are given D10 percent.

81. a. rehydration.—Contact medical control to see if rehydration should be started on the way to the hospital.

82. c. undiagnosed new onset of diabetes mellitus.—Hyperglycemia may be caused by too little or missed insulin dosing or undiagnosed new onset of diabetes mellitus.

83. b. altered mental status.—For any patient with an altered mental status, the EMT-I must rule out hypoxia and hypoglycemia first.

84. c. increased thirst and hunger.—Additional signs and symptoms include excessive urination; tachycardia; deep respirations; muscle and/or abdominal cramps; warm, dry skin, and altered mental status.

85. c. antecubital fossa—The saphenous vein should be considered when the antecubital fossa is not accessible.

86. c. a 3-year-old with epiglottitis who is crying—The additional stress of gaining vascular access may worsen the condition and raises the possibility of respiratory arrest. IO access is used in the most severe cases, such as severe shock or cardiac arrest.

87. a. pain—Pain can cause increased anxiety and fear, especially in children. For the child with a respiratory emergency, this is what you are trying to avoid.

88. a. falls—A child tends to fall on the head because the head is proportionately larger than the rest of the body. This makes head injury the most common cause of death.

89. d. a child's bones cannot protect the underlying organs as effectively as in an adult.—The softer bones make the skeleton more resistant to injury, but the underlying organs more prone to injury. The external signs of trauma are often not as apparent in children, and may be missed during the assessment.

90. b. management of the airway and ventilation.—Head injury is the most common cause of death in children. Protecting the airway and providing ventilations with high-concentration oxygen will help prevent hypoxia and help sustain neurological function.

91. d. The patient must be in stable condition, and the safety seat must be adequately secured in the ambulance when used as an immobilization device.— A child safety seat can be used as a restraining device when the patient is stable, the safety seat

can be adequately secured in the ambulance, and there is no evidence of damage to the safety seat.

92. c. normal saline and Ringer's lactate—Isotonic solutions have the same tonicity (osmolarity) as plasma and are the accepted approach for fluid therapy. Always follow local protocol.

93. d. femur and pelvis—Blood loss from the pelvis and femur can be significant in a patient of any age.

94. c. about a week—A bruise that is yellowish-green is about one week old.

95. c. Place a towel under the infant's shoulders.—Because an infant's head is large in relationship to its body, the infant's head will flex forward. A small blanket or towel placed under the infant's shoulders allows the head to naturally fall back to the neutral position.

96. a. basilar—This type of skull fracture is an extension of a linear fracture to the floor of the skull. Typically, blood vessels are disrupted and CSF or blood leaks from the ear(s) or nose. The patient may have bilateral periorbital ecchymosis or black eyes (raccoon sign), or bruising behind the ear(s), which is called Battle's sign.

97. b. sexual abuse.—Child abuse occurs when a child is injured or allowed to be injured by someone who was entrusted with care of that child. The injury can be physical, sexual, or emotional in nature.

98. a. denying a child proper nourishment—Locking or shutting a child in (for a variety of reasons) and denying medical care are additional examples of neglect.

99. b. more than 3 million reports a year.—Experts suggest that the numbers of actual child abuse cases are grossly underreported.

100. c. soft tissue injury—This includes burns, bruises, cuts, abrasions, and mouth injuries.

101. b. the same as for any other ill or injured child.— Remember to document your findings objectively.

Avoid judging the family or parent and do not take sides. Avoid confrontation, be nonjudgmental, and do not make any accusations.

102. d. defined as sudden infant death syndrome (SIDS).—The victims range in age from 2 weeks to 1 year. In many cases, the infant dies during sleep and is not discovered immediately.

103. d. all of the above—The emotional and physical reactions from the parents, caregivers, and family of a dead child will vary, and can cause them to become incapable of making decisions.

104. c. winter—Epidemiological studies reveal that more SIDS deaths occur during the winter months.

105. a. there are no symptoms.—SIDS, also called *crib death*, is the unexpected death of an infant from an unexplained etiology.

106. d. Provide psychological support to the parents or caregivers.—When signs of rigor mortis and dependent lividity are present, the EMT-I must turn her attention to providing psychological support to the child's caregivers. Do not provide false hope or reassurance.

107. a. consider the effect on the responders.—The death of a child is traumatic; very few of us are immune to the feelings engendered by such a loss. This must not be overlooked.

108. b. toddler—Toddlers and preschoolers aged 1 to 5 years may believe that their injury or illness is a punishment.

109. c. toddler—Toddlers and preschoolers aged 1 to 5 may not like to be touched by strangers (including EMS personnel) or separated from their parents or caregivers.

110. b. The patient may be more open with you.— Sometimes teens are embarrassed or afraid to say things in front of their parents or caregivers, but may tell you when the parents are not listening.

Chapter 29: Geriatrics

1. a. baking—Eating is an activity of daily living, but that does not mean the patient has to be able to bake or cook. The patient should be able to eat meals regularly, not prepare them. These meals may be partially or fully prepared (e.g., by Meals on Wheels, an in-house cafeteria, or a restaurant).

2. d. hospice programs—Hospice care emphasizes comfort measures and counseling to meet physical, spiritual, social, and economic needs. These programs also include care under medical supervision.

3. a. development of dementia—Dementia is not a normal part of aging. In fact, only 30 percent of patients over 85 years of age show a significant progressive decline in cognitive function.

4. d. increase the rate in response to stress and exercise.—Cardiac output decreases with age and affects the heart's ability to increase the heart rate at times when the body needs it (e.g., stress, illness, injury, or exercise).

5. c. reduced sight and sluggish reflexes.—Physiologic changes reduce visual abilities and slow the reflexes,

both of which increase the risk of falls and injuries associated with operating machinery and automobiles.

6. a. incontinence.—As the genitourinary system becomes less effective, incontinence and urinary tract infections occur with more frequency.

7. d. All of the above.—The elderly patient can be difficult to assess for many reasons, including vision or hearing impairment, confusion or poor history giving, and concurrent illnesses that present with confusing signs and symptoms. The EMT-I should plan on taking a little extra time with the assessment and management of an elderly patient. It is important to respect the patient's modesty and to explain what is being done, even if it takes longer.

8. a. cause the patient any additional injury.—Older patients are often cold and wear many layers of clothing, or wear supportive clothing, which can make gaining access to the body for an evaluation very challenging. Removing these layers is often necessary to perform a complete assessment. This task must be completed gently so as not cause any additional injury (e.g., skin tears, fractured ribs, bruising).

9. b. hip fractures.—Osteoporosis, often called the "silent thief," is a disease distinguished by low bone mass and the deterioration of bone tissue. The condition causes the bones to become fragile and creates a high risk of fractures, especially in the hips, spine, and wrists.

10. a. Diseases can slow the absorption of the medication, leaving too much in the system.—Geriatric patients often have concurrent illnesses that decrease their cardiac function, circulation, renal, and liver functions. This affects the rate of metabolism of drugs. When drugs cannot be metabolized as quickly as normal, the levels in the blood can become toxic.

11. d. all of the above.—Altered mental status or memory loss contributes to patients' forgetfulness about taking medication. Poor vision and lack of assistance with doses are additional reasons for noncompliance. Difficulty chewing or swallowing is also a factor.

12. d. decreased muscle and bone mass.—The most apparent effects of aging on the musculoskeletal system are decreased muscle mass and decreased bone density and strength.

13. d. pulmonary embolism—The history suggests pulmonary embolism: a patient who presents with difficulty breathing that progressively worsens, pleuritic chest pain, anxiety, leg pain, and typically no cough or fever. Often the patient with a pulmonary embolism has a history of heart failure,

recent surgery or immobilization, estrogen use or smoking.

14. d. unilateral facial paralysis.—The patient with Parkinson's disease experiences weakness and muscle rigidity, irregular gait, and a fine resting tremor. Falls are common and can result in injury. Unilateral facial paralysis is associated with Bell's palsy and stroke.

15. c. ibuprofen—This is one of the most common nonsteroidal anti-inflammatories (NSAIDs). The most serious side effect of NSAIDs is GI bleeding.

16. c. providing manual cervical immobilization.—Cervical immobilization is needed because of the mechanism of the fall. The airway is open and the patient is talking to you, so the other steps are appropriate once cervical immobilization is done.

17. d. There is not enough information to narrow down the cause of the fall.—There are many reasons for this man to have had a simple fall. His bradycardia could be responsible for the fall. However, his mentation and blood pressure do not seem significant enough for this. His recent knee surgery could explain the loss of balance.

18. c. the antidysrhythmic digitalis—With aging comes a decrease in circulation, as well as in renal and liver functions, which in turn causes a decrease in the metabolic rate and results in more drugs remaining in the system. The increased amount of drugs in the system can reach lethal levels, a condition commonly referred to as *drug toxicity*. Some of the drugs that most commonly produce drug toxicity are digitalis, lidocaine, and various beta blockers.

19. c. severe infection.—Because of a decrease in the function of the thermoregulatory system and the body's impaired ability to maintain homeostasis, even a modestly elevated or subnormal temperature is an indication for concern. This is especially true when it is associated with confusion, loss of appetite, or other behavioral changes. Consider that hypothermia in the elderly is due to a severe infection (e.g., pneumonia, urinary tract infections, and sepsis) until proven otherwise.

20. b. obtaining infectious pulmonary diseases.—The cilia in the airway act as a filter. When the filter and cough reflex become less effective, the risk of developing a respiratory illness increases. A diminished gag reflex increases the risk of aspiration.

21. a. searching for an underlying medical cause of the fall.—In addition to assessing and treating the injuries associated with the fall, the EMT-I must determine the cause of the fall. This approach can save the patient's life. The greatest life threat in a elderly patient who falls is not trauma: it is the

medical decline (e.g., stroke, MI, hypoglycemia) that caused the fall.

22. b. residential care facility.—There are more than 19,000 nursing homes in the United States. Federal regulations establish broad standards for the physical environment, medical and nursing requirements, and staffing design for three different types of nursing homes. Intermediate care facilities have independent living with limited nursing care. Residential care facilities have semi-independent living, and skilled nursing facilities have 24-hour nursing care.

23. b. They interfere with the tasks of daily living.—Injuries commonly occur with driving, falls, bending over to pick up an object, and cooking (burns or fires).

24. c. is receiving care to relieve suffering.—Palliative care is administered to relieve the suffering of a terminal condition. The care is not expected to cure the disease.

25. b. family.—If you suspect elder abuse, ask the patient when you have him away from others who may have committed the abuse.

Chapter 30: Assessment-Based Management

1. d. the decision-making process.—Assessment is critical to clinical decision making. The EMT-I must gather, evaluate, and synthesize information in order to make appropriate decisions.

2. b. classifying patients by their social status—Having a biased or prejudicial attitude is unprofessional and can cause the EMT-I to miss vital pieces of information. Assumptions and biases often short-circuit the information-gathering process.

3. a. hypoxia.—The EMT-I must consider the possibility of hypoxia first, then hypoglycemia in any ill or injured patient who presents as uncooperative. Be sure to rule out these possible causes before writing off the patient as just plain uncooperative.

4. c. the patient may not get the full medical attention deserved.—Labels, such as "another drunk" or "frequent flyer" can be very destructive to the assessment process. A label on a patient may cause you to rush and make a judgment too early in the assessment process. Remember, even regularly intoxicated patients get sick and injured once in a while.

5. c. Follow a regular sequence when performing an assessment.—The assessment process can be dynamic at times. However, in general, following a regular sequence allows a complete and smooth assessment even when distractions are present.

6. d. delegating management tasks to crew members.—When multiple crew members are present, try to avoid confusion by having each member take responsibility for specific tasks, such as obtaining vital signs, interviewing the patient, gathering scene information, and performing the physical exam.

7. c. make the appropriate patient management decisions.—The EMT-I makes a presumptive diagnosis in the prehospital setting and begins to rule out possible differential diagnoses based on the

information gathered. The definitive care and diagnosis are completed in the hospital.

8. a. give the patient presentation at the ED.—The team leader usually accompanies the patient through to definitive care. Responsibilities include having a concerned dialogue with the patient, obtaining the patient's history, performing the physical exam, giving the radio report and patient presentation at the ED, completing documentation, designating tasks, and coordinating transport.

9. d. any equipment needed to conduct the initial assessment and manage the ABCs—The primary equipment to carry to the patient's side should include the items needed to perform an initial assessment and manage life threats to the ABCs. This includes airway adjuncts, suction, stethoscope, BP cuff, bandages for bleeding control, and AED or cardiac monitor. Many advanced providers also carry in a drug box as part of their primary equipment.

10. d. equipment to conduct the initial assessment and manage the ABCs—The minimal equipment to take to any patient is the primary equipment needed to perform an initial assessment and manage life threats to the ABCs.

11. b. maintaining a calm, orderly demeanor.—Additional helpful aspects of the general approach include getting a good scene size-up and initial assessment, preplanning various examination techniques, practicing skills, and having a preplan for special situations such as respiratory or cardiac arrest.

12. c. depress the microphone button for a moment before speaking.—This helps to avoid cutting off the first few words of your transmission.

13. b. manage the patient as if the pain is cardiac pain, until proven otherwise.—Always manage the patient as if the pain is cardiac in origin until another source can be identified. Provide high-concentration oxygen, obtain vital signs, consider administering aspirin

and nitroglycerin per local protocol, get a focused history, and perform a focused physical exam.

14. d. Cardiac arrest patients are generally not transported by helicopter.—The cabin size of the aircraft limits on the number of crew members, equipment carried, and configuration of the stretcher. The noise level severely impedes the team from working on a cardiac arrest patient.

15. c. the release of digestive enzymes often worsens the condition.—Ingesting anything by mouth also increases the risk of nausea and vomiting.

16. b. treatment for shock.—Prehospital treatment of a GI bleed is the same regardless of the cause. Administer high-concentration oxygen; establish a large-bore IV, fluids, and rate as per your local protocol; consider the use of a pneumatic anti-shock garment (PASG); and give early notification to the ED.

17. d. rule out hypoxia and hypoglycemia as soon as possible.—There are many reasons why EMS may be called for a patient with an altered mental status. The first two life-threatening causes of AMS, which the EMT-I should rapidly rule out if possible, are hypoxia (administer high-concentration oxygen) and hypoglycemia (fingerstick). The mnemonic AEIOUTIPS is helpful in remembering other causes of AMS to consider.

    A = alcohol (acute or chronic)

    E = epilepsy, endocrine, exocrine, electrolytes

    I = infection (local or systemic)

    O = overdose

    U = uremia (traumatic or renal causes, including hypertension)

    T = trauma (old or new), temperature

    I = insulin (hypo- or hyperglycemia)

    P = psychoses

    S = stroke, shock, space-occupying lesion, subarachnoid bleed

18. a. doing a scene size-up—This always comes first. Pulmonary complaints may be associated with a variety of toxin exposures. Ensure a safe environment for all EMS providers before initiating patient contact.

19. d. ensuring that the scene is safe, completing a scene size-up, and evaluating the MOI.—The foundation of excellent trauma patient care consists of evaluating the MOI to understand the pathology of what happened, combined with a detailed physical exam for non-life- or limb-threatening injuries and making the appropriate decision regarding application of a cervical collar.

20. c. rapidly determine if the patient's symptoms are life-threatening.—Allergic reactions must be assessed thoroughly for the potential of progression into anaphylaxis.

21. b. modify your approach according to the age of the patient.—Use common sense in cases in which the child's chronological age does not match the apparent emotional age. Adjust your approach to the assessment as needed for you and the patient.

22. c. comprehension of existing BLS or ALS treatment protocols.—Accurate information is critical to decision making because decisions are only as good as the information they are based on.

23. b. be organized and systematic in your approach.—Your general approach to a patient should be made with a calm, orderly demeanor. You should have a preplan to avoid the appearance of confusion. Be sure to have all the essential equipment with you.

24. d. be concerned about all of the above.—When assessing the elderly patient, it is essential to care for emergent problems first, but it is also necessary to assess the patient's medical, psychosocial, and functional problems and capabilities.

25. a. Protocols are used as guidelines for care.—The EMT-I must also understand when and how to deviate from a protocol if the patient's conditions warrants. Contact medical control when the patient's presentation does not fit the protocol.

26. c. Attempt to insert an OPA and be prepared to suction if the patient vomits.—A lot is happening on this call. The patient is in critical condition. The first responders on the scene are trying to do the right thing, but are falling short. Although the patient is very close to the hospital, many tasks must be accomplished before you can transport him. The patient is unresponsive and gasping. The airway must be managed first! Attempt to place an oral airway and begin bag-mask ventilations.

27. d. administer high-concentration oxygen and encourage the patient to breathe deeper and faster.—This type of call can be complicated by not getting the full story or history of what happened right away or at all. The patient may also be unreliable for providing a history. This physical exam and vital signs with the information provided suggest that the patient has inadequate ventilations because of injured ribs. Encourage the patient to breathe deeper and faster despite the pain, and administer high-concentration oxygen.

28. b. She is in anaphylactic shock.—This patient has respiratory distress with signs and symptoms of shock from a sting with a known allergic reaction. This call has a few potential complications for the EMT-I: the patient is critical, access is difficult due to location and the crowd around her, and transport may be delayed because of the difficult access.

These distractions can make it difficult for the EMT-I to complete a thorough assessment.

29. b. Perform a focused neuro exam for signs of stroke.—The patient is conscious with neurological signs of a possible stroke: loss of consciousness, confusion, and inability to speak. Because there was a loss of consciousness, hypoxia and hypoglycemia should also be ruled out as quickly as possible. Administer high-concentration oxygen and obtain a blood glucose reading.

30. c. black widow spider—Many bites or stings are painful. Some are potentially dangerous. Assessment findings depend on the organism involved. Insect bites and stings can cause local (redness and swelling) and/or systemic (muscle spasms and abdominal pain) reactions. In this case, the signs and symptoms correlate with those of a black widow spider bite. Always ensure your own safety first before attempting to provide patient care.

Appendix B:
Tips for Preparing
for a Practical Skills Examination

EMT-I courses are designed to cover specific objectives as outlined in the DOT National Standard Curriculum. The curriculum also suggests that EMS educators take the option of enriching these courses with more material if they or their medical directors so choose. What prohibits many educators from enriching their courses is limited time and resources.

During an EMT-I course, many educators teach the core curriculum and provide enrichment material as time, resources, and experience permit. Near the end of an EMT-I course, it is typical for educators to change their style of teaching and start preparing students for the exam. That is, they provide examples of the material to be tested on state and national exams and give tips on how to take the written exams. Teachers may also hold one or more practice skills sessions and a mock practical exam to help the students prepare. Limited time and resources often do not allow for as much practice time for skills as students would like. Therefore, we have included some tips here to help you get ready as you prepare for the practical skills exam.

If you have not done so already, obtain a copy of the skills testing sheets to be used for *your* practical skills exam and carefully read the instructions well before the day of the exam. Note that each exam skill sheet identifies some items as critical pass or fail items; these are usually bolded for easy identification. Critical items include taking or verbalizing BSI or scene safety, as well as other key tasks. National Registry skills sheets also list "Critical Criteria" at the bottom of each skills sheet. This is a list of items that were not performed but should have been. When an evaluator checks one of these items, the candidate will fail the station.

Often the course instructor will hand out a set of the skills testing sheets to be used for the state and/or registry exam during or near the end of the course, and will give students an opportunity to practice the skills in lab using the testing sheets. We strongly recommend that you take every opportunity provided during the course to do this. In addition, find one or more other students or experienced EMT-Is to practice skills with. While you demonstrate the skill, have another person use the testing sheet to evaluate your performance. Be tough on each other—in a friendly way! Pay close attention to the critical failure items and then focus on obtaining every point available.

Before the day of the practical skills exam, make certain you are familiar with the exam location. Arrive 15 minutes early on the day of the exam. Bring a copy of the skills sheets with you to review while you are waiting. On the testing day, be patient and prepared to be at the testing site for most of the day. Practical skills testing typically takes a lot of time. In addition to bringing the skills sheets to review, bring a book, a drink, lunch, and plenty of patience.

On the day of the practical exam, if you have the option of choosing the order of the testing stations, go with one of two recommended strategies. The first one: If you are a little nervous and you want to build your confidence, start with a short skill station like bleeding control and shock. This is a skill that you successfully completed in the EMT-B practical exam. From there, continue to build your confidence by selecting the stations that you feel you can complete without difficulty.

The second recommended strategy is to select the most difficult stations and complete them first. For most people, the assessment stations seem the most difficult because they have the most steps and take the longest to complete. Once you have finished these stations, you can breathe a little easier while completing the remaining stations.

If you do not have the option of choosing the order of skills to be tested, do not worry; at this point you have prepared and are ready for each skill station no matter what the order. During the exam, the evaluators are instructed not to tell you whether you passed or failed a skill station until you have finished testing at all the stations, so don't expect them to. The reasoning underlying this is that if you fail a station early in the testing, you may become distracted or flustered and fail another.

Once in a station, you will be read a set of instructions and given an opportunity to ask questions for clarification and to check the equipment provided. We recommend that you do this, especially if you are the first candidate of the day coming into a station. The evaluator has been instructed to make sure that the equipment is functioning properly and that there are no distractions for the candidates. The evaluators are not there to trip you up—but occasionally a blood pressure cuff turns out to be broken and was not detected before the exam started.

While in the patient assessment station, we recommend that you ask if the injuries or significant signs that you are supposed to detect are going to be visible with moulage or by another method. This is a common problem area. Verbalize the steps and tasks you complete as if you were talking to a new partner. After a long day of testing, evaluators become fatigued just like you do. If an evaluator happens to have his or her head turned while you are performing a critical step, he or she will still hear you verbalizing it.

If you should have to repeat a station, know the retest policy and don't overreact. You have spent a lot of time training and should persevere rather than throwing it in because of one bad day! Remember, we humans do make mistakes occasionally. The key is how you learn from your mistakes, correct them, and move forward.

Lastly, get some sleep before the examination. Try to get a good night's rest for two nights before, in addition to the night immediately before the exam. Many people are very nervous about test taking and do not sleep well the night before the exam, no matter what they have done to prepare and relax. Getting a good sleep two nights before does help.

Best of luck, and be prepared!

—Kirt and Bob